1986

PERGAMON INTERNATIONAL LIBRARY
of Science, Technology, Engineering and Social Studies

*The 1000-volume original paperback library in aid of education,
industrial training and the enjoyment of leisure*

Publisher: Robert Maxwell, M.C.

Community Mental Health and the
Criminal Justice System

PGPS–57

———— Publisher's Notice to Educators ————

THE PERGAMON TEXTBOOK
INSPECTION COPY SERVICE

An inspection copy of any book suitable for use as a course text for
undergraduate or graduate students will gladly be sent for consideration for adoption without obligation. Copies may be retained for a
period of 30 days from receipt and returned if not suitable. When a
particular title is adopted or recommended for adoption for class
use and the recommendation results in a sale of 12 or more copies,
the inspection copy may be retained with our compliments. If after
examination the lecturer decides that the book is not suitable for
adoption but would like to retain it for his personal library, then
our Educators' Discount of 10% is allowed on the invoiced price.

PERGAMON GENERAL PSYCHOLOGY SERIES

Editor: Arnold P. Goldstein, *Syracuse University*
Leonard Krasner, *SUNY, Stony Brook*

Community Mental Health and the Criminal Justice System

Editor
John Monahan

Program in Social Ecology
University of California, Irvine

PERGAMON PRESS INC.

New York / Toronto / Oxford / Sydney / Braunschweig / Paris

U.S.A.   Pergamon Press Inc., Maxwell House, Fairview Park,
                  Elmsford, New York 10523, U.S.A.

U.K.   Pergamon Press Ltd., Headington Hill Hall, Oxford
                  OX 3 OBW, England

CANADA   Pergamon of Canada, Ltd., 207 Queen's Quay West,
                  Toronto 1, Canada

AUSTRALIA   Pergamon Press (Aust.) Pty. Ltd., 19a Boundary
                  Street, Rushcutters Bay, N.S.W. 2011, Australia

FRANCE   Pergamon Press SARL, 24 rue des Ecoles,
                  75240 Paris, Cedex 05, France

WEST GERMANY   Pergamon Press GMbH, 3300 Braunschweig,
                  Postfach 2923, Burgplatz 1, West Germany

Copyright © 1976. Pergamon Press Inc.

Library of Congress Cataloging in Publication Data

Monahan, John, 1946-   comp.
    Community mental health and the criminal justice system.

    (Pergamon general psychology series)
    Includes index.
    1. Psychology, Forensic—Addresses, essays, lectures.
2. Community mental health services—Addresses, essays, lectures.
3. Criminal justice, Administration of—Addresses, essays, lectures.
I. Title.
[DNLM: 1. Community mental health services—Collected
works.   2. Criminology—Collected works.   HV7431
M734c]
RA1148.M66   1975   362.2'2   74-28001
ISBM 0-08-018758-7 (pbk.)
ISBN 0-08-018759-5

Printed in the United States of America

To my parents, brothers, and sister

Contents

The Editor

John Monahan (Ph.D., Indiana University) is currently an assistant professor in the crossdisciplinary Program in Social Ecology at the University of California, Irvine. Dr. Monahan has frequently testified before the legislatures of California and other states on matters regarding public policy in the area of psychology and law. He has published widely in journals of psychology, psychiatry, criminology and law, and is on the editorial boards of the *American Journal of Community Psychology* and *Criminal Justice and Behavior*. He is the coeditor of two additional books, *Violence and Criminal Justice* and *Rape: A Critical Anthology*.

Contributors

Marc F. Abramson, M.D.
Courts and Correction Unit
San Mateo County Mental Health Services
County Government Center
Redwood City, California

James F. Alexander, Ph.D.
Department of Psychology
University of Utah
Salt Lake City, Utah

Morton Bard, Ph.D.
Graduate School and University Center
City University of New York
New York City, N.Y.

Allan Beigel, M.D.
Associate Professor of Psychiatry
University of Arizona College of Medicine
Tucson, Arizona

Arnold Binder, Ph.D.
Professor and Director
Program in Social Ecology
University of California
Irvine, California

Jerald T. Dade, Ph.D.
Assistant Professor
Department of Psychology
DePaul University
Chicago, Illinois

James J. Driscoll, Ph.D.
Associate Professor and Chairman
Department of Psychology
University of Louisville
Louisville, Kentucky

Ellsworth Fersch, J.D., Ph.D.
Lecturer, Department of Psychology
    and Social Relations
Harvard University
Cambridge, Massachusetts

Susan Frank, M.S.W.
Woodburn Center for Community Mental Health
Annandale, Virginia

Maurice Guberman
Asst. Chief Probation Officer
Norfolk County, Mass.
Box 109
Dedham, Massachusetts

Joseph Hickey, ED.D.
Assistant to the Commissioner
Connecticut Department of Corrections
Hartford, Connecticut

John J. Hughes, M.S.W.
Associate Professor of Social Welfare
George Mason University
Fairfax, Virginia

Honora A. Kaplan, J.D.
Laboratory of Community Psychiatry
Harvard Medical School
Boston, Massachusetts

Francis J. Kelly, ED.D.
Professor of Education
Boston College
Boston, Massachusetts

Nora Klapmuts, B.A.
Associate Director, Information Center
National Council on Crime and Delinquency
Hackensack, New Jersey

Lawrence Kohlberg Ph.D.
Professor of Education and Social Psychology
Harvard University
Cambridge, Massachusetts

Philip A. Mann, Ph.D.
Scott County Community Health Center
Davenport, Iowa

Leah B. McDonough, Ph.D.
Chief, Courts and Corrections Unit
San Mateo County Mental Health Services
Redwood City, California

A. Louis McGarry, M.D.
Laboratory of Community Psychiatry
Harvard Medical School
Boston, Massachusetts; State Director
    of Legal Medicine
Massachusetts Department of Mental Health
Boston, Massachusetts

Robert G. Meyer, Ph.D.
Associate Professor and Director
Psychology Clinic
University of Louisville
Louisville, Kentucky

John Monahan, Ph.D.
Assistant Professor
Program in Social Ecology
University of California
Irvine, California

Rudolf H. Moos, Ph.D.
Social Ecology Laboratory
Department of Psychiatry
Stanford University and Veteran's Hospital
Palo Alto, California

Martha Newkirk, R.N.
Coordinator of Youth Service Program
Program in Social Ecology
University of California
Irvine, California

Michael Nietzel, Ph.D.
Department of Psychology
University of Kentucky
Louisville, Kentucky

Bruce V. Parsons, Ph.D.
Clinical and Administrative Director
Downtown Unit
Salt Lake Community
    Mental Health Center
Salt Lake City, Utah

Edward J. Rolde, M.D.
Assistant Professor of Psychiatry
Harvard Medical School
Boston Massachusetts; Director
    of Legal Medicine
Massachusetts Mental Health Center
Boston, Massachusetts

Charles F. Schanie, M.A.
Department of Psychology
University of Louisville
Louisville, Kentucky

Peter Scharf, ED.D.
Assistant Professor
Program in Social Ecology
University of California
Irvine, California

Saleem A. Shah, Ph.D.
Chief, Center   for   Studies
    of Crime and Delinquency
Department of Health, Education and Welfare
National Institute of Mental Health
Rockville, Maryland

David E. Silber, Ph. D.
Department of Psychology
George Washington University
Washington, D.C.

Irving A. Spergel, D.S.W.
Professor, School of Social Service Administration
University of Chicago
Chicago, Illinois

Ernst A. Wenk, M.CRIM.
Associate Director Research Center
National Council on Crime and Delinquency
Hackensack, New Jersey

Preface

Collaboration with the criminal justice system is one of the most rapidly growing activities of community mental health practice. The theory of community mental health provides ample justification for such collaboration, and financial support is becoming increasingly available. On the federal level, for example, funds for criminal justice-related work continue to increase, while support for other potential consultees dwindles. When ideological fervor meets financial backing, the resultant burst of activity is predictable.

A creative interaction between mental health and criminal justice professionals, however, has been hampered by the lack of a comprehensive "handbook" which explicated theory, guided practice and sharpened issues. This book is an attempt to fill that gap. I have gathered together twenty-one exemplary reports of recent intervention and research projects, including several theoretical papers. The selections have been presented in a conceptually meaningful format by arranging them on a hierarchy of prevention. Thus, the first part of the book considers primary prevention programs which involve intervention in the community, the second deals with secondary prevention, which involves intervention in the criminal justice system, and the third considers treatment (sometimes called tertiary prevention). The final part of the book addresses itself to the legal and ethical issues invariably raised by mental health—criminal justice interaction.

The selections have been carefully chosen from among the vast recent literature in the area and three of the chapters were written specifically for this volume. The introductions to each part of the book review the relevant literature and place each selection into perspective. A prime criterion in the selection or invitation of chapters was that they reflect a *community* orientation. The insanity defense, competency to stand trial, civil commitment and other traditional clinical topics are not directly considered. While these topics are indeed worthy of discussion, they have been extensively dealt with elsewhere, and they do not reflect the concern with prevention which characterizes community mental health.

This work is, of necessity, addressed to an audience as heterogeneous as the fields of community mental health and criminal justice themselves. Its primary target population, however, is comprised of those psychologists, psychiatrists and social workers in a position to actively engage in consultation or research with those in the criminal justice system, as well as graduate and undergraduate students in community mental health courses.

It is also the editor's hope that this work find a place on the bookshelves of those on the criminal justice side of the consultative relationship. Police officials, judges, lawyers, probation officers and correctional personnel may glean from the projects reported here some ideas on how they might utilize community mental health resources to their own advantage.

I am grateful to many colleagues for their encouragement and assistance in the preparation of this book. My fellow faculty in the Program in Social Ecology, especially Arnold Binder, Gilbert Geis and Peter Scharf, were as supportive and helpful as ever. Kenneth Heller of Indiana University generously provided very constructive feedback. Debra Crawford and Lana Farnsworth ably assisted in preparing the materials. The book would not have been completed if my wife, Linda, had not taken on more than her share of family responsibilities to allow me the time to work on it.

J.M.

Introduction

The period from the mid-1960s to the mid-1970s has not been an easy time for those working in either the mental health of the criminal justice systems. Professionals in the mental health field have seen a tremendous and often confusing expansion of their roles. Community treatment facilities burgeoned over night and state hospital populations dwindled as quickly. Psychologists, psychiatrists and social workers found themselves challenged by paraprofessionals and castigated by a community which demanded an active role in determining the allocation of its mental health resources.

Criminal justice agents found themselves in even more of a social vortex. Urban riots and campus disorders thrust police practices into the glaring spotlight of the media. Real-life courtroom drama – and sometimes spectacle – held the interest of the nation as formerly only fiction could. The powder-keg of our correctional practices was ignited at Attica and elsewhere. The ranks of convicted felons began to include not only "common criminals" but those at the pinnacle of government. "Pardon" was formerly thought to be something Presidents gave; now it is something they also receive.

In this tumultuous context, the mental health and criminal justice systems began to reach out to one another, each believing that the other possessed skills and resources that could be of use. The mental health professional began to realize the psychological impact of the criminal justice system on those who came into contact with it, and the professional in criminal justice began to more freely acknowledge his need for assistance in fulfilling the demands made of him by society (Shah, 1972). Gradually, the

1

mental health worker stepped out of his traditional role as an "expert witness" in commitment, competency and insanity cases and began applying behavioral science principles to all facets of criminal justice work. The vehicle which provided the impetus and theoretical justification for adopting this activist stance was the community mental health movement (e.g., Zax and Specter, 1974).

COMMUNITY MENTAL HEALTH

Despite great variations in theory and technique, mental health treatment has traditionally been provided in what might be called the *waiting mode* of service delivery. Rappaport and Chinsky (1974) describe the characteristics of the waiting mode:

1.   Service is rendered by an "expert" or authority who is highly educated in a mental health profession.
2.   Service is rendered in the expert's office or in a hospital.
3.   The expert passively waits for the client to find him. The expert does not initiate contacts.

In the beginning of the last decade, a growing number of mental health professionals began to question the adequacy of this form of care delivery for dealing with the volume and diversity of psychological problems in the population. The deficiencies of the waiting mode were painfully evident. The clients it reached were a highly select group, primarily composed of those fitting the YAVIS syndrome (Young, Attractive, Verbal, Intelligent, and Successful) (Schonfield, 1964). The class bias toward those who could afford private treatment and who were culturally disposed to define their problems in psychological terms was the most glaring deficiency of the model, but far from the only one. The reliance upon highly trained professionals to deliver service created a severe manpower shortage, and the emphasis on long-term individual psychotherapy further reduced the number of clients who could be seen. Treatment focused on the neuroses of the upper and middle classes, while more difficult — and in many ways more important — problems, such as the abuse of alcohol and other drugs, and anti-social aggression, went unattended. Finally, since the traditional mode of service delivery relied on waiting until the client's difficulties were severe enough to motivate him or her to seek expert help, the opportunity to intervene early in the development of a problem, when help might be most effective, rarely presented itself.

The community mental health movement arose in response to these deficiencies. In contrast to the waiting mode, community mental health employs what might be called the *seeking mode* of service delivery, characterized by Rappaport and Chinsky (1974) as:

1. Service can be delivered by a number of persons, professionals as well as trained paraprofessionals.
2. Service is delivered where it is most needed and where the consumers are, which generally is not in the expert's office or hospital.
3. Mental health personnel can actively seek out new roles for themselves and offer their services to others.

Heller and Monahan (1975) discuss community mental health in terms of three core principles. In their view, the primary characteristic of community mental health is a strong emphasis on the *prevention,* rather than the treatment, of psychological disorder (Bloom, 1971, 1973). Prevention is commonly discussed as being of three types (Caplan, 1970). Primary prevention attempts to prevent a disorder from ever occurring. Secondary prevention aims at the early identification of cases and prompt provision of service so that disorders can be resolved before they become severe. Tertiary prevention strives to reduce the impairment that results from a disorder which has already occurred. As Cowen (1973) has pointed out, however, "tertiary prevention" is really what most people call "treatment." The term "prevention" should be read to include only its primary and secondary varieties.

The second essential element of community mental health, according to Heller and Monahan (1975), is a *population perspective,* a concern for the psychological functioning of the total membership of a given locale. This public health analogy takes the population, rather than the individual, as the unit of care (Caplan, 1970). There are two aspects to a population perspective: (a) identifying and intervening in populations (i.e. people) at risk of developing psychological disorder, and (b) identifying and intervening in risk-producing situations. Thus, community mental health professionals are not bound by the social forces and class biases which lead only certain subgroups to define their problems as "mental health" in nature and to seek out psychotherapy. The adoption of a population perspective allows community mental health personnel to seek out populations at risk of developing psychological disorder (regardless of how they originally defined their problems), and to offer their services, and it allows for attempts at the modification of pathogenic environmental conditions.

Finally, both the emphasis on prevention and the adoption of a population perspective are actualized in community mental health by a commitment to *institutional change*. The assumption is that a major portion of the factors giving rise to psychological disorder are environmental in nature and transmitted through the institutions of society. Stress created by psychologically malfunctioning community institutions and agencies can lead to psychological problems experienced by community members, or can exacerbate already existing problems. Further, community agencies and institutions not part of the mental health system (such as educational, welfare, religious, occupational and criminal justice agencies) frequently encounter persons in psychological distress. They are the "primary care givers" of society, and how they handle a person in distress may make a great difference in that person's future adjustment. The way to prevent psychological disorder, therefore, and the way to reach the problems of the entire population, is by insuring that societal institutions are responsive to the social and psychological needs of the community.

Application to the Criminal Justice System

When mental health professionals left their couches for the community, one of the first community institutions to which they offered their services was the criminal justice system. It is not difficult to see why. Many problems lie on the border of the mental health and criminal justice systems, and rather than fighting for jurisdiction, a cooperative approach would appear more fruitful. Probably no community agency encounters more persons in a state of psychological crisis than the agencies of the criminal justice system (Howard, 1974). Wolfgang (1975), in this regard, notes that a *majority* of urban males will have at least one contact with the criminal justice system during their lifetimes.

Further, the criminal justice system deals with large segments of the population who are unlikely ever to come to the attention of a "waiting mode" mental health professional. For example, drug abuse or sexual behavior on the part of one juvenile might be seen by his parents as indicating psychological difficulties and they might seek psychotherapy for him. Other parents might define the identical behavior in disciplinary terms and petition the child to juvenile court as "incorrigible." The way the parents have been led to define problems in the family, rather than any characteristics of the child's behavior, may determine whether he spends one hour a week with a therapist or has a lengthy stint in juvenile hall. By consulting with the appropriate juvenile justice agencies, the community mental health professional might be able to reach families independent of the way they originally define their problems. It should be emphatically stressed that this is not to say that the mental health system "owns" certain problems — juvenile delinquents, sex offenders, drug users, "mentally disturbed" criminals, etc.— and that the criminal justice system "owns" others, such as "normal" adult offenders. Little is gained, and much may be lost, by designating an individual as "sick" rather than "bad." Jurisdictional disputes over whether a given class of problems should fall under the control of the mental health or the criminal justice system are ultimately counterproductive distractions from the central question of what should be done to alleviate these problems. We are not dealing with mental health problems, or with criminal justice problems, but rather with *human* problems.

The efforts of community mental health personnel to affect criminal justice agencies in order to prevent the occurrence of psychological problems in the population have taken many forms. The selections which comprise the present volume, and the introductions to each part, detail the nature and implications of these collaborative ventures. Several impressions arise from the literature, however, which cut across the type of project or the level of intervention.

If a mental health professional wishes to be accepted by a criminal justice agency and have a project succeed, it appears absolutely essential to demonstrate the *convergence of interests* between himself and the personnel of the criminal justice agency. In Morton Bard's family crisis intervention program, for example, "there is no intention to convert the police officer into a social worker or psychotherapist. Rather, it is to demonstrate that the functioning of the police officer can be enhanced if he is given knowledge and skills realistically consistent with his daily functioning" (Bard and Berkowitz, 1969, p. 214). Thus, the mental health professional fulfills his preventive mental health mission and policemen live longer. If the already burdened personnel of the criminal justice system are made to feel that additional burdens are being placed on them – that now they must "give therapy" as well as keep the peace – the program will surely fail. What is necessary is to assure criminal justice personnel that mental health collaboration will help them perform better a job *that they are already doing,* e.g., intervening in family disputes, or any of the other "social service" activities which comprise the majority of police work (Cumming, Cumming and Edel, 1965).

Another impression shared by many in the field is that meaningful collaboration can take place only in an *atmosphere of mutual respect.* To continue using consultation with the police as an example, the police officer "does not want to be talked down to. He feels that his daily experience on the beat brings him into contact with as many emotionally disturbed people as the mental health worker. He has something to teach the professional person, just as the latter has something to teach the policeman. He may not have the 'book learning' and 'theory', but he has had a wealth of practical experience and would like this recognized" (Freeman, 1969, p. 221). The same could be said of the lawyer, probation officer or correctional official. Formal training for mental health professionals interested in interacting with criminal justice agencies might go far in insuring the attitudes necessary for program success (Suarez, 1972; Brodsky, 1973; Gormally and Brodsky, 1973; Sadoff, 1974; Monahan, 1974).

The Central Issues

The interaction between the community mental health and criminal justice systems, while still in its exploratory and formative stages, has progressed far enough that two substantive issues are beginning to come into focus. The future of collaborative efforts may well depend on their resolution.

The first issue is an empirical one. While there is much intuitive appeal to notions such as the prevention of crime and psychological disorder, diversion to mental health programs, and the treatability of offenders, the actual effects of such efforts are more difficult to document. Preliminary data on some programs suggest a measure of success (e.g., screening police recruits and some forms of family crisis intervention), while the evaluation of other efforts has been largely negative (e.g., predicting and treating violent offenders). The great majority of programs in the interface of mental health and criminal justice have not been evaluated at all. While the difficulties associated with program evaluation in the "real world" are not to be underestimated, the methodology to evaluate virtually any program is currently available (Bloom, 1972; Rossi and Williams, 1972; Weiss, 1972a, 1972b; Caporaso and Roos, 1973; Heller and Monahan, 1975; Campbell, in press). Without meaningful and sophisticated evaluation, community mental health interaction with criminal justice agencies will undoubtedly fade away with little to show for itself but glowing press releases. With such evaluation, it may have substantial and lasting impact.

The second issue central to collaboration between mental health and criminal justice agencies is a moral and ethical one. No topic evokes more heated emotions than coerced intervention in the lives of those who have not been convicted of a crime, and the rights of those targeted for such intervention (Kittrie, 1971; Robinson, 1974).

Szasz (1970), for example, states that the purpose of community mental health "seems to be the dissemination of a collectivistic mental health ethic as a kind of secular religion" (p. 33). Its values are "collectivism and social tranquility" (p. 224), and its goal is to make people "uncomplainingly submissive to the will of the elites in charge of Human Engineering" (p. 224).

At least three factors appear to be involved in the charge by Szasz and others that community mental health programs violate the rights of those involved in them. One is the issue of the *medical model* of psychological disorder. Szasz (1963) holds that medical analogies are inappropriate in individual psychotherapy and certainly more inappropriate in community mental health. A second issue concerns *coerced intervention.* The fear is that prevention and treatment programs will be launched in the interest of "mental health" against the wishes of those involved in them. Finally, it is charged that community mental health is actually a *political movement,* which simply disguises its political goals in mental health terminology.

Heller and Monahan (1975) consider these objections to community mental health and conclude that, while there is unfortunate evidence to substantiate each, there is no *necessity* that these antilibertarian factors must encumber community practice. Thus, while some community practitioners undoubtedly adhere to outdated medical analogies, many do not, and the "Nader Report" on mental health centers (Chu and Trotter, 1974) explicitly recommends that the use of the medical model in community practice be discontinued. Likewise, while some community mental health professionals have advocated coerced treatment (e.g., Bellak, 1971), others have argued equally strongly for voluntary programs (e.g., Monahan 1973a; 1973b; Geis and Monahan, in press; Denner and Price, 1973). Finally Heller and Monahan (1975) state that community mental health *must* be, at least in part, a political enterprise. The problems of the community are often political problems, and alleviating those problems is of necessity a political as well as a psychological venture. Even individual psychotherapy is not without its political ramifications (Halleck, 1971). To be apolitical is to be irrelevant. The problem lies in being *deceptively* political. Community mental health personnel must be open about the public policy aspects of their work, and not hide behind objective-sounding mental health terminology.

The issues of empirical evaluation and civil liberties are the most pressing ones confronting community mental health as it interacts with the criminal justice system. It is this author's belief, however, that community mental health professionals can rise to the challenges confronting them, and based on a solid empirical and ethical foundation, can make far-ranging and long-lasting contributions to the criminal justice system, and, thereby, to the psychological functioning of the community.

REFERENCES

Bard, M. and Berkowitz, B. A community psychology consultation program in police family crisis intervention: preliminary impressions. *International Journal of Social Psychiatry*, 1969, **15**, 209-215.

Bellak, L. The need for public health laws for psychiatric illness. *American Journal of Public Health*, 1971, **61**, 119-121.

Bloom, B. Strategies for the prevention of mental disorders. In Division 27 of the American Psychological Association (Ed.) *Issues in community psychology and preventive mental health*. New York: Behavioral Publications, 1971, pp. 1-20.

Bloom, B. Mental health program evaluation. In S. Golann and C. Elisdorfer (Eds.) *Handbook of community mental health*. New York: Appleton-Century-Crofts, 1972, pp. 819-839.

Bloom, B. *Community mental health*. Morristown, New Jersey: General Learning Press, 1973.

Brodsky, S. *Psychologists in the criminal justice system*. Urbana, Illinois: University of Illinois Press, 1973.

Campbell, D. Methods for the experimenting society. *American Psychologist*, in press.

Caplan, G. *The theory and practice of mental health consultation*. New York: Basic Books, 1970.

Caporaso, J. and Roos, L. *Quasi-experimental approaches: Testing theory and evaluating policy*. Evanston, Illinois: Northwestern University Press, 1973.

Chu, F. and Trotter, S. *The madness establishment*. New York: Grossman, 1974.

Cowen, E. Social and community interventions. *Annual Review of Psychology*, 1973, **24**, 423-472.

Cumming, E., Cumming, I. and Edel, L. Policeman as philosopher, guide, and friend. *Social Problems*, 1965, **12**, 276-286.

Denner, B. and Price, R. (Eds.) *Community mental health: Social action and reaction*. New York: Holt, Rinehart and Winston, 1973.

Freeman, M. Community mental health education with police. In A. Bindman, and A. Spiegel (Eds.) *Perspectives in community mental health*. New York: Aldine, 1969, pp. 218-222.

Geis, G. and Monahan, J. The social ecology of violence. In T. Lickona (Ed.) *Man and morality*. New York: Holt, Rinehart and Winston, in press.

Gormally, J. and Brodsky, S. Utilization and training of psychologists for the criminal justice system. *American Psychologist*, 1973, **28**, 926-928.

Halleck, S. *The politics of therapy*. New York: Science House, 1971.

Heller, K. and Monahan, J. Unpublished text in community mental health, 1975.

Howard, J. Law enforcement in an urban society. *American Psychologist*, 1974, **29**, 223-232.

Kittrie, N. *The right to be different*. Baltimore: Johns Hopkins University Press, 1971.

Monahan, J. The psychiatrization of criminal behavior. *Hospital and Community Psychiatry*, 1973, **24**, 105-107. (a)

Monahan, J. Abolish the insanity defense? — Not yet. *Rutgers Law Review*, 1973, **26**, 719-741(b).

Monahan, J. Toward undergraduate education in the interface of mental health and criminal justice. *Journal of Criminal Justice* 1974, 2 61-65.

Rappaport, J. and Chinsky, J. Models for delivery of service: an historical and conceptual perspective. *Professional Psychology*, 1974, **5**, 42-50.

Robinson, D. Harm, offense, and nuisance: Some first steps in the establishment of an ethics of treatment. *American Psychologist*, 1974, **29**, 233-225.

Rossi, P. and Williams, W. (Eds.) *Evaluating social programs: Theory, practice and politics*. New York: Seminar Press, 1972.

Sadoff, R. Comprehensive training in forensic psychiatry. *American Journal of Psychiatry*, 1974, **131**, 223-225.

Schonfield, W. *Psychotherapy: The purchase of friendship*. Englewood Cliffs, N.J.: Prentice-Hall, 1964.

Shah, S. The criminal justice system. In S. Golann and C. Eisdorfer (Eds.) *Handbook of community mental health*. New York: Appleton-Century-Crofts, 1972, pp. 73-106.

Suarez, J. Psychiatry and the criminal law system. *American Journal of Psychiatry*, 1972, **129**, 293-297.

Szasz, T. *Law, Liberty, and Psychiatry*. New York: Macmillan, 1963.

Szasz, T. *The manufacture of madness*. New York: Harper and Row, 1970.

Weiss, C. (Ed.) *Evaluating Action Programs*. Boston: Allyn and Bacon, 1972. (a)

Weiss, C. *Evaluation Research: Methods for Assessing Program Effectiveness*. Englewood Cliffs, New Jersey: Prentice Hall, 1972.(b)

Wolfgang, M. Contemporary perspectives on violence. In D. Chappell & J. Monahan (Eds.) *Violence and criminal justice*. Lexington, Mass.: Lexington Books, 1975.

Zax, M., and Specter, G. *An Introduction to Community Psychology*, New York: Wiley, 1974.

Part I
Primary Prevention—Intervening in the Community

Primary prevention, writes Bernard Bloom (1971) is "the great task still before us in the field of community mental health." While primary prevention was the *raison d'etre* given by John Kennedy for launching the federal involvement in community mental health in 1963, the subsequent history of the movement has not lived up to its mandate. Resources at many mental health centers are still deployed solely in providing traditional treatment services (Chu and Trotter, 1974). Even more significantly, research in the field has largely neglected prevention. Cowen (1973) notes that less than three percent of the articles published in the first seven years of the *Community Mental Health Journal* had "prevention" in the title, and Golann's (1969) bibliography classified only two percent of the literature as concerned with primary prevention. Roen (1971) has urged patience with this situation, due both to the youthfulness of the field and the intrinsic difficulties of prevention research.

In this volume's first selection, Monahan addresses himself to the prevention of a problem of concern to both the psychological and legal communities: violence. Until now, efforts to prevent violence have centered around isolating potentially violent individuals. Monahan's review of the data on psychiatric and psychological prediction, however, leads him to suggest a different preventive tack, the identification of potentially violent *situations*. The current surge of interest in environmental psychology bodes well for the development of new strategies of violence prevention.

In the second selection, Spergel addresses himself to the primary prevention of another problem at the interface of mental health and criminal justice: juvenile delinquency. He considers historical and contemporary efforts at delinquency prevention, and some crucial policy issues in developing community-based prevention programs. On the question of the effectiveness of such programs, he concludes that "firm and satisfactory answers still elude us."

In this regard, Berleman, Seaberg and Steinburn (1972) have reported a thorough and sophisticated evaluation of a large-scale delinquency prevention experiment in the open community. A group of central-city junior high school boys was provided with one to two years of intensive social services (insight-oriented group discussions, parent groups, summer camp, consultation with teachers, etc.). When compared with a randomly assigned control group on measures of disciplinary problems in school and police records, however, no differences were discovered. These researchers state that previous community-based delinquency prevention experiments had similar findings, and they conclude that "to help inner-city youths develop less destructive life styles may require radically different intervention strategies, more comprehensive and system focused, as well as focused on the individual" (p. 344).

REFERENCES

Bloom, B. Strategies for the prevention of mental disorders. In Division 27 of the American Psychological Association (Ed.) *Issues in community psychology and preventive mental health.* New York: Behavioral Publications, 1971, pp. 1-20.

Berleman, W., Seaberg, J. and Steinburn, T. The delinquency prevention experiment of the Seattle Atlantic Street Center: A final evaluation. *The Social Service Review,* 1972, **46**, 323-346.

Chu, F. and Trotter, S. *The madness establishment.* New York: Grossman, 1974.

Cowen, E. Social and community interventions. *Annual Review of Psychology,* 1973, **24**, 423-472.

Golann, S. *Coordinate index reference guide to community mental health.* New York: Behavioral Publications, 1969.

Roen, S. Evaluative research and community mental health. In A. Bergin and S. Garfield (Eds.) *Handbook of psychotherapy and behavior change.* New York: Wiley, 1971, pp. 776-811.

1

The Prevention of Violence *

JOHN MONAHAN[1]

Violence, like cancer, is a frightening word. It evokes images of glistening switchblades and angry mobs, sounds of pounding flesh and screams. Fear of it leads people to constrict their lives, to look over their shoulders, bolt doors and be in before dark. Like cancer, violence is something nearly everyone wishes to prevent. Like cancer, too, violence has perversely resisted all attempts at eradication.

I would like to review and critically examine the current state of affairs regarding the ability of psychiatrists and psychologists to prevent outbreaks of violence. As current attempts toward the prevention of violence are almost solely restricted to intervening in the behavior of those predicted to be violent, the accuracy of those predictions will be carefully scrutinized. From this analysis of current prevention efforts, an alternate and possibly more fruitful strategy for prevention will be proposed and defended. First, however, we must briefly consider precisely what is meant by the term "violence," and how society makes use of efforts to predict and prevent its occurrence.

*This chapter was written especially for this volume.

[1]The author is grateful to Gilbert Geis, Kenneth Heller, Jonas Rappeport, Henry Steadman, Saleem Shah and Gary Evans for their incisive comments on an earlier version of this chapter, and to Patricia Guttridge for her editorial assistance. Some parts of this material were presented in modified form to the Pacific Northwest Conference on Violence and Criminal Justice, Issaquah, Washington, 1973, and to the Western Psychological Association, San Francisco, California, 1974.

DEFINITIONS OF VIOLENCE AND DANGEROUSNESS

While Sarbin (1967) cogently distinguishes between violence and dangerousness ("Violence denotes action; danger denotes a relationship"), virtually all others hold the terms synonymous. Some define violence to include only injury or death to persons (e.g., Rubin, 1972), while others include the destruction of property (e.g., Mulvihill and Tumin, 1969). Violent *thoughts* are considered dangerous by some "because patients with fears and fantasies of violence sometimes act them out" (Ervin and Lion, 1969). In the District of Columbia, dangerousness is defined in terms of acts "which result in harm to others, or cause *trouble* or *inconvenience* to others" (Comment, 1965). A federal court once ruled that writing a bad check was a sufficiently "dangerous" behavior to justify commitment (Overholser v. Russell, 1960).

The Model Sentencing Act defines two types of dangerous offenders: "(1) the offender who has committed a serious crime against a person and shows a behavior pattern of persistent assaultiveness based on serious mental disturbances and (2) the offender deeply involved in organized crime" (Board of Directors, NCCD, 1973, p. 456). The Act comments that in no state would such offenders total more than 100 at any given time. One may wonder, however, about the harmlessness of an offender who has committed a serious crime against a person and shows a behavior pattern of persistent assaultiveness *without* having a serious mental disturbance. Is society's legitimate need for protection any less in the case of crime by the socially deprived than by the psychologically depraved? Note that if one considers all repetitive violent offenders to have a serious mental disturbance, one has reduced the notion of mental disturbance to a meaningless and redundant tautology.

The working definition of violence adopted by the National Commission on the Causes and Prevention of Violence (Mulvihill and Tumin, 1969) was "overtly threatened or overtly accomplished application of force which results in the injury or destruction of persons or property or reputation, or the illegal appropriation of property." Megargee (1969) notes that such a definition would include as violence accidental homicide, homicide in self-defense, injury on the football field, "or the newspaper reporter who exposes graft at the expense of someone's reputation" (p. 1038). He states that two issues confound the framing of a completely acceptable definition of violence. The first of these is legality. By ignoring legality and focusing on the act itself, the Commission has unwittingly characterized as violent various legal injuries to people. The alternative of defining violence in terms of illegal acts, however, "is to classify as nonviolent the behavior of Nazi genocidists or Roman gladiators . . ." (p. 1039). The second nemesis of obtaining an acceptable definition of violence is the question of intentionality. The Commission's definition includes unintentional or accidental violence. The alternative of specifying that violence can only be intentional or conscious would not hold well with those of psychoanalytic bent. An initial difficulty, therefore, confronting mental health professionals desirous of preventing violence is the lack of definitional consensus. Violence, as Skolnick (1969, p. 4) points out, "is an ambiguous term whose meaning is established through political processes." Etymology may reveal more about its nature than can be found in legal statutes or psychiatric reports: "dangerous" derives from a 13th century word meaning "difficult to deal with or please" (Steadman 1973b).

VIOLENCE PREVENTION AND CURRENT SOCIAL POLICY

The prevention of violence is currently synonymous with the prediction of violence. Preventive efforts consist of early case identification and the provision of immediate treatment (i.e., secondary prevention, Caplan, 1970).

Society has allocated the task of identifying the violence-prone to those in the mental health and criminal justice systems. At least seventeen states include a prediction of dangerousness as part of their civil commitment criteria (Kittrie, 1971), resulting in approximately 50,000 persons each year involuntarily detained for society's protection and their own treatment (Rubin, 1972). Of the 600,000 persons who will be apprehended and accused of index crimes against persons (homicide, aggravated assault, rape and robbery) in a year, five percent to 10 percent will be given a mental health examination to advise the court about their potential for dangerous behavior, and an additional 10,000 persons will annually be confined as dangerous "mentally ill offenders," including "sexual psychopaths" and those found not guilty by reason of insanity (Rubin, 1972). In addition, the judicial choice of probation or prison for "normal offenders" can be heavily swayed by formal or informal assessments of dangerousness, as can decisions about suitability for community rehabilitation programs or fitness for granting bail (Foote, 1970; Dershowitz, 1970). Predictions of violence likewise play a crucial role in deciding the transfer of a case from juvenile to adult court (Fox, 1972).

While predictions of violence are often critical in deciding who will be detained for the protection of society, they are equally influential in deciding when that detention will end. The indeterminate sentence is perhaps the most extreme example of reliance on predictions of violence in determining length of incarceration. The individual is incarcerated for an unspecified or vaguely specified amount of time, e.g., one to 15 years, on the basis of his assumed dangerousness, and released when authorities predict that he is no longer dangerous. Parole decisions in more determinate sentences also rely heavily upon predictions of violence (Wenk, Robison and Smith, 1972). In general, whenever a form of correctional or mental health treatment is applied to an assumed dangerous person, his release from the treatment institution (prison, civil mental hospital or hospital for the criminally insane) is predicated on a negative prediction of dangerousness. The only way to know when the treatment of a dangerous person is over is to know when he is no longer dangerous.

The Model Sentencing Act of the National Council on Crime and Delinquency proposes that those found to be "dangerous offenders" could be given an extended term of up to 30 years in prison. Yet the President of that organization recently called the identification of dangerous persons "the greatest unresolved problem the criminal justice system faces" (Rector, 1973, p. 186).

PREDICTING VIOLENCE: A REVIEW OF THE EMPIRICAL LITERATURE

The last few years have witnessed a remarkable increase in the number of experimental and naturalistic studies aimed at validating the ability of behavioral scientists (primarily psychiatrists and psychologists) to predict violence.[2] This literature is even more remarkable in that every study has led to similar conclusions.

Wenk, Robison and Smith (1972) reported three massive studies on the prediction of violence undertaken in the California Department of Corrections. The first study, begun in 1965, attempted to develop a "violence prediction scale" to aid in parole decision making. The predictor items employed included commitment offense, number of prior commitments, opiate use, and length of imprisonment. When validated against discovered acts of actual violence by parolees, the scale was able to identify a small class of offenders (less than three percent of the total) of whom 14 percent could be expected to be violent. The probability of violence for this class was nearly three times greater than that for parolees in general, only five percent of whom, by the same criteria, could be expected to be violent. However, 86 percent of those identified as potentially violent, did not, in fact, commit a violent act while on parole.

---

[2] It is one of the more established pieces of psychiatric folklore that the triad of firesetting, enuresia and cruelty to animals is clinically predictive of violence (e.g., Hellman and Blackman, 1966). A recent survey reviewed 1500 references to violence in the behavioral science literature, interviewed 779 professionals who deal with problem youth and retrospectively analyzed 1055 cases to ascertain the best childhood predictors of adult violence. The authors report that four "early warning signs" of violence were identified: fighting, temper tantrums, school problems (including truancy) and an inability to get along with others (Justice, Justice and Kraft, 1974). No prospective studies using these predictors are reported.

The second study reported by Wenk *et al.* (1972) was undertaken in 1968 also in regard to parole decision making. On the basis of actual offender histories and psychiatric reports, 7712 parolees were assigned to various categories keyed to their potential aggressiveness. One in five parolees was assigned to a "potentially aggressive" category, and the rest to a "less aggressive" category. During a one-year follow-up, however, the rate of crimes involving actual violence for the potentially aggressive group was only 3.1 per thousand (5/1630), compared with 2.8 per thousand (17/6082) among the less aggressive group. Thus, for every correct identification of a potentially aggressive individual, there were 326 incorrect ones.

The final study reported by Wenk *et al.* (1972) sampled 4146 California Youth Authority wards. Attention was directed to the record of violence in the youth's past, and an extensive background investigation was conducted, including psychiatric diagnoses and a psychological test battery. Subjects were followed for 15 months after release, and data on 100 variables were analyzed retrospectively to see which items predicted a violent act of recidivism. The authors concluded that the parole decision-maker who used a history of actual violence as his sole predictor of future violence would have 19 false positives in every 20 predictions, and yet "there is no other form of simple classification available thus far that would enable him to improve on this level of efficiency" (p. 399). Several multivariate regression equations were developed from the data, but none was even hypothetically capable of doing better than attaining an eight to one false positive to true positive ratio.

Kozol, Boucher and Garofalo (1972) have recently reported a 10-year study involving 592 male offenders, most of whom had been convicted of violent sex crimes. At the Massachusetts Center for the Diagnosis and Treatment of Dangerous Persons, each offender was examined independently by at least two psychiatrists, two psychologists and a social worker. These clinical examinations, along with a full psychological test battery and "a meticulous reconstruction of the life history elicited from multiple sources — the patient himself, his family, friends, neighbors, teachers, employers, and court, correctional and mental hospital records" (p. 383) formed the data base for their predictions.

Of the 592 patients admitted to their facility for diagnostic observation, 435 were released. Kozol *et al.* recommended the release of 386 as nondangerous, and opposed the release of 49 as dangerous (with the court deciding otherwise). During a five year follow-up period, eight percent of those predicted not to be dangerous became recidivists by committing a serious assaultive act, and 34.7 percent of those predicted to be dangerous committed such an act.

While the assessment of dangerousness by Kozol and his colleagues appears to have some validity, the problem of false positives stands out. Sixty-five percent of the individuals identified as dangerous did not, in fact, commit a dangerous act. Despite the extensive examining, testing and data gathering they undertook, Kozol *et al* were wrong in two out of every three predictions of violence. (For an analysis of the methodological flaws of this study, see Monahan (1973c) and the rejoinder by Kozol, Boucher and Garofalo (1973)).

The Patuxent Institution in Maryland is similar in purpose to Kozol's Massachusetts Center. Data has recently become available on its first ten years of operation (State of Maryland, 1973). Four hundred and twenty-one patients, each of whom received at least three years of treatment at Patuxent are considered. The psychiatric staff opposed the release of 286 of these patients on the grounds that they were still dangerous (with the court releasing them anyway). The staff recommended the release of 135 patients as safe (with the court concurring). The criterion measure was any new offense (not necessarily violent) appearing on F.B.I. reports during the first three years after release.

Of those patients released by the court against staff advice, the recidivism rate was 46 percent if patients had been released directly from the hospital, and 39 percent if a "conditional release experience" had been imposed. Of those patients released on the staff's recommendation and continued for outpatient treatment on parole, seven percent recidivated.[3] Thus, after at least three years of observation and treatment, between 54 and 61 percent of the patients predicted by the staff to be dangerous were actually safe. As with the Kozol *et al.* (1972) study, some predictive validity does seem to accrue to the psychiatric predictions (seven percent recidivism compared with 39 to 46 percent recidivism). Still, the majority of those patients predicted dangerous were actually not so. In addition, it is possible that variables other than psychiatric predictions accounted for the differential recidivism rates. Those who remained until the staff considered them "cured" were, in all likelihood, older than those released by the courts against staff advice. The fact they had a lower rate of recidivism may in part be accounted for by their simply being older.

Credence is lent to this observation by the fact the mean age of those

---

[3] The Patuxent study (State of Maryland, 1973) also makes reference to an 81 percent recidivism rate for those individuals who were recommended for commitment to Patuxent, but who never received treatment because the courts decided not to commit them. This figure is derived from a study by Hodges (1971). The methodological inadequacies of Hodges investigation were severe enough to force one psychiatric commentator to conclude that "this study presents no evidence that justifies its overblown conclusions or the existence of Maryland's [indeterminate sentence] law" (Stone, 1971).

recommended by the staff for commitment to Patuxent, but whom the court did not commit, was 23 years, while the mean age of those who received treatment and were recommended for release by the staff was 30.

In 1966, the U.S. Supreme Court held that Johnnie Baxstrom had been denied equal protection of the law by being detained beyond the maximum sentence in an institution for the criminally insane without the benefit of a new hearing to determine his current dangerousness (Baxstrom v. Herold, 1966). The ruling resulted in the transfer of nearly 1000 persons "reputed to be some of the most dangerous mental patients in the state (of New York)" (Steadman, 1972) from hospitals for the criminally insane to civil mental hospitals, or their direct release into the community. It also provided an excellent opportunity for naturalistic research on the validity of the psychiatric predictions of dangerousness upon which the extended detention was based.

There have been at least eight published follow-up reports on the Baxstrom patients (Hunt and Wiley, 1968; Steadman and Halfon, 1971; Halfon, David and Steadman, 1972; Steadman and Keveles, 1972; Steadman, 1972, 1973a; Steadman and Cocozza, 1973, in press). All concur in the finding that the level of violence experienced in the civil mental hospitals was much less than had been feared, that the civil hospitals adapted well to the massive transfer of patients, and that the Baxstrom patients were being treated the same as the civil patients. The precautions that the civil hospitals had undertaken in anticipation of the supposedly dangerous patients — the setting up of secure wards and provision of judo training to the staff — were largely for naught (Rappeport, 1973). Only twenty percent of the Baxstrom patients were assaultive to persons in the civil hospital or community at any time during a four-year follow of their transfer. Further, only three percent of Baxstrom patients were sufficiently dangerous to be returned to a hospital for the criminally insane during four years after the decision (Steadman and Halfon, 1971). Steadman and Keveles (1972) followed 121 Baxstrom patients who had been released into the community (i.e. discharged from both the criminal and civil mental hospitals). During an average of two and one-half years of freedom, only nine of the 121 patients (eight percent) were convicted of a crime, and only *one* of those convictions was for a violent act.

The Supreme Court decision in the Baxstrom case prompted a similar group of "mentally ill offenders" in Pennsylvania, who had likewise been kept in a hospital after the original judicial authority for their confinement had terminated, to sue for their release. The federal district court agreed with the plaintiffs, held the relevant section of Pennsylvania's Mental Health Act to be unconstitutional, and ordered all such patients transferred to civil hospitals for re-evaluation (*Dixon v. Attorney General of the Commonwealth of Pennsylvania,* 1971). Thornberry and Jacoby (1974) have just completed a four-year follow-up on the 438 patients released into the community on the basis of the Dixon decision. Only 14 percent of the former patients were discovered to have engaged in behavior injurious to another person during that time. The youngest patients, those under 35 years old, had the highest rates of violence on release (23 percent). While the oldest patients, those over 65 years old, had the lowest rates (3 percent).

Table 1 The Prediction of Violence

Study	% True Positives	% False Positives	N Predicted violent	Follow-up Years
Wenk *et al* (1972) Study 1	14.0	86.0	?	?
Wenk *et al* (1972) Study 2	0.3	99.7	1630	1
Wenk *et al* (1972) Study 3	6.2	93.8	104	1
Steadman (1973)	20.0	80.0	967	4
Kozol *et al* (1972)	34.7	65.3	49	5
State of Maryland (1973)	46.0	54.0	221	3
Thornberry & Jacoby (1974)	14.0	86.0	438	4

One might also note Megargee's (1970) extensive review of the use of psychological tests to predict violent behavior. He was unable to find any test which could predict violence adequately in the individual case. "Indeed, none has been developed which will adequately *post*dict, let alone *pre*dict, violent behavior" (p. 145). None of the testing literature of the past few years would modify his statement.

The conclusion to emerge most strikingly from these studies is the great degree to which violence is overpredicted (see Table 1).[4] Of those predicted to be dangerous, between 54 percent and 99 percent are false positives — people who will not, in fact, commit a violent act. Indeed, the literature has been consistent on this point ever since Pinel took the chains off the supposedly dangerous mental patients at La Bicetre in 1792, and the resulting lack of violence gave lie to the psychiatric predictions which had justified their restraint. Violence is vastly overpredicted whether simple behavioral indicators are used or sophisticated multivariate analyses are employed, and whether psychological tests are administered or thorough psychiatric examinations are performed. It is also noteworthy that the population used in each of the research studies reviewed here was highly selective and biased toward positive results — primarily convicted offenders, "sexual psychopaths" and adjudicated delinquents. The fact that even in these groups, with substantially higher base-rates for violence than the general population, violence cannot be validly predicted bodes very poorly for predicting violence among those who have not committed a criminal act.

We are left with the central moral issue: how many false positives — how many harmless men and women — are we willing to sacrifice to protect ourselves from one violent individual? "What represents an acceptable trade-off between the values of public safety and individual liberty?" (Wenk et al., 1972, p. 401). No one insists that prediction be perfect. We do not, after all, require absolute certainty for convicting the guilty, only proof "beyond a reasonable doubt". That means that we are willing to tolerate the conviction of some innocent persons to assure the confinement of a much larger number of guilty criminals (Dershowitz, 1970). But we insist on a process that minimizes erroneous confinement. How can this prized principle of our jurisprudence be squared with the fact that, where the prediction of violence is concerned, we are willing to lock up many to save ourselves from a few? Clearly, an individual should have as much right to remain unmurdered, unmugged, and unraped as he or she does to avoid unjust incarceration as a falsely positive case of dangerousness. Yet the stark facts of current efforts to

---

[4]The objection might be raised that violence sometimes *can* be validly predicted. The husband who needs to be physically restrained by policemen from his wife's throat and who is yelling "I'll kill her" might be an example. While predicting violence in such a situation would be reasonable, it should be noted that a mental health professional would probably have no greater predictive powers than anyone else (in the present example, no greater than the policemen or the wife); and, more importantly, that the prediction would be valid only in the extremely short run (i.e., a matter of minutes or hours). As soon as the immediate situation had passed (e.g., the husband had "cooled off"), predictive validity would probably decline rapidly and the typical pattern of overprediction would set in.

predict and prevent violence lead inexorably to the conclusions of Wenk and his colleagues:

> Confidence in the ability to predict violence serves to legitimate intrusive types of social control. Our demonstration of the *futility* of such prediction should have consequences as great for the protection of individual liberty as a demonstration of the *utility* of violence prediction would have for the protection of society (1972, p. 402).

PSYCHOLOGICAL FACTORS INVOLVED IN THE OVERPREDICTION OF VIOLENCE

To gain an adequate appreciation of the nature of the overprediction of violence by psychiatrists and psychologists, it may be worthwhile to speculate on the factors which lead to this unfortunate situation. Attempts to improve the accuracy of prediction may benefit from an analysis of the processes underlying overprediction. Seven factors are described below which might cumulatively account for the current state of the (in) validity of predictions of violence (Monahan, 1975).

1. *Lack of corrective feedback.* The legal or mental health official who erroneously assesses violence seldom has a chance to learn of his error and modify his subsequent predictions accordingly. Those predicted to be violent are generally incarcerated on the basis of the prediction, and thus there is little opportunity to confirm or disconfirm the judgment (Dershowitz, 1969; 1970). It is not difficult to convince oneself that the predicted offender *would have been* violent had the state not preventitively detained him. A lack of violence after release is attributed to the success of "treatment", rather than to the lack of anything to be treated in the first place.

2. *Differential consequences to the predictor.* If one overpredicts violence, the result is that individuals are incarcerated needlessly. While an unfortunate and, indeed, unjust situation, it is not one likely to have significant public ramifications for the individual responsible for the overprediction. But consider the consequences for the predictor of violence should he err in the other direction — *under*prediction. The correctional official or mental health professional who predicts that a given individual will not commit a dangerous act is subject to severe unpleasantness should that act actually occur. Often he will be informed of its occurrence in the headlines ("Freed Mental Patient Murders Mother") and he or his supervisors will spend many subsequent days fielding reporters' questions about his professional incompetence and his institution's laxity (see the case described in Monahan, 1974a). "There may be no surer way for the forensic psychiatrist to lose power than to have a released mental patient charged with

a serious crime in the district of a key legislator" (Steadman, 1972). Given the drastically differential consequences of overprediction (i.e., "type 1 errors") and underprediction (i.e., "type 2 errors") for the individual responsible for making the judgment, it is not surprising that he or she should choose to "play it safe" and err on the conservative side.

3. *Differential consequences to the subject.* The prediction of dangerousness may often be nothing more than a convention to get someone to treatment. If the ticket to secure involuntary treatment is a diagnosis of dangerousness, many psychiatrists and psychologists appear willing to punch it. Once in treatment, the assessment of dangerousness is forgotten (Rubin, 1972). Monahan and Cummings (1974), for example, have demonstrated in a laboratory context that individuals are more likely to be predicted dangerous when that prediction will lead to mental hospitalization than when it will lead to imprisonment. To the extent that states tighten their criteria for involuntary civil commitment from "need for treatment" to "dangerous to others", one should expect predictions of dangerousness to increase. Overprediction, therefore, may be less a comment on any lack of scientific acumen and more a testimony to the ability of officials to subvert the intent of the law to accomplish what they think is "best" for the patient.

An alternate form of using the prediction of dangerousness as a ploy for other purposes is suggested by the Morris and Hawkins (1970) observation that when dangerousness is invoked, it often is for retributive purposes. There are some, e.g., "mentally disordered sex offenders", for whom the law requires "treatment" rather than "punishment" (Kittrie, 1971). By diagnosing such persons as dangerous, however, one may satisfy tacit retributive demands by insuring that the treatment they receive will involve at least as much incarceration as punishment would have. Foote puts it more strongly: he holds the concept of dangerousness to be "devoid of meaningful content and a convenient handle for political repression" (1970, p. 8).

4. *Illusory correlation.* An illusory correlation is a type of systematic error of observation in which observers report seeing relationships between classes of events where no relationship actually exists (Chapman and Chapman, 1969). Sweetland (1972) has demonstrated how this phenomenon influences the assessment of dangerousness. Psychiatrists were surveyed to determine which personality traits they considered to be most characteristic of dangerous and nondangerous persons. Following this, naive subjects were asked to examine personality descriptions which were made up of these characteristics and which were paired with the diagnoses "dangerous" or "nondangerous". In one condition of this study, a zero correlation was present between the items designated by the psychiatrists as indicating a dangerous person and the diagnostic formulations with which these items were paired. Subjects were asked after the presentation to describe what they

had observed. The results indicated that even when there was a zero correlation, the subjects responded as if they had observed a relationship in the materials. They consistently recalled that certain of the characteristics had appeared more frequently with the diagnosis of "dangerous", when, in fact, they were uncorrelated. These systematic errors of observation were consistent with the subjects' prior expectations about which characteristics implied dangerousness.

The poor ability of mental health professionals to predict violence, therefore, can be partially explained by their reliance upon stereotypic prior expectations as to what constitutes a predictor of violence, rather than valid correlations. Predictor variables which, in fact, bear no relationship to violence will continue to be used, because those who believe in them will find (illusory) support for their beliefs by selectively attending to the data: they will see only what they wish to see. The relationship between violence and mental illness, for example, appears to be an illusory correlation (see below).

5. *Unreliability of the criterion.* We have already noted the plethora of definitions which have been advanced for the designation of a violent act. In addition to the handicap of definitional vagary, research on the prediction of violence is actually research on the prediction of *discovered* and reported violence. Undetected violence and police discretion in certifying acts of violence necessarily decrease the reliability of the event being predicted. "The problem, then, is this: Most of the violent behavior we would wish to predict probably never comes to our attention, and the part that does is far from a representative sample" (Wenk *et al.,* 1972, p. 401). A prediction of violence may itself be reactive — it may influence the later certification of a violent act. Those at whom a finger has been pointed may be scrutinized more carefully than others, and the prophecy may thus fulfill itself.

6. *Low Baserates.* A vexing statistical problem further complicates the prediction of violence. The problem has to do with the low baserates of violence in society, e.g., an annual murder rate of 8.9 per 100,000 (Kelley, 1973).

If the baserate of an event is high, predicting that event without many false positives is relatively easy. If nine out of 10 people commit murder, one could simply predict that everyone will commit murder and be correct 90 percent of the time. As the baserate become lower, however, the problem of false positives becomes more salient. Livermore, Malmquist and Meehl (1968) address themselves to this problem in discussing dangerousness as a criteria for involuntary civil commitment.

> Assume that one person out of a thousand will kill. Assume also that
> an exceptionally accurate test is created which differentiates with 95
> percent effectiveness those who will kill from those who will not. If
> 100,000 people were tested, out of the 100 who would kill, 95

would be isolated. Unfortunately, out of the 99,000 who would not kill, 4995 people would also be isolated as potential killers. In these circumstances, it is clear that we could not justify incarcerating all 5090 people. If, in the criminal law, it is better that ten guilty men go free than that one innocent man suffer, how can we say in the civil commitment area that it is better that 54 harmless people be incarcerated lest one dangerous man be free? (p. 84)[5]

7. *Powerlessness of the subject.* Finally, the gross overprediction of violence may be so easily tolerated because those against whom predictive efforts are mounted are generally powerless to resist. Prisoners or mental patients (who became or remained such due to overprediction) are unlikely to arouse a public outcry in their defense. As Geis and Monahan (in press) have recently put it:

> The persons involved as patients or prisoners almost invariably are located in social positions where they do not have adequate political or financial resources to protest effectively against what is being done to them. That is, they lack things such as ready media access and funds to hire good lawyers . . . If society's aim is really to isolate the violent and the violence-prone and protect the innocent, then why are those who allow faulty fuel tanks to continue to be installed in the planes they market, and those who are or ought to be responsible for things such as an unconscionably high national infant mortality rate (Gross, 1967, p. 24) not similarly 'diagnosed' and 'rehabilitated?'

The fact that the provision of free legal services to mental hospital patients results in drastically increased discharge rates (Kumasaka, Stokes, and Gupta, 1972) supports a social power interpretation of predictive efforts.

SOCIAL POLICY IMPLICATIONS OF THE INABILITY TO IDENTIFY DANGEROUS PERSONS

The prediction of violence, of course, has importance only as an initial step in society's action in behalf of what it considers its own protection. Those predicted to be violent are involuntarily detained to prevent the occurrence of the undesired act. The law normally requires conviction of a crime before subjecting a citizen to incarceration on the basis of a prediction of dangerousness. (Being denied bail on the grounds of alleged dangerousness is a form of preventive detention in which a crime has been charged, but not

[5]For a lucid discussion of why individuals generally ignore baserates in making intuitive predictions, see Kahneman and Tversky (1973).

proven (Foote, 1970; Dershowitz, 1970)) The fact that dangerousness is greatly overpredicted would suggest grave caution in relying upon such predictions as a principle means for deciding who should be detained or when detention should end (e.g., indeterminate sentencing) (see Monahan and Cummings, in press). Given that past behavior tends to be the single best predictor of future behavior (Mischel, 1968), one might generally weigh evidence of previous violence more heavily than clinical or judicial predictions (*cf.* Speiser, 1970).

There is one group in society, however, for which preventive detention is sanctioned even in the absence of a conviction or allegation of a violent act — the "mentally ill" (Dershowitz, 1970; Monahan, 1973a). This is, no doubt, due to the widespread public belief that the psychologically disturbed are intrinsically more violence-prone than the rest of us (Rabkin, 1972). This belief is frequently reinforced by the media, which takes great pains to report when an offender is an ex-mental patient, or has even seen a private psychologist or psychiatrist, but which never reports when a criminal does not have a previous psychiatric history.

The research literature on violence and psychological disorder, however, does not support public opinion. The most extensive review of the area, citing scores of studies, concluded that "an individual with a label of mental illness is quite capable of committing any act of violence known to man, but probably does not do so with any greater frequency than his neighbor in the general population" (Gulevich and Bourne, 1970, p. 323; see also Mulvihill and Tumin, 1969, p. 444).

The lack of ability to predict dangerousness, combined with the similar baserates for violence among the psychologically disturbed and "normals," suggests that there is no empirical basis to support the preventive detention of those psychologically disturbed persons who have not committed a violent act (Monahan, 1973d). A similar conclusion was reached by Pennsylvania's Task Force in Commitment Procedures (1972) studying revisions of that state's mental health laws: "since the capacity to predict dangerous conduct is no greater in the case of mentally ill persons than others, preventive detention is no more justified in the case of mental illness than elsewhere". Likewise, one cannot argue for the preventive detention of the mentally ill on the therapeutic grounds that they can be helped by psychiatric treatment, since no form of psychiatric treatment has yet been empirically demonstrated to have an enduring effect on reducing violent behavior (Monahan, 1973b; Geis and Monahan, in press).

The overprediction of violence has even more sobering implications for attempts at prevention by the early identification of violence-prone children. Former President Nixon asked the Department of Health, Education, and Welfare to study the proposals of Arnold Hutschnecker, a psychiatrist who had formerly been the president's physician. Hutschnecker suggested that psychological tests such as the Rorschach be administered to all six-year-olds in the United States to determine their potential for criminal behavior, followed by "massive psychological and psychiatric treatment for those children found to be criminally inclined". Such a program, Hutschnecker said, was "a better short-term solution to the crime problem than urban reconstruction. Teenage boys later found to be persisting in incorrigible behavior would be remanded to camps . . ." (Maynard, 1970). While some comfort may be taken in the fact that these proposals were resoundingly condemned by officials of all mental health disciplines, it is nonetheless disconcerting that they ever reached the level they did.[6]

A PROPOSED STRATEGY FOR VIOLENCE PREVENTION: IDENTIFYING VIOLENCE – ELICITING SITUATIONS

The conclusion suggested by the literature on the prediction of violence is that violence-prone individuals cannot be identified without erroneously identifying a much larger number of non-violent persons. The factors we have hypothesized to account for this state of affairs are not especially conducive to facile improvement. I do not wish to imply, however, that the task of predicting and preventing acts of violence is necessarily hopeless. At least part of the inability to predict violent acts may lie with the theoretical paradigms and research strategies which have constricted the psychological and psychiatric fields until very recently. Efforts to predict and modify violent behavior, like efforts to predict and modify all types of problems, have been almost exclusively focused on identifying *persons* who are likely to perform the behavior in the future (Mischel, 1968). It is becoming increasingly documented, however, that behavior is a joint function of personal characteristics and characteristics of the *situation* with which a person immediately interacts (Mischel, 1973; Bandura, 1973). This recognition that behavior is at least in part situationally determined opens a new perspective on the prediction and prevention of violence. Rather than attempting to

[6]Perhaps even more amazingly, Hutschnecker (1973) has recently recommended a psychiatric overseer for the President. "I cannot help think if an American President had a staff psychiatrist, perhaps a case such as Watergate might not have a chance to develop. A President has a personal physician to watch over his physical health. Why could a man of outstanding leadership not have a physician watching over his and his staff's mental health?" Hutschnecker also states that staff psychiatrists to Presidents Lincoln and Wilson might have been able to prevent both the Civil War and World War I. Like Juvenal, one can only wonder who will guard the guardians (see Szasz's retort, 1973). Recent history suggests that the nation is better protected by a Special Prosecutor than by the President's analyst.

identify and modify violence-prone persons, energy could be expended in the attempt to identify and modify situations conducive to violence (*cf.* Wenk and Emrich, 1972, p. 196). An ecological analysis (Moos and Insel, 1973) could shed light on the situational context in which violent crime occurs. Attempts to prevent violence could then take one of the following forms: (1) modification of the situation, (2) modification of one's response to the situation, or (3) avoidance of the situation.

In attempting to prevent the crime of violent rape, for example, a hypothetical ecological analysis of a given community might reveal that a sizeable proportion of past rapes occurred in certain areas of the community with poorly-lit streets, where public transportation was unavailable, and when hitch-hiking. Preventive efforts based on this analysis might then include modifying the environment by providing increased lighting and public transportation, and a publicity campaign to advise women to avoid hitch-hiking situations (*cf.* the notion of "target hardening", Mulvihill and Tumin, 1969, p. 776). Such preventive tactics are obviously not panaceas. Care would have to be taken not to induce community paranoia. There is always the possibility that would-be rapists will merely relocate their activities in another environmental context. But to the extent that rape is situationally determined and "perceived opportunity" gives rise to sexual assault, such a strategy might have a significant impact.

As another example, a situational analysis of violence on policemen reveals that 22 percent of the police killed nationally and 40 percent of police injuries occur when intervening in family disputes (Bard, 1971). Knowing, then, that family crisis situations are conducive to violence against the police, preventive efforts in the form of modifying police responses to these situations may prove fruitful. Training police to effectively deal with such violence-eliciting situations has already been mounted on a large scale with considerable success (Bard, 1971; Driscoll, Meyer and Schanie, 1973).

The tack being suggested has implications for the broader realm of public policy as well. Surely among the contexts most conducive to lethal violence is the easy accessibility of a gun during a heated argument. "Can there be any doubt that a significant decrease in the availability of weapons would do infinitely more about violence prevention than screening the population for 'low violence threshold,' and without the need for doctors to become policemen-in-disguise?" (Coleman, 1974).

Likewise, the presence of drunken drivers on the highway provides a situational gauntlet which tens of thousands of innocent persons run unsuccessfully each year. This massive slaughter to which we have become numbed might be partially abated if the criminal justice system began treating drunk driving as the social menace it is, rather than as something akin to having a burned-out tail light. Considering that more Americans are killed on the highway *each year* than in the entire ten year involvement in Vietnam, and that research has consistently found that *at least* 50 percent of traffic fatalities are alcohol-related, our tolerance for this group of *demonstrably dangerous persons* in our midst is nothing short of incredible (Shah, in press).[7]

Finally, the settings which breed violence are to be found in corporate board rooms as well as on urban street corners. "If you want to talk about violence," Nader (1970, p. 10) has said, "don't talk of Black Panthers. Talk of General Motors." Legislative efforts to curb death-dealing corporate irresponsibility will go much farther in preventing violence than legislated psychotherapy for those unfortunate enough to be identified as "violence-prone" (Geis and Monahan, in press).

A situational approach to violence prevention[8] is most compatible with a community mental health orientation to the delivery of psychological services (Cowen, 1973; Catalano and Monahan, in press; Monahan, 1974c). It is a "system-centered" approach rather than a "person centered" one (Bloom, 1971), and as such is less likely to result in "blaming the victim" for his own plight (Caplan and Nelson, 1973). It shifts the emphasis from early case identification (i.e., secondary prevention) to the modification of those factors which give rise to violence (i.e., primary prevention). In addition, a situational approach to violence prevention can draw from the rapidly growing literature on environmental psychology in the design of intervention programs (Craik, 1973; Moos, 1973; Insel and Moos, 1974; Monahan, 1974b; Heller and Monahan, 1975; Price, 1974).

Efforts by mental health professionals to prophesy the perpetrators of violence appear to be doomed. Efforts to identify and intervene in situations conducive to violence may lead to appreciable gains in preventive efficiency and would obviate the seemingly insurmountable problem of unjustly interfering in the lives of innumerable false positives. Ultimately, it may be

---

[7] It is interesting to note in this regard that while the media consistently overreports the relationship between violence and mental illness, it severely under reports other relationships. Waller and Worden (1973), in a study of newspaper coverage of automobile crashes, found that "alcohol is mentioned in only 11 percent of the fatal crashes and 2 percent of the nonfatal ones, although it is known to be a factor in at least five times as many fatal crashes and about eight times as many nonfatal ones" (p. 7).

[8] It should be clear that the present discussion has limited itself to the immediate or *proximal* situations which are conducive to violence. A comprehensive approach to violence prevention must also address itself to those *distal* situations and environmental contexts which foment violence (e.g., poverty, bigotry). While difficult to argue without degenerating into a tired rhetoric, it is nonetheless true that, in the long run, social justice is a prerequisite to social tranquility.

possible to classify both persons and situations in a typology of violence. One might eventually be able to predict that persons of a given type will commit a violent act if they remain in one environment, yet will be nonviolent if placed into a different situational context. Appropriate interventions at both the person and system level could then be planned. While working for an empirically valid and morally acceptable scheme for the prevention of violence, however, we would do well to be guided by the admonition of Benjamin Franklin: "They that can give up essential liberty to obtain a little temporary safety, deserve neither liberty nor safety."

REFERENCES

Bandura, A. *Aggression: A social learning analysis.* Englewood Cliffs, New Jersey: Prentice-Hall, 1973.

Bard, M. The role of law enforcement in the helping system. *Community Mental Health Journal,* 1971, **7**, 151-160.

Baxstrom v. Herold, *U.S. Reports,* 1966, **383**, 107.

Bloom, B. Strategies for the prevention of mental disorders. In *Issues in community psychology and preventive mental health.* New York: Behavioral Publications, 1971.

Board of Directors, National Council on Crime and Delinquency. The nondangerous offender should not be imprisoned: a policy statement. *Crime and Delinquency,* 1973, **19**, 449-456.

Caplan, G. *Theory and practice of mental health consultation.* New York: Basic Books, 1970.

Caplan, N. and Nelson, S. On being useful: The nature and consequences of psychological research on social problems. *American Psychologist,* 1973, **28**, 199-211.

Catalano, R. and Monahan, J. The community psychologist as social planner. *American Journal of Community Psychology,* in press.

Chapman, L. and Chapman, J. Illusory correlations as an obstacle to the use of valid psychodiagnostic signs. *Journal of Abnormal Psychology,* 1969, **74**, 271-280.

Coleman, L. Perspectives on the medical research of violence. Paper presented at the annual meeting of the American Orthopsychiatric Association, San Francisco, April, 1974.

Comment, Liberty and required mental health treatment. *University of Pennsylvania Law Review,* 1965, **114**, 1067-1070.

Cowen, E. Social and community interventions, *Annual Review of Psychology,* 1973, **24**, 423-472.

Craik, K. Environmental psychology, *Annual Review of Psychology*, 1973, **24**, 403-422.

Dershowitz, A. Psychiatrist's power in civil commitment, *Psychology Today*, 1969, **2**, 43-47.

Dershowitz, A. Imprisonment by judicial hunch: The case against pretrial preventive detention. *The Prison Journal*, 1970, **1**, 12-22.

Dixon v. Attorney General of the Commonwealth of Pennsylvania, *Federal Supplement*, 1971, **325**, 966.

Driscoll, J., Meyer, R. and Schanie, C. Training police in family crisis intervention. *Journal of Applied Behavioral Science*, 1973, **9**, 62-68.

Ervin, F. and Lion, J. Clinical evaluation of the violent patient. In D. Mulvihill and M. Tumin (Eds.) *Crimes of violence: Staff Report submitted to the National Commission on the Causes and Prevention of Violence*. U.S. Government Printing Office, 1969, Vol. 13, pp. 1163-1188.

Foote, C. Preventive detention — What is the issue? *The Prison Journal*, 1970, **1**, 3-11.

Fox, S. Predictive devices and the reform of juvenile justice. In S. Glueck and E. Glueck (Eds.) *Identification of predelinquents*. New York: Intercontinental Medical Book Corporation, 1972.

Geis, G. and Monahan, J. The social ecology of violence. In T. Lickona (Ed.) *Morality: A handbook of moral development and behavior*. New York; Holt, Rinehart and Winston, in press.

Gross, M. *The doctors*. New York: Dell, 1967.

Gulevich, G. and Bourne, P. Mental illness and violence. In D. Daniels, M. Gilula and F. Ochberg, (Eds.) *Violence and the struggle for existence*. Boston: Little, Brown, 1970.

Halfon, A., David, M. and Steadman, H. The Baxstrom Women: A four-year follow up of behavior patterns. *The Psychiatric Quarterly*, 1972, **45**, 1-10.

Heller, K. and Monahan, J. Community mental health. Unpublished manuscript, 1975.

Hellman, D. and Blackman, N. Enuresis, firesetting, and cruelty to animals: A triad predictive of adult crime. *American Journal of Psychiatry*, 1966, **122**, 1431-1435.

Hodges, E. Crime prevention by the indeterminate sentence law. *American Journal of Psychiatry*, 1971, **128**, 291-295.

Hunt, R. and Wiley, E. Operation Baxstrom after one year. *American Journal of Psychiatry*, 1968, **124**, 974-978.

Insel P. and Moos, R. Psychological environments: Expanding the scope of human ecology. *American Psychologist*, 1974, **29**, 179-188.

Justice, B., Justice, R. and Kraft, J. Early warning signs of violence: Is a triad enough? *American Journal of Psychiatry*, 1974, **131**, 457-459.

Kahneman, D. and Tversky, A. On the psychology of prediction. *Psychological Review*, 1973, **81**, 237-251.

Kelly, C. *Crime in the United States — 1972*. Washington, D.C.: Government Printing Office, 1973.

Kittrie, N. *The right to be different.* Baltimore: John Hopkins University Press, 1971.

Kozol, H., Boucher, R. and Garofalo, R. The diagnosis and treatment of dangerousness. *Crime and Delinquency,* 1972, **18**, 371-392.

Kozol, H., Boucher, R. and Garofalo, R. Dangerousness. *Crime and Delinquency,* 1973, **19**, 554-555.

Kumasaka, Y., Stokes, J. and Gupta, R. Criteria for involuntary hospitalization. *Archives of General Psychiatry,* 1972, **26**, 399-404.

Livermore, J., Malmquist, C. and Meehl, P. On the justifications for civil commitment. *University of Pennsylvania Law Review,* 1968, **117**, 75-96.

Maynard, R. Doctor would test children to curb crime. *Los Angeles Times,* April 5, 1970, Sect. A, p. 9.

Megargee, E. The psychology of violence. In D. Mulvihill and M. Tumin (Eds.) *Crimes of violence: A Staff Report submitted to the National Commission on the Causes and Prevention of Violence.* U.S. Government Printing Office, 1969, Vol. **13**, pp. 1037-1116.

Megargee, E. The prediction of violence with psychological tests. In C. Speilberger (Ed.), *Current topics in clinical and community psychology.* New York: Academic Press, 1970.

Mischel, W. *Personality and assessment.* New York: Wiley, 1968.

Mischel, W. Toward a cognitive social learning reconceptualization of personality. *Psychological Review,* 1973, **80**, 252-283.

Monahan, J. The psychiatrization of criminal behavior. *Hospital & Community Psychiatry,* 1973, **24**, 105-107. (a)

Monahan, J. Abolish the insanity defense? – Not yet. *Rutgers Law Review,* 1973, **26**, 719-741. (b)

Monahan, J. Dangerous offenders: A critique of Kozol, *et al. Crime and Delinquency,* 1973, **19**, 481-420. (c)

Monahan, J. Dangerousness and civil commitment. Testimony before the (California) Assembly Select Committee on Mentally Disordered Criminal Offenders. December 13, 1973. (d)

Monahan, J. In defense of civil liberty – despite fear of violence. *Los Angeles Times,* February 3, 1974, Part VI, p. 3. (a)

Monahan, J. Community mental health as applied environmental psychology. Paper presented to the annual meeting of the American Psychological Association, New Orleans, August, 1974. (b)

Monahan, J. Toward undergraduate education in the interface of mental health and criminal justice. *Journal of Criminal Justice,* 1974, **2**, 61-65.(c)

Monahan, J. The prediction of violence. In D. Chappell and J. Monahan (Eds.) *Violence and criminal justice.* Lexington, Mass.: Lexington Books, 1975.

Monahan J. and Cummings, L. The prediction of violence as a function of its perceived consequences. *Journal of Criminal Justice,* 1974, **2**, 239-242.

Monahan, J. and Cummings, L. Social policy implications of the inability to predict violence. *Journal of Social Issues,* in press. (b)

Moos, R. Conceptualizations of human environments. *American Psychologist,* 1973, **28,** 652-665.

Moos, R. and Insel, P. *Issues in social ecology.* Palo Alto: National Press, 1973.

Morris, N. and Hawkins, G. *The honest politicians' guide to crime control.* Chicago: University of Chicago Press, 1970.

Mulvihill, D. and Tumin, M. (Eds.). *Crimes of violence: a Staff Report submitted to the National Commission on the Causes and Prevention of Violence.* U.S. Government Printing Office, 1969.

Nader, R. Quoted in white-collar crime, *Barron's.* March 30, 1970, pp. 1, 10.

Overholser v. Russell, *Federal Reporter,* (2nd. ed.), 1960, **282,** 195.

Price, R. Etiology, the social environment and the prevention of psychological dysfunction. In P. Insel and R. Moos (Eds.) *Health and the social environment.* Lexington, Massachusetts: D.C. Heath, 1974.

Rabkin, J. Opinions about mental illness: A review of the literature. *Psychological Bulletin,* 1972, **78,** 153-171.

Rappeport, J. A response to "Implications from the Baxstrom experience." *Bulletin of the American Academy of Psychiatry and the Law,* 1973, **1,** 197-198.

Rector, M. Who are the dangerous? *Bulletin of the American Academy of Psychiatry and the Law,* 1973, **1,** 186-188.

Rubin, B. Prediction of dangerousness in mentally ill criminals. *Archives of General Psychiatry,* 1972, **27,** 397-407.

Sarbin, T. The dangerous individual: An outcome of social identity transformations. *British Journal of Criminology,* July 1967, 285-295.

Shah, S. Some interactions of law and mental health in the handling of social deviance. *Catholic University Law Review,* in press.

Skolnick, J. *The politics of protest.* New York: Simon and Schuster, 1969.

Speiser, L. Preventive detention: The position of the American Civil Liberties Union. *The Prison Journal,* 1970, **1,** 49-52.

State of Maryland (Department of Public Safety and Correctional Services). Maryland's Defective Delinquency Statute – A Progress Report. Unpublished manuscript, 1973.

Steadman, H. The psychiatrist as a conservative agent of social control. *Social Problems,* 1972, **20,** 263-171.

Steadman, H. Implications from the Baxstrom experience. *Bulletin of the American Academy of Psychiatry and the Law,* 1973, **1,** 189-196. (a)

Steadman, H. Some evidence on the inadequacy of the concept and determination of dangerousness in law and psychiatry. *The Journal of Psychiatry and Law,* Winter, 1973, 909-426. (b)

Steadman, H. and Cocozza, J. The criminally insane patient: Who gets out? *Social Psychiatry,* 1973, 8, 230-238.

Steadman, H. and Cocozza, J. *Careers of the criminally insane: Excessive social control of deviance.* Lexington, Mass: Lexington Books, 1974.

Steadman, H. and Halfon, A. The Baxtrom patients: Backgrounds and outcome. *Seminars in Psychiatry,* 1971, 3, 376-386.

Steadman, H. and Keveles, G. The community adjustment and criminal activity of the Baxstrom patients: 1966-1970. *American Journal of Psychiatry,* 1972, **129**, 304-310.

Stone, A. Discussion of Hodge's "Crime prevention by the indeterminate sentence." *American Journal of Psychiatry,* 1971, **128**, 295.

Sweetland, J. "Illusory correlation" and the estimation of "dangerous" behavior. Unpublished dissertation, Indiana University, 1972.

Szasz, T. The dominion of psychiatry. *The New York Times,* August 5, 1973, p. E-15.

Task Force in Commitment Procedures, Commonwealth of Pennsylvania. Pennsylvania Department of Public Welfare, 1972.

Waller, J and Worden, J. Application of baseline data for public education about alcohol and highway safety. Office of Alcohol Countermeasures, U.S. Department of Transportation, Bethesda, Md., 1973 (Mimeo).

Wenk, E. and Emrich, R. Assaultive youth: An exploratory study of the assaultive experience and assaultive potential of California Youth Authority Wards. *Journal of Research in Crime and Delinquency,* 1972, **9**, 171-196.

Wenk, E., Robison, J. and Smith G. Can violence be predicted? *Crime and Delinquency,* 1972, **18**, 393-402.

2
Community-Based Delinquency-Prevention Programs: An Overview*[1]

IRVING A. SPERGEL

Recent years have witnessed the development of a social movement to deal with deviants in the context of the community. The movement, in its physical and social sense, has been from outlying or rural to urban areas; from large to small institutions; from custodial, corrective, rehabilitative, even therapeutic milieus to family arrangements or special facsimiles thereof, from isolation and stigma to more normal and equal involvement in the mainstream of community living. Service patterns for the aged, the mentally ill, the mentally retarded, children in need of protective care, drug addicts, public aid recipients, and others have been affected by the effort to involve deviants more fully in the control and development of their own destiny. The latest outcast to become the beneficiary of changing professional, public, and legislative thinking and morality is the delinquent. For example, Massachusetts has already implemented its recent decision to close correctional institutions for youth and deal with them in community facilities (11).

The following is a discussion of selected policy and program issues that face or will face policy makers and administrators in developing community-

*Reprinted from *Social Service Review,* 1973, **47**, 16-31, with permission. Copyrighted by the University of Chicago Press.

[1]This article is based on a paper presented at a conference held at Boston College, Newton, Massachusetts, June 28, 1972, and sponsored by the Commonwealth of Massachusetts Joint Correctional Planning Commission, Department of Youth Services, Boston College Law School and Department of Sociology, Fordham University Institute for Social Research, and the National Program for the Development of Strategies for Juvenile Delinquency Prevention of the Department of Health, Education and Welfare.

based programs. Interorganizational and political or interest-group constraints consitute the framework of the analysis. The discussion is organized into three major sections: policy and program rationales, past and present programs, and program effectiveness. However, the complex issues of the decision to close down residential institutions in the first instance will not be addressed.

POLICY AND PROGRAM RATIONALES

The problem of developing community-based institutions and programming for and with delinquents in the open community requires consideration of three types of questions: What is a community-based program, and who is a delinquent or predelinquent? What is the rationale of the program, or what is the connection between the program and the social or community problem to be solved? What are the objectives of the program, and how are they to be achieved?

Definition. The terms *community-based program* and *delinquent* or *delinquency* require some explanation and ideally, agreen-upon definitions. In fact, the terms are used to identify variable elements and qualities. Meanings are often implicit, and one man's community or delinquent is often not the same as another man's. For example, the term *community* may suggest a geographical area, a collection of people, an organization of local groups and institutions, or a desirable state of relationship between people and institutions. Discussions or debates on community problems may focus on one or more of the following related elements: power or negotiating capability; voluntary association, participation, self-determination, or community control; service-delivery systems; common or comprehensive interests; social change and/or its effects. The terms *neighborhood* and *community* may be used interchangeably.

Suggested for purposes of the present discussion is the following geographically oriented definiton: A community is a collectivity of individuals and groups, often located within a specific geographic area, and variously organized and differentiated by sex, age, race, ethnicity, status, interest, need, and purpose. The area tends to be identified both locally and externally, not always sharply or consistently, on the basis of administrative, historical, physical, political, economic, social, and cultural considerations.

A greater problem arises in the definition of *community-based program.* For most administrators it probably refers to a program run on a decentralized basis, still governed by established agency interests, but more sensitive to the needs of individuals defined as delinquent; the program also involves local citizens in some way. It is important, however, to think of community-based programs in political as well as administrative terms. One must consider such questions as: For whom is the program primarily run? Who makes key policy decisions? What is the character of community participation in and identification with the program?

Organizations and agencies may differ further in certain distinctive ways. In somewhat oversimplistic and general terms, community programs for delinquents may vary along certain strategic dimensions of intervention, such as goals and locus of decision making. Organizations may be concerned with providing effective services, yet be status quo oriented, with decisions made by professional workers, bureaucrats, and established group representatives. Organizations may also be concerned with limited forms of community development and protection, and still be status quo oriented, but with decisions made by interests identified as highly local or indigenous. Other organizations may be change oriented; that is, certain professional workers and reformers, even within the establishment, may run programs seeking institutional changes on behalf of a deprived or stigmatized population; however, local citizens may not be involved in key decisions. On the other hand, organizations and their programs may be run for, by, and with local community people, even by the disadvantaged or deviant sector or their direct representatives, to bring about institutional change (13; 14). In reality, of course, community-based programs are different blends of these orientations, which produce varying strategies of service provision, community development, advocacy, and conflict. At one extreme, community participation may indicate little or no policy and administrative involvement and, at the other, complete control and staffing of programs by local adults and/or offenders (1; 2).

The definition of *delinquency* is critical for the development of a community-based program. The term is just as variable and complex as community. In fact, it may be even more variable within a community than across the juvenile-justice system. There appears to be no across-the-board operational definition of delinquents or predelinquents in community-based programs. It is not at all clear what a community program to prevent or to treat delinquents really is or should be.

Some agencies established specifically to deal with delinquents may seek to avoid isolating or stigmatizing certain youths by serving mainly nondelinquents. The process of working with youth in delinquency-control programs may nevertheless contribute to negative labeling and delinquency-creating process. Several years ago, a public delinquency-prevention agency in a large city utilized its suddenly expanded budget to work with a variety of street-corner groups heretofore not served. A number of youths who did not participate in antisocial acts but hung out occasionally on street corners were identified, screened, and referred for service. In consequence, the police began to pay more attention to them. Several who ordinarily might have escaped agency and police attention were picked up for minor offenses, for example, breaking a window or unlawful assembly. The illustration is used not to suggest that community agencies should not ordinarily maintain open intake and include delinquents and nondelinquents, but to raise questions about program definition and attendant problems of purpose and client labeling.

The definition of the delinquency problem and, in part, the character of the program and its rationale are determined on the basis of organizational interests under market conditions. Organizations may be concerned primarily or only peripherally with services for delinquents. Programs may be derived largely as an effort to bolster the agency's capacity to achieve other purposes, for example, general services to community, institutional change, or community development. Delinquency-prevention or delinquency-control programs may come to be more an arena for general competition among institutional interests or service suppliers than a specific means to identify or solve a problem that derives primarily from individual youth and family needs and from the breakdown of basic urban structures and processes. Under these conditions, it is not hard to predict that community-based programs can ignore or aggravate rather than ameliorate or control delinquency problems. Delinquents or predelinquents, however defined, may become targets for community attention and agency services that contribute more to the growth and status of organizations than to the solution of problems of individual or collective delinquency.

Program rationale. While there may be some limit on definitions of the delinquency problem, there seems to be no limit on the number of rationales for programming, that is, for what to do about the problem. The logic of problem analysis somehow is never rigorous enough to provide a clear or an interrelated set of program objectives and solutions. Organizational and professional ideology and particularistic access to resources appear to determine the connection between the problem and the program. The market for solutions to the delinquency problem seems unlimited, particularly if agencies or community groups promise quick and dramatic results. While the problem of delinquency among youngsters under sixteen years old may be assessed as growing worse, either in the ghettos or in the suburbs, in relation to drug use, gang behavior, and run-aways, the cures are unclear, multiple, and competing. Everybody gets into the act of explaining the problem and providing answers to it. The causes of delinquency include everything from family breakdown and inadequate ego development to a defective juvenile-justice system and the collective powerlessness of ghetto people. The solutions also vary, from long-term therapy to revolution and counterrevolution. The individual and the community as complex but interacting and interdependent entities seem not to exist. The delinquent, the gang, the agency, the community "power structure," and specific community conditions become targets for fragmented attack or change according to particular interest-group perspectives and remedies. Everyone wants a piece of the action. Nobody wants the whole thing, or is even concerned with it.

Program objectives and means. Once an agency or community group has selected its delinquent population or delinquency-generating condition and established its rationale and the general intent of its program, the problem of relation between goals and objectives, ends and means, arises. While the agency may set out in pursuit of stated objectives, very quickly and tenaciously it may settle down to pursuit of means or, in current parlance, the efficient service-delivery system. The system aspects, usually in terms of methods and procedures, may become dominant. Even when the system is open and flexible, even when explicit guidelines for the worker are not initially established, whatever it is that has to be done becomes in due course the end as well as the means. Agency operational problems and daily activities consume administrative energies. Organizational maintenance rather than goal achievement becomes the test of survival. The agency purpose seems to be to build a better mouse trap, but who gets trapped and what happens to the object of entrapment, manipulation, control, or change is unclear and perhaps of secondary importance.

Basic program decisions are usually not centrally made and are susceptible to many influences. Indeed, the separation between the internal and the external structure of a community-based program is difficult to make. Furthermore, environmental influences are not consistent or reinforcing; usually they are in a state of flux.

Organizations have conflicting approaches, norms, and practices in regard to delinquents. The impact of varied community forces on a given delinquency-control or treatment program is therefore not clearly predictable. For example, the police, the district attorney, and certain citizen groups are primarily concerned with control of delinquent behavior and protection of the community. Their objectives and practices are defined in official, legitimate, middle-class, and often traditional terms. The outreach or streetworker program may be concerned primarily with social and recreational development of the gang and its members; the counseling agency may be interested primarily in interpersonal, educational, or employment problems of the individual; the employer is concerned mainly with the extent to which the delinquent can contribute to certain objectives of production and profit; still other organizations, including churches, social agencies, and civil-rights and militant groups, are concerned with delinquents as a way to change the community or societal system so that institutions will work better and produce less delinquency and other types of social problems. Delinquents themselves may be organized into gangs, nonprofit associations, economic development corporations, or social-action groups. The various organizations represent, in a sense, different communities of interest. Each views and utilizes delinquents quite differently. Each not only tailors its program to meet the needs of delinquents, but also adapts to the needs of other interest groups in the immediate community. Furthermore, the organization must adapt to the larger societal system of influences, in which federal funding policies, public values, and technological change, as well as time itself, are important variables.

PAST AND PRESENT PROGRAMS

While considerable organizational and technical innovation has occurred in recent years, it is possible to question whether the basic nature of the problem of delinquency and the general community response to it have changed.

Historical perspective. The problems of delinquency and the response of community agencies and groups to these phenomena appear to have some historical continuity, is not indeed some cyclical characteristics. Some knowledge of history helps us to build on past experience in a clear and rational way lest we find ourselves reinventing programs that have been tried and found wanting. The phenomena of urban gangs and community response to them will serve as examples. In Chicago there are striking similarities between the Ragen Colts of an earlier era and the Black P. Stone Nation of today. The Ragen Colts, organized in 1912 by Frank Ragen in the Back of the Yards area of Chicago, was reputed to be composed of three thousand young toughs. The gang considered itself an athletic club. The gang and its members were involved in a long series of delinquent and criminal activities, which have been described as follows:

> Their headquarters at 5412 South Halsted Street was a reputed hangout for South Side gangsters. Thomas Shields, a beer runner wanted by the police, was killed in their clubhouse and a black man was executed there by two Colts.

> Fifty Colts broke up a speech by "anti-papist" crusader Eli Erickson in 1922 and sent him running from the Viking Temple. Later, trying to improve their image, they offered to help Illinois Governor J.C. Walton stamp out the Ku Klux Klan activity in 1923.

> Several Colts developed into distinguished citizens. One was Hugo Bezdek, head football coach at the University of Chicago. Many other members did not, however. Danny Stanton, one of Al

Capone's hottest gunmen, was in this category. He died on a saloon floor after a shootout.

Chicago police repeatedly tried to eliminate the Ragen Colts, but were hampered by a special injunction obtained from City Hall which barred them from the clubhouse. The Ragen Colts were not the only gang to receive protection from high officials, however. Many gangs had political patrons or protectors. Ward heelers and even aldermen sponsored the groups because gangs were useful in getting out the vote on election days. Gangs often did this thru intimidation, bribery, or fraud.

The Ragen Colts finally disbanded in 1927 after a member was shot in an internal dispute. Their demise left a power vacuum on the South Side, which the Taylor Colts filled for a while. They were quickly eclipsed by the 42nd Street Gang, a group unmatched for sheer terror [5: 14].

The Blackstone Rangers and other Chicago gangs of the 1960s and early 1970s seem to possess similar characteristics and to elicit remarkably similar community responses, highlighted in the following brief description:

The leaders of the Blackstone Rangers . . . (Bull) Hairston, then Jeff (Black Prince) Fort, gained control thru their organizational abilities and personal charm . . .

The Rangers popped into the news in 1964 when 49 of the most battle-hardened members of Woodlawn's 12 fighting gangs marched thru the South Side carrying motorcycle chains . . .

In 1965 the Rangers reorganized with 1,500 members and a board of directors called the Main 21 . . .

The Rangers [along with other gangs] soon expanded into citywide coalitions, calling themselves nations.

Between 1968 and 1970, a total of 209 youth-gang killings were recorded by the police. What proportion could be attributed to the Rangers' involvement is unknown. During this period the Black P. Stone Nation, formerly the Rangers, was the largest and most influential gang in Chicago. Violence was a means to profit:

The violence that gangs used to become powerful, however, created problems in the neighborhoods. Small businessmen were finding it hard to exist. City agencies compiled a confidential report of extortion activities of youth gangs in 1970 . . .

The Stones asked an auto dealer to supply them with several cars. The dealer couldn't afford to let the gang break his windows because of high insurance costs, so he arranged financing for the vehicles. When the payments stopped, he did not ask the Stones for money . . .

Black radio and T.V. personality Daddy-O-Daylie was threatened by the Cobra Stones . . . He would not pay, denounced them as "black monsters" and hired a bodyguard . . .

Four teenagers introduced themselves as Stones, told a foreman on a Woodlawn construction site that he had to pay or be shot. A woman tavern owner left the state after a group of Stones told her the same . . .

The Black P. Stone organization has continually denied that extortion as well as drug peddling and gun running were ever sanctioned by the gang's leadership [5: 18-19].

Like the Ragen Colts, the Black P. Stone Nation had organized community support for some of its activities. While support did not come from City Hall, it came from certain aldermen and state and congressional representatives. One of the leaders of the gang was a guest at a Washington reception for President Nixon's inauguration. The Stones got out the vote for several candidates for local and state elections. Two members ran and won office as members of an advisory council to a model-cities program in the Woodlawn community.

Major support for the Stones, however, came from local neighborhood organizations, including the Woodlawn Organization, a Presbyterian church, Operation Breadbasket, and the Office of Economic Opportunity. The Stones joined welfare-rights groups in a march on the state legislature. They assisted the police and won a commendation for their role in the prevention and control of riots, especially after the assassination of the Reverend Martin Luther King, Jr. They joined an association of black social-action organizations in demonstrations against building contractors and unions to obtain more opportunities for black and other minority groups.

In 1972 five of the organization's top leaders, including Jeff Fort, were sentenced to long terms in federal prison for fraud and conspiracy in relation to their conduct of a youth manpower program funded by the Office of Economic Opportunity. The organization still remains, however, the single largest and most powerful gang in Chicago.

In large cities the underlying social, economic, and political dynamics generating delinquency and associated phenomena may not have changed much in the past fifty or sixty years, or perhaps certain precipitating factors recur at various times. Even some of the current community-oriented approaches to dealing with the problem seem remarkably similar to those of an earlier period. In the 1930s the Chicago Area Project devised various community-based delinquency-control and delinquency-prevention programs. The key principle was organization of local community interest and leadership in behalf of the welfare and development of predelinquent and delinquent youths. Saul Alinsky — originally a worker for the project — claimed that social agencies had been too building centered, had depended primarily on professional and bureaucratic rationale and expertise, and had focused on individual rather than community problems and collective responsibilities. These grassroots efforts emphasized the legitimate aspirations, norms, values, and skills of local people.

Many of today's so-called innovations are reverberations of approaches developed in these early projects. The Alinsky approach emphasized political style and conflict strategies and tactics. Adult leaders, some of whom were former prisoners, worked with street gangs. Counseling and jobs were stressed. The Back of the Yards Council opened an estimated thirty recreational centers and dozens of storefronts as self-governing recreational clubs. Other highly progressive or radical ideas were tried, with apparent success. Born describes the work of the Back of the Yard Council as follows:

> Children were given priority in all neighborhoods projects. Instead of sending them to juvenile court, the council formed its own court. It consisted of the deviant child's parents, [the director of the council], clergymen, a probation officer, and a policeman.
> The humilation of appearing before the court was enough to straighten out most errant children. The community slowly came under tight control as a result of close cooperation between community leaders and residents in trying to properly raise the children. By the mid 1950s, the neighborhood juvenile crime rate there had dropped from the highest to one of the lowest in the city [5: 15].

Probably forces other than the community organization were also operating during this period. The population in the Back of the Yards area was stabilized; economic and social status of first- and second-generation white ethnics rose. Local community cohesion was intensified as the surrounding area on the South Side witnessed a massive influx of black and brown residents to the expanding ghettos. The area-project idea in its community dimension did not "catch on" immediately outside of Chicago. At the present time, while a score of local community committees under the aegis of the Chicago Area Project still exist, it is questionable whether they have continued to be successful at either community organization or delinquency control. It is possible that the Chicago Area Project, now largely under state government auspices, has become too simplistic, routinized, and perhaps apolitical in dealing with urban problems more complex than those of an earlier period.

After World War II, social agencies appeared to take the leadership in various delinquency-prevention and delinquency-control efforts. Emphasis was no longer on community participation and control but on the provision of social services, usually under the aegis of large public and voluntary agencies. But change again occurred in the late 1950s and early 1960s. First, the Ford Foundation, through its Grey Areas Projects, sought to increase coordination of public agencies and schools and thereby to improve the quality of social-development and educational opportunities for ghetto youth. A little later the President's Committee on Juvenile Delinquency and Youth Development, assuming a structural basis for delinquency, funded a number of large-city projects. These programs, under reform-minded leadership, were established within the framework of public and voluntary agencies. Based in part on the Cloward-Ohlin "opportunity" thesis(6), a variety of "innovative" programs were created, particularly for education, training, job-development, and social action. However, many of these programs, in response to changing federal funding patterns, quickly shifted emphasis from delinquency to poverty, from the needs of delinquent youths to the needs of the mass of poor youths and their families in the ghettos. The Office of Economic Opportunity and the Department of Labor, aided by the civil-rights movement, stimulated the change. The focus turned to institutional and political mechanisms in order to deal with a variety of interrelated civil-rights, social, and economic problems. Opportunities could be created only as the existing structures of agency and local-government decision making were changed. Community participation and control efforts were initiated. Controversy about "maximum feasible participation" was precipitated.

In the late 1960s, the national political pendulum swung back: control of delinquency-prevention programs devolved again upon city and public agencies and, to some extent, upon the state, particularly with the implementation of model-city and safe-street legislation. There was a return to more specific concern with delinquency and greater emphasis on services.

Yet all these different approaches in various shapes, sizes, and intensities are present in urban communities today, but there is a great lack of clarity about their relationships. Interacting with the development of the above community approaches have been programs spawned through urban renewal, mental health, and educational and general social welfare legislation, as well as the impact of the ghetto riots of the mid-1960s.

Present programs. Community-based programs today seem increasingly directed to overlapping populations of delinquents and nondelinquents. They seek various goals: to divert youth from the juvenile-justice system; to provide a variety of social, economic, and cultural opportunities for youth; to improve the effectiveness and efficiency of direct-service programs; to avoid "bad labeling" of vulnerable youth; to diminish the distance between youth and adult generations; to deal with problems of racism, poverty, housing, employment, education, and social services; or to be concerned with youth involvement, participation, and control (8; 18). Perhaps two general program approaches have evolved: innovative service and institutional change. The service-oriented programs have included street work and new approaches to counseling and guidance — for example, guided group interaction and behavior modification; special education, training, tutoring; decentralized job referral, placement, development; "hot line" and crisis intervention in relation to drug use, suicide, pregnancy, and abortion; legal aid, medical services, and economic-development activities — through drop-in, multi-service, or more general community-center arrangements.[2] These programs are operated under the auspices of youth-service and social agencies; benevolent or voluntary associations; church and businessmen's organizations; independent grass-roots and social- or economic-development organizations; schools; police departments, courts, or probation agencies; park departments; or housing projects. They may be in relatively small isolated units or in large complex structures. Professional and paraprofessional workers, citizen volunteers, youth, and adults may be involved at different levels and in varying policy-making and staffing arrangements.

In partial contrast to these service-dominated programs, it is possible to identify certain institutional-change approaches or even adversary approaches to programs. These programs emphasize change or more appropriate development of organizational policies and practices; mobilization of youth and/or adults for collective action; use of local advisory councils and policy-making groups; and various forms of political and parapolitical activity. These activities involve leadership development and training, planning, legal proceedings, mass education, protest, and street action. In the

---

[2]Not included for purposes of this discussion is community-based residential care, which includes group homes, foster homes, hostels, and open-shelter facilities for temporary emergencies, such as runaway centers.

instances in which these institutional-change programs have operated outside established or traditional agencies and community organizations, they have tended to be more experimental, controversial, and militant. The guiding spirits and staff members of these efforts, whether they are well or poorly organized, include reform-minded professional workers, bureaucrats, citizen volunteers, youth, and even the clientele themselves.

Many of the more complex and relatively stable community-based programs seem able to incorporate both service and institutional-change approaches. Indeed, impressionistic evidence suggests that, whereas one program may emphasize a service approach and another a militant institutional-change approach, in due course a convergence takes place. The well-balanced and viable organization apparently is required to pursue both types of objectives, often in some interactive manner. One writer has recently observed that these programs represent "a return to the political clubhouse style of help, with social workers instead of politicians dispensing the aid," but that they go "far beyond the clubhouse into the realm of the institutional ombudsman, functioning as the watchdogs of public agencies" (9: 49).

PROGRAM EFFECTIVENESS

How effective have these community-based programs been? To what extent, for example, have particular programs diverted youth from the juvenile-justice system? Firm and satisfactory answers still elude us. The failure to obtain clear answers may be due to various factors: defective program methods or delivery systems, insensitive evaluative instruments or defective research designs. It is possible that delinquency is a function of general urban, industrial, class-stratification, or cultural processes, as suggested above, and that no specific institutional changes or particular programmatic efforts will make much difference unless they are part of broad, large-scale structrual efforts. Perhaps we also expect too much in light of our limited knowledge, limited expenditure of resources, and rapidly changing urban conditions. On the other hand, we have been reasonably successful in achieving certain modest and preliminary or intermediate objectives. Community-based "innovative" programs have proved to be effective mechanisms for reaching large numbers of adolescents, many of whom were not served in established agencies. For example, the visibility and accessibility of service centers for adolescents have been important in attracting teen-agers. Such programs have been successful as first-aid stations in handling crisis situations. They have been useful mechanisms of training, job referral, and job development. They have provided opportunities for social, educational, cultural, and political development of street-oriented youth, but the relation of these varied results to delinquency prevention, reduction, or control remains obscure (3; 4; 7; 10; 12; 17). It is true that evaluations have been restricted almost exclusively to service programs. It is possible that current efforts at institutional change — for example, through diversion of delinquent youngsters from the juvenile system and avoidance of "bad labeling" processes at schools — will lead to positive and measureable results, but we cannot be sure yet.

We can identify the failures of community-based programs more readily than we can the successes. The reasons for the failures are becoming clearer. Some community-based programs may be non-programs. They may accomplish little, or serve simply to aid in confining youth to certain ghettos, subcommunities, or public-housing sites. It is possible for a part of a community to be so encapsulated and isolated that it becomes for many purposes an institutionalized environment. A highly deprived, barricaded, and coercive community can be created as functionally equivalent to an institution. An unanticipated consequence of closing down correctional institutions could be dumping delinquents into and further barricading such communities.

It is also possible to develop programs of a group or counseling character that are "successful" within or even outside four walls, yet relatively isolated from significant aspects of the community surrounding them. A program may not be effectively interactive with the community. It may not serve to reintegrate youth into important role structures. For example, the use of group-interaction approaches and social or recreational activities per se in the open community with highly delinquent youth and with gangs has proven generally unproductive. Several recent gang studies have shown no positive relationship between reduction of delinquent behavior and street-gang work efforts (3; 4; 7; 10; 12; 17). Indeed, there may be a negative association between gang delinquency and intensive street work. Delinquency may increase as the worker spends more time with the gang and the gang becomes more cohesive. The problem of delinquency may not be amenable to planned worker intervention unless the gang structure is modified or even dissolved. This is not to denigrate street work or outreach efforts as long as the focus moves beyond counseling and group activities and toward integration of individual delinquents into legitimate community subsystems, such as education or employment (15).

We have learned or should have learned by now that programs on behalf of youth, especially delinquent youth, will not succeed unless there is significant community support. If the police, established agencies, politicians, and active community groups do not want them, certain programs may be denied resources or may be attacked and made to fail (16). Youth clientele cannot be served successfully under these circumstances. Viable working relationships, especially with police, schools, and employment resources, must be established. To ignore these subsystems or to attack them frontally may be a grievous error. In exceptional situations, of course, such attacks may be necessary if humanitarian and social-development objectives are to be achieved. If this route is selected or required, powerful allies should be available and the possibilities of success should be relatively high.

Institutional-change programs based largely on the organized or unorganized inputs of delinquents usually do not succeed. Despite wishes, fantasies, and propaganda to the contrary, the primary involvement of delinquents in social or political action is not tolerated by the community, and it usually results in strong counter-mobilization. The ingredients of failure include manipulation of community leaders and program personnel by gang leaders for delinquent or highly personalized purposes. Civil-rights militants and radical professional workers or bureaucrats interested in social causes and general community problem solving may be viewed by delinquents as exploiting, and in turn may be "conned" and exploited by delinquents. Programs that undersell or oversell the potential of youth leadership do not succeed. Youths, let alone delinquents, will not participate for long in activities that do not meet their interests or needs at a given stage of their development. Also programs for education, social action, economic development, and other goals may fail because youths lack organizationl "know how," motivation, or capacity, as well as adequate adult support, supervision, or consultation.

Perhaps the major cause of program failure is interorganizational and community conflict. Youth programs and problems, especially those concerned with delinquency, become public issues that are readily politicized. They become sources of agency and community-group development, prestige, power, and funding. In such instances, the key problem may not be youth-adult or intergenerational conflict but adult-adult or interorganizational conflict. Furthermore, the source of the conflict may lie only partically in issues of community participation and control, racism, unemployment, poor education, and inadequate social service system. It may well be based mainly in defective national social policy and planning in regard to youth development. There appears to be no set of interrelated goals, objectives, and priorities for the social development of the youth of the nation. Each organization concerned with youth, including delinquents, operates essentially on a short-term, crisis, fragmented basis. The national commitment and policy to provide those opportunities and services required for each youth to achieve his social potential do not yet exist. Even the identification of needs of various categories of socially handicapped youth has not yet been achieved on a community or national basis. Particularistic organizational priorities and programs continue to be emphasized; they have produced a crazy-quilt patchwork of programs to deal with community and national problems of delinquency.

Ideally, community-based programs of delinquency prevention should be related to each other in a socially ordered and effective way. The freedom of community groups, agencies, and independent youth groups to deal with youth problems must be safeguarded, but it probably also should be functionally limited. The question of local organizational autonomy and funds to sustain it must be viewed within a larger framework of what makes sense on a community and national basis for the social development of youth. Issues of national policy and planning must be identified and must take precedence over local and idiosyncratic community interests, which in turn are more important than particularistic organizational interests. These levels are interacting, of course, but the overall goal- and standard-setting responsibility of the federal government has to be more fully developed.

While the economic interdependence of various sectors of American society has been recognized and national economic and fiscal policies gradually but firmly established, the social needs of youth, including delinquents, and the interdependence of various groups of society dealing with youth have not yet been adequately recognized and national goals and policies have not been formulated in regard to them. Technological development, the rapidity of social change, the complexity of human and social problems, and the limits on economic resources demand a more systematic approach to problem solving. It may be that a major break with the past is appropriate and required at this time. A new and rational approach to delinquency prevention and control would require as a first step that the federal government take a strong stand and establish general, coordinated criteria for youth development as a framework for community-based programming.

REFERENCES

1. Altshuler, Alan A. *Community control.* New York: Pegasus, 1970.
2. Arnstein, Sherry R. A Ladder of Citizen Participation. *Journal of the American Institute of Planners* 35 (July 1969): 216-24.
3. Berleman, William E., Seaberg, James R. and Steinburn. Thomas W. The delinquency prevention experiment of the Seattle Atlantic Street Center: A final evaluation. *Social Service Review* 46 no. 3 (September 1972): 323-46.
4. Block, Richard. The Chicago Youth Development Project: An Evaluation Based on Arrests. Master's thesis. University of Chicago, 1967.
5. Born, Peter W. *Street gangs and youth unrest.* Chicago: Chicago Tribune Educational Service Department, 1971.
6. Cloward, Richard A. and Ohlin, Lloyd E. *Delinquency and opportunity.* New York: Free Press, 1960.

7. Empey, LaMar T., and Lubeck, Steven G. *The Silverlake Experiment.* Chicago: Aldine Publishing Co., 1971.

8. Gemignani, Robert J. "National Strategy for Youth Development and Delinquency Prevention." Washington, D.C.: Youth Development and Delinquency Prevention Administration. Department of Health, Education, and Welfare, 1971.

9. Jones, Hettie. Neighborhood Service Centers. In *Individual and group service in the mobilization for youth experience.* edited by Harold H. Weissman, pp. 33-53. New York: Association Press, 1969.

10. Klein, Malcolm W. *Street gangs and street workers.* Englewood Cliffs, N.J.: Prentice-Hall, 1971.

11. Massachusetts. Department of Youth Services. "Programs and Policies of the Department of Youth Services." Mimeographed. Boston: Department of Youth Services, 1972.

12. Miller, Walter B. The impact of a 'Total Community' community delinquency control project. *Social Problems,* **10,** (Fall 1962): 181-91.

13. Perlman, Robert and Gurin, Arnold. *Community organization and social planning.* New York: Council on Social Work and Education. John Wiley & Sons, 1971.

14. Spergel, Irving A. *Community problem solving: The delinquency example.* Chicago: University of Chicago Press, 1969.

15. ———. Street Gang Work. In *Encyclopedia of Social Work.* edited by Robert Morris. 2: 1486-94. New York: National Association of Social Workers, 1971.

16. ———. Community action research as a political progress. In *Community organization: Studies in constraint,* edited by Irving A. Spergel, pp. 231-62. Beverly Hills, Calif.: Sage Publications, 1972.

17. Spergel, Irving A., Turner, Castellano, Pleas, John and Brown, Patricia. *Youth manpower: What happened in woodlawn.* Chicago: School of Social Service Administration. University of Chicago, 1969.

18. U.S. Department of Health, Education, and Welfare. Youth Development and Delinquency Prevention Administration. *Delinquency Prevention through Youth Development.* Washington, D.C.: Department of Health, Education, and Welfare. 1972.

Part II
Secondary Prevention—Intervening in the Criminal Justice System

Secondary prevention aims at reducing the prevalence of psychological disorder in the population by the early identification of cases and prompt provision of services. This necessitates intervening in the criminal justice system so that the cases encountered by criminal justice personnel can be easily identified and effectively treated.

Secondary prevention efforts in this area revolve principally around law enforcement officers, for it is they who, in the course of their work, most frequently encounter problems susceptible to secondary prevention efforts. Not only is the policeman the first to encounter many cases of psychological disturbance (and so is an invaluable asset for early identification), but he is often in a position to provide competent service or referral. This is in distinction to the formal "treatment" phase of the criminal justice system, which may be many years and judicial appeals away.

In the first paper in this section, Mann provides both a conceptual and practical guide for establishing a consultation program with a police department. He delineates three phases of consultation — entry, familiarization and implementation — and demonstrates how a successful program can be mounted. Elsewhere, Mann (1973) has fully described his own police consultation project, and made special note of the consultant's role in reducing the threat of violence in police-student encounters (Mann and Iscoe, 1971). Reiser (1972) also provides a comprehensive overview of what he terms "the police department psychologist" and Schwartz and Liebman (1973) review many projects in this area.

Among the most potentially fruitful activities of a mental health consultant is the screening of police recruits. McDonough and Monahan, in this book, describe one such project aimed at the "quality control" of law enforcement officers. As they state, "a police population screened of potential psychological casualties and selected for emotional suitability for law enforcement work would seem to go far in preventing disruptive police-community incidents and in fostering police-community solidarity." Mills (1972) also reports an extensive and ingenious program in police selection and several recent projects and reviews can be found in Snibbe and Snibbe (1973).

After recruits are selected, they must be trained. Rolde, Rersch, Kelly, Frank and Guberman (Chapter 5) report on a successful training program for law enforcement officers that would seem to have great potential for being adopted elsewhere. Especially noteworthy was the fact that the attitudes and behavior of the agencies doing the training seemed to change as much as did the attitudes and behavior of the officers.

Hughes' paper (Chapter 6) focuses on training police recruits for work in the urban ghetto. His well-conceptualized program provides a comprehensive model for training in this exceedingly important and especially difficult area. Other projects attempting to improve the relationships between the police and community can be found in Johnson and Gregory (1971) and Sikes (1973).

Bard's training program in family crisis intervention is surely the most well known in the field. In the present selection (Chapter 7), Bard places his program in the context of a theory of police functioning. Most importantly, Bard notes that role-identity confusion among the officers was avoided. Training in family crisis intervention made the officers better policemen, not amateur therapists. (See also Zacker and Bard, 1973; and Bard, in press). Driscoll, Meyer and Shanie (Chapter 8) discuss the disappointing evaluation of Bard's project and suggest that psychosocial variables, rather than crime statistics, are more appropriate measures of success. Basing their family crisis program on social learning principles, Driscoll and his colleagues report substantial impact on crisis situations. A comprehensive review of domestic crisis intervention projects is presented by Liebman and Schwartz (1973).

The final selection (Chapter 9) in this section, by Binder, Monahan and Newkirk, describes a delinquency prevention program based in a police agency. Juvenile early offenders are voluntarily referred to a short-term intervention program aimed at altering counterproductive patterns of family interaction and involving community agencies in the provision of preventive services. A more lengthy discussion of juvenile diversion strategies can be found in Klapmuts (in press).

The second section of this part concerns community mental health interaction with legal and judicial agencies. Beigel (Chapter 10) describes various aspects of a collaborative endeavor by the judicial system, law enforcement agencies and a mental health center to resolve problems at the interface of mental health and criminal justice. Procedures to reduce unnecessary civil commitments, a court clinic and an alcoholism program are examples of what his program has accomplished. Other consultation projects with judges are described in Geis and Tenney (1968), McDonough and Anderson (1969), and Nir and Cutter (1973).

Nietzel and Dade (Chapter 11) report an experimental bail reform project and see it as a demonstration of community psychology's potential impact on the criminal justice system. Nonfinancial release was as effective as bail in ensuring the appearance of the accused at trial.

Abramson (Chapter 12) is more sanguine about the potential benefit of consulting with public defenders. He notes that "if a mental health consultant wishes to function in some part of the criminal justice system, his time might be better spent with police, judges or probation officers, instead of with attorneys playing stylized, ritualized adversary prosecution or defense rules." He does, however, note several factors which could positively affect consultation in this area.

REFERENCES

Bard, M. The unique potentials of the police in interpersonal conflict management. *International Journal of Group Tensions,* in press.

Geis, G. and Tenney, C. Evaluating a training institute for juvenile court judges. *Community Mental Health Journal,* 1968, **4**, 461-468.

Johnson, D. and Gregory R. Police-community relations in the United States: a review of recent literature and projects. *Journal of Criminal Law, Criminology and Police Science,* 1971, **62**, 94-103.

Klapmuts, N. Diversion from the justice system. *Crime and Delinquency Literature,* in press.

Liebman, D. and Schwartz, J. Police programs in domestic crisis intervention: a review. In J. Snibbe and H. Snibbe (Eds.) *The policeman in transition: A psychological and sociological review.* Springfield, Illinois: Charles C. Thomas, 1973.

Mann, P. *Psychological consultation with a police department.* Springfield, Illinois: Charles C. Thomas, 1973.

Mann, P. and Iscoe, I. Mass behavior and community organization: Reflections on a peaceful demonstration. *American Psychologist,* 1971, **26**, 108-113.

McDonough, L. and Anderson, T. Courts and corrections unit. In H. Lamb, D. Heath, and J. Downing (Eds.) *Handbook of community mental health practice.* San Francisco: Jossey-Bass, 1969, pp. 322-348.

Mills, R. New directions in police selection. Paper presented to the Annual Convention of the American Psychological Association, 1972.

Nir, Y. and Cutter, R. The therapeutic utilization of the juvenile court. *American Journal of Psychiatry,* 1973, **130**, 1112-1117.

Reiser, M. *The police department psychologist.* Springfield, Illinois: Charles C. Thomas, 1972.

Schwartz, J. and Liebman, D. Mental health consultation in law enforcement. In J. Snibbe and H. Snibbe (Eds.) *The urban policeman in transition: A psychological and sociological review.* Springfield, Illinois: Charles C. Thomas, 1973.

Sikes, M. Police-community relations: The Houston experience. In J. Snibbe and H. Snibbe (Eds.) *The urban policeman in transition: A psychological and sociological review.* Springfield, Illinois: Charles C. Thomas, 1973.

Snibbe, J. and Snibbe, H. (Eds.) *The urban policeman in transition: A psychological and sociological review.* Springfield, Illinois: Charles C. Thomas, 1973.

Zacker, J. and Bard, M. Effects of conflict management training on police performance. *Journal of Applied Psychology,* 1973, **58**, 202-208.

3
Establishing a Mental Health Consultation Program with a Police Department *

PHILIP A. MANN

"If the liberal and intellectual communities are to have any impact on the police, if they are to play any role in reducing the growing political alienation of many police, they must show some recognition that the police force is also composed of human beings, seeking to earn a living. They must be willing to engage in a dialogue with the police concerning their problems."

Seymour Martin Lipset (1969)

About half of the requests for assistance which urban police departments receive involve domestic and family problems (Cumming, Cumming, and Edell, 1965). Among the lower class particularly, the police and courts together constitute a primary avenue for bringing patients to treatment (Miller and Mishler, 1959). It is hardly necessary to document the increasing recognition of the importance of police work in community life, but it is also too easy to polarize their position as the standard bearers of "law and order" and to overlook their important humanitarian functions. The importance of the mental health aspects of police work is being increasingly recognized as community mental health centers develop their programs (Bard and Berkowitz, 1967).

*Reprinted from *Community Mental Health Journal,* 1971, 7, 118-126, with permission. Copyrighted by Behavioral Publications, New York, 1971.

However, these facts contrast dramatically with the limited preparation and training which police officers usually have in mental health and behavioral science. Mental health consultation is one way of attempting to meet the needs of policemen in this important area.

The author undertook to offer mental health consultation services to an urban police department as part of a community mental health center project to bolster and coordinate mental health resources in a neighborhood with a high prevalence of social and mental discord. In this paper three phases of the consultation process are identified and described. These are entry, familiarization, and implementation.

ENTRY

Even though mental health consultation is not psychotherapy, resistance on the part of consultees is always to be expected (Rhodes, 1960). In the case of the police there are a number of reasons to expect that the consultant would encounter more than usual resistance. For example, Cohen (Undated, p. 35) describes a consultation project with the police in which the ideological differences between consultants and policemen were a persistent source of difficulty. To some extent these differences may have their roots in the kinds of socioeconomic backgrounds from which policemen and mental health professionals come (Lipset, 1969). Furthermore policemen have been stereotyped as authoritarian and suspicious of outside intervention, both of which could serve to heighten resistance.

However, there is also reason to believe that these potential sources of resistance could stem from differences in perceptions of the role and objectives of the consultant, which in turn arise from differences between policemen and mental health professionals in their own role expectations and operational patterns.

Recognizing this it seemed insufficient for the consultant merely to pass along his knowledge and concepts to the policemen. Rather, an important aspect of entering the consulting relationship was for the consultant to understand the concepts, viewpoints, and operational patterns of the police.

Actually entry proved to be easier than these preconceptions had led the consultant to imagine. The consultant initiated the relationship by contacting the Chief of Police. In the initial contact the consultant described the proposal for consultation to the police department as part of the project to coordinate mental health resources within a high-risk neighborhood.

A number of factors can be identified which seemed to help in the entry process. It became clear in the first contact that the consultant was more acceptable to the police because he came from a community agency than would have been the case had he come from a university base. The idea of having an "outside" consultant was more acceptable because the police had built up some positive expectations through a previous good experience with a consultant on a research study of traffic accidents. The police had some positive motivation for seeking consultation because they could acknowledge frankly their needs and limitations in the mental health area. Finally the fact that they were being included in on a project that involved other agencies rather than being singled out for attention reduced some of the pressure they might have felt otherwise and made it less necessary for them to react defensively. (See Sikes and Cleveland, 1968, for a different strategy.) The next step, familiarization, was a critical bridge between gaining entry to the system and implementing consultative activities (Jarvis and Nelson, 1967).

FAMILIARIZATION

Representatives from the police department were invited to attend a series of biweekly meetings of community agency workers. Although the content of these meetings was concerned with behavior problems in the community, they frequently focused on problems of interagency cooperation and initially the police received a disproportionate share of criticism. The response of the policemen was admirable in that they honestly pointed out the legal limitations of their role, which contributed to some of the criticisms, and admitted their mistakes when this was appropriate. In most instances the police were not the only ones at fault in these difficult situations and their candor made it easier for the rest of the group to recognize errors that others had made in the instances discussed. As a consequence of these interchanges the policemen gained more respect and understanding from the other members of the group, which seemed to meet an important need for them.

Since the consultant and other staff members of the community mental health center were the group leaders in these meetings, this provided an opportunity for the policemen to observe mental health professionals in a setting other than the police department and to become more familiar with their modes of operation, as well as giving the consultant and the agency workers a better understanding of police work.

Concurrently the consultant accompanied policemen on their rounds, riding in a patrol car, to familiarize himself with their "front-line" activities and to become visible and familar to the policemen in that setting. An additional familiarization activity involved the consultant meeting each week with the senior captain of the department to review all of the cases of family difficulties, assaults, and mentally ill persons that were handled by the department the previous week. These reviews helped the consultant to become better informed about police activities and when particularly difficult or questionable cases arose, the officers who handled these cases were asked to discuss the case with the consultant, and suggestions for improved handling of such cases were worked out in these meetings. After this process, it was possible to describe the social-psychological aspects of police work so as to illuminate the issues raised earlier concerning work-role related sources of resistance.

THE POLICE DEPARTMENT AS A BEHAVIOR MEDIATING INSTITUTION

Historically, communities have established a number of institutions for mediating human behavior (Rhodes, in press). As a part of the legal-correctional institution, the police have both historical and legal sanction for their interventions in the behavior of members of the community. The community expects the police to assume a major responsibility for controlling behavior.

Role Pressures

In ways that are not obvious to the ordinary citizen the community exerts a variety of pressures on the police department that necessarily influence the work of the individual policeman. Whereas the policeman himself may not be aware of the sources of these pressures, he nevertheless experiences them and may react to them in a variety of ways.

Both the law and community sentiment demand that policemen play an essentially conservative role in society. Thus it is natural for policemen to be more sensitive to the disturbing aspects of behavior than to the disturbed features of the persons with whom they come in contact. An important difference in the orientations of policemen and mental health workers is that the mental health professional is primarily concerned with the individual. His responsibility to society usually comes into play only in those rare instances when his patient may be dangerous to himself or others and he must then institute such measures as increasing hospital security or obtaining a commitment order for his patient. The policeman, on the other hand, whose primary commitment is to the protection of society, responds first to whatever threat the behavior of the individual may pose to the social order, and only after that threat is under control may he give attention to the needs of the individual.

This is not to say that the policeman is not sensitive to the psychology of the individual, but rather that the hierarchy of priorities differs for the roles of policemen and mental health professionals in this regard. In fact the individual police officers with whom the author has worked have proven to be more sensitive to individual psychology than stereotypes of policemen suggest. Such a misconception may be due in part to a failure to separate the social role of policeman from the personality of the individual who may fill that role. It is usual to assume a fairly close fit between the needs of an individual and the satisfactions that his social role makes available to him, but it is a mistake to assume perfect congruency in this respect for policemen, just as it would be a mistake to overlook the problem of countertransference for the mental health professional in the therapist's role.

Uncertainty and Judgment

In enforcing the law the policeman is constrained to do so according to the way his contacts with the prosecuting attorney and the courts have instructed him that it should be enforced. But in other areas of his work the policeman is required to make a number of judgments concerning the cases with which he deals, and this happens frequently in areas where he has the least training and preparation. It is in the area of assessing suicidal or homicidal potential, deciding whether a person should be detained for this reason, and in knowing how to handle such persons, that the policeman is the least confident of the criteria for making a decision.

To be sure, a number of police officers develop the ability to make these judgments through experience, but acquiring knowledge in this way alone leaves considerable room for error. At the same time, the penalties for an incorrect decision can be quite severe. On the one hand such situations are among the most dangerous that policemen face (Bard and Berkowitz, 1967); on the other hand the policeman can be sued for false arrest, or become subject to severe criticism when he errs in making such judgments. Thus the experienced policeman must consider constantly the possible consequences of the decisions that he makes to himself, to the police department, and to society at large, as well as to the individual with whom he is confronted.

Given the ambiguity and stress under which policemen must make decisions, and the pressures for making them correctly, it should not be surprising that police officers sometimes attempt to adopt a few simple rules for making such judgments, and to adhere to them rigidly (Rokeach, 1960). This trait might be considered authoritarianism by behavioral scientists; it is called "discipline" by police supervisors.

The policeman's contacts with behavior problems are usually lonely, spontaneous confrontations, in contrast to those of the mental health professional that take place in the context of a protective and supportive agency structure. Consequently the policeman's routine for handling behavior problems is frequently based on self-reliance and expediency, and the idea of interdisciplinary cooperation is one with which he is likely to have had little experience. It should be clear, then, that an imposed clinical point of view would not have direct relevance to the policeman's work, and that such information could tend to confuse an already ambiguous area unless it is modified to be applicable to the social role of police work. Otherwise the policeman's aloofness towards outsiders would seem to be justified.

IMPLEMENTATION

The familiarization phase gradually merged into more active implementation of consultative activities. The sequence of these activities evolved naturally as the policemen articulated a need for them. The sequence of expressed need should be distinguished from the hierarchy of needs which an outsider might impose.

Crisis Intervention

The first activity was crisis intervention. The mental health center has a 24-hour emergency telephone service and was in the process of establishing a crisis intervention service with a walk-in clinic. The policemen were told that they could call the telephone service at any time for advice and assistance from the person on duty. In fact, they consistently called and asked for the consultant in person, which underscores the highly personal nature of the consultation relationship. All of the early contacts with the consultant were initiated by policemen with whom the consultant had previously become personally acquainted.

These contacts ranged from the police asking for help in arranging for a psychiatric examination as part of an emergency commitment procedure, to asking the consultant's direct assistance in managing a difficult, emotionally disturbed person. Occasionally the policemen would call the consultant for advice while in the course of trying to deal with a person who was contemplating suicide, but more frequently they would ask the consultant to come to the police station to help them in dealing with a very disturbed, usually psychotic, person.

The consultant gradually changed his handling of these requests in a deliberate way. Initially, the consultant went to the police station, interviewed the person, and made an assessment. An attempt was then made to work out a solution in mutual discussion with the person and police officers. Since many of these persons were highly paranoid, this approach of openness and honest participation seemed to be the only workable one. The entire process was conducted in view of other police officers, so that the consultant served as a model for the policemen for handling other cases on their own. In addition, this procedure had a dramatic impact in demonstrating to the police that persons who were so bewildering to them could be dealt with on a constructive basis.

Later the consultant began to work with the policemen themselves in helping them to handle the case without the consultant actually seeing the person involved. This gave the policemen an opportunity to employ some of the techniques they had seen demonstrated and helped to bolster their confidence in dealing with such cases.

Training

As a consequence of these experiences in learing and of becoming more aware of their needs in this area, the police requested the consultant to participate in the training program for police recruits. Training sessions consisted of eight to ten hours with groups of six to eight police recruits. After a brief introduction to the program of the mental health center and the role of the policeman in dealing with behavior problems, representative cases from the police department's own files were presented to the recruits. They were given the kind of information they would receive from a call to the police station and were asked to assess the kinds of behavior they might expect to encounter in such situations, to determine the cues to which they would be especially sensitive, and to decide how they would deal with the situation. After they had proposed their solutions, discussions were held in which the assumptions that had led to their solutions were scrutinized, questioned, and modified. Although these discussions began dealing with cases of suicidal, homicidal, and psychotic behavior, they gradually moved into the area of human relations in general. By this time the consultant had become sufficiently familiar with police activities to be able to discuss with the recruits their responsibilities as policemen in dealing with varieties of behavior.

As a consequence of this training program, the consultant was asked to participate in other training activities. One was a program of in-service training for command-level officers. It became clear that the behavior of individual policemen is strongly influenced by the attitudes and examples set for him by command-level officers. Training for police recruits can be wasted if the command officers do not have a similar awareness of an orientation to dealing with behavior problems.

The consultant was also asked to participate in human relations training which was being conducted by representatives of the city government's Human Relations Commission. This was an area about which the policemen were very concerned, but one in which they felt they lacked understanding and effective techniques. These additional training concerns led into discussions between the consultant and police administrators on program planning.

Program Planning

After being involved in the activities described above for some time, the consultant began to enter discussions with police administrators around program concerns. Whether such discussions could have been initiated earlier is doubtful. The consultant referred to these concerns repeatedly throughout the relationship, but did not push them. These concerns did come up in the training sessions but only when other items had been cleared from the agenda and trust in the consultant had been established were the police ready to discuss these issues.

One problem that was recognized was the policeman's limited awareness of community resources for assisting with behavior and social problems. Whereas he is usually acquainted with hospital emergency rooms, he does not generally have an opportunity to learn about resources for emergency housing, financial aid, and other social services. Plans were made to include this information in training programs, and a handbook was made up that included the specific resources and responsibilities of various community agencies, the names of people to be contacted in those agencies, and suggested procedures for working cooperatively with them. It should be emphasized that this handbook was a much more specific and straightforward document than the usual "image-oriented" booklet that is published by community organizations for general use. The major impact of the handbook was that it provided the basis for more frequent and meaningful contact between workers in various agencies.

The police administration also began to voice some concern about influencing the attitudes and behavior of their own men. Whereas the department had a good training and supervisory system, one mistake by an officer in these times could precipitate a barrage of criticism, protest, or riot. Discussion of this point began with the recognition that there could be no absolute guarantees against an individual officer making a mistake, but steps could be taken to reduce the risk.

A potent force for norm setting and reality testing among policemen arises immediately following a crisis situation. In a manner analogous to Festinger's (1954) social comparison process, policemen get together to discuss the situation and ventilate their feelings after such events as a high-speed chase in which shots are fired at fleeing suspects or the subduing of a violent psychotic person. It is a time of heightened emotional excitement and attitudes are checked out with each other with intensity. The attitudes that are formed and reinforced under such circumstances would seem to be very strong, but it also would seem to be a time of increased influencibility according to crisis theory (Rapoport, 1962).

The best solution seemed to be along the lines of crisis units composed of policemen, mental health workers, ministers, and others who could not only be more effective in terms of the service they could render than the individual policeman, but could also serve to broaden the kind of information that would be fed into postcrisis social comparison processes. Problems of manpower and coordination prevented immediate implementation of a formal program of this kind, but it did become more common for the police to involve others in attempting to deal with crises. These others might include workers from other social agencies who were already working with the subject in crisis. They might be representatives of black community groups in the case of a white officer attempting to work with a black subject who did not trust white people. In other cases they might be friends or acquaintances who knew and were trusted by the person.

Finally, the police administration expressed dismay and impatience in trying to answer criticisms from black citizens. Their major complaint was that the criticisms were usually general, and that unless they had specific information they were powerless to correct any wrong doing that a police officer might have committed. They felt that they presented their position clearly and rationally and could not understand why the situation did not improve. The consultant helped them to understand that the criticism of the police was based on what the police symbolized as well as what the police did. He pointed out that often the people doing the criticizing were representing others, and they were as much committed to defending their position as the police were pressured into absorbing criticism for the entire societal structure that gave impetus to the complaints. This point of view helped the police to feel that the criticism was less personal and left them free to respond to it more sympathetically and less defensively. Feeling less personally frustrated, they were able to continue the necessary dialogue about these issues.

CONCLUSIONS

The consultation experience described here demonstrates that the consultant must be willing to meet the consultee group on their own ground and see the issues from their point of view. Mental health consultation can provide an important and needed service to policemen, and in time can have a rather broad influence. It is essential that the consultant be willing to tolerate a lack of immediate response and deal with those issues that the consultees are ready to address as they arise. Involvement in crisis situations is important to establishing the consultation relationship and increasing the effectiveness of influence processes. A crusading attitude on the part of the consultant is nearly certain to produce failure in a consultation program.

REFERENCES

Bard, M. and Berkowitz, B. Training police as specialists in family crisis intervention: A community psychology action program. *Community Mental Health Journal,* 1967, **3**, 315-317.

Cohen, L.D. *Consultation: A community mental health method, report of a survey of practice in sixteen southern states.* Southern Regional Education Board, updated.

Cumming, Elaine, Cumming, I. and Edell, L. Policeman as philosopher, guide and friend. *Social Problems,* 1965, **12**, 276-286.

Festinger, L. A theory of social comparison processes. *Human Relations,* 1954, **7**, 117-140.

Jarvis, P. E. and Nelson, S. Familiarization: A vital step in mental health consultation. *Community Mental Health Journal* 1967, **3**, 343-348.

Lipset, S. M. Why cops hate liberals and vice versa. *Atlantic Monthly,* 1969, **223**, No. 3, 76-83.

Miller, S. M. and Mishler, E. G. Social class, mental illness, and American psychiatry. *Milbank Memorial Fund Quarterly,* 1959, **37**, 174-199.

Rapoport, Lydia. The state of crisis: Some theoretical considerations. *The Social Service Review,* 1962, **36**, No. 2.

Rhodes, W. C. *Training in community mental health consultation in the schools.* American Psychological Association, Chicago, 1960.

Rhodes, W. C. Community structures for the regulation of human behavior. In Golann, S., and Eisdorfer, C. (Eds.) *Handbook of community psychology and mental health.* New York: Appleton Century Crofts (in press).

Rokeach, M., *The open and closed mind.* New York: Basic Books, 1960.

Sikes, M. P. and Cleveland, S. E., Human relations training for police and community. *American Psychologist,* 1968, **23**, 766-769.

4
The Quality-Control of Community Care-Takers:
A Study of Mental Health Screening in
a Sheriff's Department [*][1]

LEAH B. McDONOUGH and JOHN MONAHAN

The criminal justice system is one of the primary community structures for the regulation of human behavior (Rhodes, 1972). Mental health professionals, in their desire to improve the functioning of community caretakers, have become increasingly involved with the legal system in recent years. Efforts have been concentrated on that aspect of criminal justice which most proximately relates to the community — law enforcement. Mental health consultation with the police has taken the form of inservice training (Friedman, 1969; Mann, 1970), family crisis management (Bard and Berkowitz, 1967), community relations workshops (Johnson and Gregory, 1971), and case and program consultation (Mann, 1971; McDonough and Anderson, 1969).

Given the volume and importance of mental health interactions with the police, it is surprising that so little effort has been placed on the quality-control of the basic commodity of any police system: the policeman himself. A police population screened of potential psychological casualties and selected for emotional suitability for law enforcement work would seem to go far in preventing disruptive police-community incidents and in fostering police-community solidarity. In addition, subsequent mental health consulta-

*Reprinted from *Community Mental Health Journal,* 1975, in press, with permission. Copyrighted by Behavioral Publications, New York, 1974.
[1]The authors wish to express their appreciation to Dr. Lincoln Moses of the Stanford University Department of Statistics for his suggestions concerning the analysis of the data.

tion and training of the police would appear to be considerably facilitated by insuring a police population amenable to such efforts.

A recent review of mental health screening of police applicants (Smith, 1971) indicates that while the use of some form of mental health screening has greatly increased in the past 20 years, and has official sanction to be incorporated into the selection of *all* law enforcement officers (The President's Commission on Law Enforcement and the Administration of Justice, 1967), research on the validity of the screening procedures has been minimal. Further, the majority of the research which does exist falls so far short of the minimally acceptable standards of experimental design that the mental health professional desirous of initiating a police screening program is left with little more than clinical intuition on which to base his selection procedures.

The available literature suggests that present screening efforts involve one or more of four components:

1. *The psychiatric interview.* Psychiatrists routinely interview all applicants for some police departments, and their impressions are incorporated into the regular selection procedure (e.g., Shev and Wright, 1971).

2. *Psychological tests.* The most frequent type of mental health screening of police applicants involves the use of one or more paper-and-pencil psychological tests, such as the MMPI and intelligence tests (e.g., Blum, 1964).

3. *Situational tests.* Recently some mental health personnel have attempted to go beyond paper-and-pencil testing and to create a microcosm of a natural field event a future policeman might encounter (Mills, McDevitt and Tonkin, 1966; Mills, 1969).

4. *Background data.* In their evaluation of potential law enforcement officers, some mental health professionals have given weight to psychologically relevant life-history variables, such as number of marriages, number of times fired from previous jobs, etc. (e.g., Levy, 1966).

No research at all is available on the utility of situational tests to predict future success in a law enforcement career, and only impressionistic accounts exist with regard to the psychiatric interview. There are some data, however, relevant to psychological testing and background data.

Levy (1966) retrospectively surveyed the personnel records of 5000 policemen and compared those who remained on the force with those who had been fired. She found that officers who had been fired were younger at the time of appointment, were more educated, had a greater number of marriages, shorter work histories and more vehicle citations than officers who remained on the force (see also Cross and Hammond, 1951).

Blum (1964) used a battery of psychological tests including the MMPI, Rorschach, Strong Vocational Interest Blank, Draw-a-Person, F-scale and Otis

Intelligence Test to predict police behavior seven years later along a number of dimensions (including commendations, terminations, promotions, etc.). Of the 324 correlations he obtained, only 36 reached $r = .20$, and only 3 reached $r = .40$ (MMPI scales: Sc, F and Pt).

The most recent major study of the prediction of police effectiveness is that of Baehr, Furcon and Froemel (1969). Using primarily tests which they themselves developed, the authors conclude "that the ideal attributes for success are all related to stability — stability in the parental and personal family situations, stability stemming from personal self-confidence and the control of emotional impulses, stability in the maintenance of cooperative rather than hostile or competitive attitudes and stability deriving from a resistance to stress and a realistic rather than subjective orientation toward life" (pp. IX-9). One difficulty with the Baehr et al (1969) study is that the subjects had been on the police force for some time when the psychological assessment took place. Extrapolation of their results to the prediction of future performance, of recruits who have not yet been socialized into police mores is somewhat tenuous (Smith, 1971). Another difficulty in trying to generalize from Baehr's study is the criteria of "good performance." What may be considered good in one department or assignment, e.g., a high number of arrests, may be less valued in another. Problem-solving may be considered a higher level of police performance than making an arrest.

The present study attempts to evaluate the mental health screening procedures in a large county sheriff's department. The study has the advantages of (1) employing several mental health screening procedures, including the psychiatric interview, many psychological tests and several background variables, (2) utilizing a variety of relevant criterion measures including supervisor ratings, personnel files and status in the department, and (3) evaluating the relationship between the predictors and the criteria in a more statistically sophisticated manner than has typically been the case in previous research.

METHOD

Background

The sheriff's department in a county of about 500,000 provides law enforcement services for the unincorporated areas of the county. In the late 1950s there were several incidents of deputy sheriffs arousing community concern by their aberrant behavior (e.g., reckless shooting, burglary). A decision was made to require mental health screening of all applicants to the sheriff's department in an effort to screen out potential sources of trouble.

Since 1959, every applicant has been screened by a team of mental health professionals.

Besides the sheer increase in numbers (there were 61 deputies in 1959, and 190 in 1972), the role of the deputy sheriff began to expand greatly soon after screening was initiated. In addition to the normal police functions of patrol, detective work and serving as bailiffs, civil service revisions made the running of the county jail part of the deputy sheriff's duty. All deputies were expected to change assignments and rotate from patrol to jail duty. In addition, about this time the jail opened an "honor camp" based on a therapeutic community concept. The deputies were expected to engage in group and individual counseling with the inmates, with consultation from mental health personnel. This was a marked shift in the deputies' role definition. Several years later, a work furlough facility was opened which allowed a man serving a jail sentence to leave the jail daily to continue his normal job. Here, also, the deputies were expected to be "counsellors" and run large group meetings to assist in the management of the facility.

Finally, a small section of the county changed from a rural area to a largely black community of about 20,000 people. Areas of tension and hostility developed. In time, at the request of the community, the sheriff established a separate sub-station for this community, in close liaison with their municipal council, and with a lieutenant who was in effect the chief of police for the area. The deputies assigned to this substation were clearly expected to be in closer touch with the citizens than had previously been the case and to be skilled in community relations.

The Selection of Police Recruits

Although the procedures have varied slightly over the years, the basic pattern has been constant. The applicant passes a physical agility test and takes a written Civil Service test before the mental health evaluation. An extensive background investigation is then conducted (enquiries to wives, employers, neighbors, etc.). The results of the mental health and background investigations are made known to an Oral Board, consisting of at least two law enforcement personnel and someone from Civil Service, which interviews each candidate. The Oral Board rating is added to the individual's Civil Service score to determine his rank on an eligible list. At times there was a cut-off score or passing grade on the Civil Service test, at other times the Civil Service score, no matter what it was, was simply added to the Oral Board Score to determine ranking. Applicants were generally hired in order of their ranking for as many openings as were available.

The Mental Health Screening Procedures

Some slight variations took place from year to year. Thus, the results of the first mental health screening were not presented to the Oral Board, to increase experimental precision. Since then, purity of design has given way to pressure to have the data presented to the Oral Board. For the first two screenings (100 applicants) only an applicant whose psychological test data aroused some concern was interviewed by a psychiatrist. Since then, every applicant has been interviewed. The psychological test battery has also undergone some revision. Tests which were used briefly and dropped included a sociometric rating by fellow applicants, the Strong Vocational Interest Blank, and the Edwards Personal Preference Scale. However, the screening typically proceeded in three phases:

Psychological Testing. In a group setting, the applicants were administered the MMPI, CPI, Rorschach, F-scale, Otis IQ test, Draw-A-Person, and instructed to write a 10 minute essay on "Why I Want to be a Deputy Sheriff." They were also given a specially developed demographic questionnaire which inquired into their birth order, presence of a father in the home during their childhood, etc.

Psychiatric Interview. Each applicant was interviewed by a psychiatrist for approximately one hour. At times, the psychiatrist had access to the psychologist's data. At other times, the interview was done independently.

Reports and Input. The examining psychologist reviewed the test data, then the background file, including the Civil Service test score, and wrote a report for the Oral Board. The examining psychiatrist likewise reported his interview findings. One of these mental health professionals was present at the Oral Board hearing, to answer any questions about the reports, but did not have voting power.

Outcome Measures

Three criteria were employed to assess the validity of the overall mental health ratings and validity of their components.

1. *Status in Department.* A basic criterion of the deputy's performance is his remaining on the job. Four categories were used to assess status at the time of the follow-up: Fired; Still employed but not promoted; Resigned; and Promoted. Included in the fired group were men who were allowed to resign but who would have been fired and/or faced criminal charges if they had not resigned.

2. *Personnel File.* At the time of the follow-up, each deputy's personnel file was reviewed and rated by a psychologist. The data in the file included

regular civil service evaluations, commendations, letters from citizens, suspensions, reprimands, criminal charges and notices of legal or financial problems.

3. *Supervisor Evaluations.* Obtaining specific criteria against which to measure a deputy's performance presented problems. Numerous conferences with sheriff's department personnel resulted in a set of 35 statements which were considered indicative of good police performance. In addition, there was a "general" overall rating. Each man was rated on a five point scale (poor to superior) on each of these 36 items, by two officers who had functioned in a supervisory role with him. The two ratings were completed independently, at the time of the follow-up. The 35 statements were grouped into nine a priori clusters for the analysis.

The specific scoring procedures for the predictor and criteria variables are detailed in the following section.

RESULTS

The subjects for this study were screened between February 1960 and October 1965. A total of 372 men were screened, of whom 91 were hired and are included here. The follow-up took place during January of 1966. The mean number of months on the job at the time of the follow-up was 24.8, with the range being between three and 66.

Status in the Department

For the criterion of status in the department a total of 54 predictor variables were analyzed. The variables and their scoring were as follows:

a. *Psychiatric evaluation.* The psychiatrist assigned a global rating to the candidate on a four point scale. The points were defined as:
    1. grossly unsuited for the job
    2. doubtful candidate
    3. acceptable
    4. eminently suited, strong addition to the department
b. *Psychological evaluation.* The psychologist assigned a global score to the candidate, on the same scale as above, based on all of the data.
c. *Psychological test scores.* The 13 MMPI scale scores (T-scores, K-corrected) and 18 CPI scores were each included in the analysis, along with a rating on a four-point scale (from pathological to well-integrated) of the Rorschach and Draw-A-

Person. Also, the F-scale raw score, Otis IQ score and score on the Civil Service examination were employed. The essay on "Why I Want to be a Deputy Sheriff" was scored on a four-point scale ranging from poor motivation and articulation to superior motivation and articulation.

d.   *Demographic data.* Included in the analysis were indices of the applicant's birth order, whether his father was out of the home during the applicant's childhood, the highest grade he completed in school, whether or not he went to college (O = never went, 1 = has less than an associate degree, 2 = AA, 3 = BA), his age at application and type of military service.

For the analysis of status in the department, the data was analyzed by means of Bonferroni multiple t-tests (Miller, 1966). These tests provide pairwise comparisons between each possible combination of means. The necessary percentage points were computed by interpolation in Federighi's tables (Federighi, 1959).

Rather than presenting the analysis on all 54 variables, we shall present the means and analyses for the psychiatric evaluation, the psychological evaluation, and only those psychological test scores and demographic data scores which significantly differentiated between at least one pair of means. The mean data and analyses are presented in Table 1.

It can be seen that while the global psychological evaluation significantly distinguished between some of the groups, the psychiatric evaluation did not. Most of the psychological tests and background variables also did not predict status in the department. Thus none of the MMPI scales, the F-scale or the Draw-A-Person differentiate the groups.

The conclusion which can most strongly be derived from this analysis is that 'general intelligence' (as evident in amount of college, IQ, and Civil Service score) is the best predictor of whether or not an applicant will eventually be promoted in the department. To predict whether an applicant will be a sufficient source of trouble to be fired, the personality factors evidenced in the Rorschach, CPI Re and So scales, and psychological global rating are most important.

Personnel File

The data from each individual's personnel file were reviewed by a psychologist and a score on a four-point scale was assigned. The four points were defined as follows:

1.   *Poor.* This rating included notices of some serious difficulties of either a legal, personal or job-related nature (e.g., arrests, brutality, extortion), a combination of lesser difficulties (e.g.,

Table 1 Status in the Department

Variable	Mean Group Score				Pairwise Comparisons					
	Fired (1)	Still Employed (2)	Resigned (3)	Promoted (4)	1 - 2	1 - 3	1 - 4	2 - 3	2 - 4	3 - 4
Psychiatric evaluation	2.8	2.8	2.7	3.2	*					
Psychological evaluation	1.9	2.6	2.8	2.8			*			
Rorschach	2.1	2.7	3.0	3.1		*	**			
Highest Grade	12.1	12.4	12.4	13.3			**			
CPI Responsibility scale	36.7	32.6	34.8	32.0	*					
CPI Socialization scale	43.5	38.5	37.3	39.4	*	*				
College	0.3	0.6	0.5	1.2			**		**	
Civil Service Score	62.4	64.5	68.6	76.7			**	~	**	
Otis IQ	106.7	109.7	112.3	119.5			*		**	

* = p < .05
** = p < .01

all tests are two-tailed

drunk driving and extensive credit problems) or serious errors in judgment (e.g., discharging a gun inappropriately).

2. *Below Standard.* This category included a poor driving record, drunk or asleep on duty, excessive force, noncompliance with supervision, accepting gifts, and an inability to relate to his co-workers or the public.

3. *Average.* An officer was rated as average if no mention of any of the above incidents was made in his file. It is possible that officers in this category were better than "average," but had no official action recognizing it.

4. *Superior.* This rating was given to officers whose record contained none of the events listed in Poor and Below Standard, yet did contain official commendations, or letters from citizens attesting to their superior abilities at police work.

For the analysis of the personnel file ratings, the data from the psychiatric evaluation, psychological evaluation, psychological test scores and background variables were entered into a step-wise multiple regression program. Variables were entered into the equation in order of increasing importance, and the equation was terminated when additional steps did not substantially increase the multiple correlation. The resulting equation was forthcoming:

Personnel file score is estimated by:

(weight of variable 1) (variable 1) + (weight of variable 2) (variable 2) + (weight of variable 3) (variable 3) + a constant.

Variable 1 is the psychological global score (weight = .37), variable 2 is the CPI dominance scale (weight =-.03), variable 3 is the CPI sociability scale (weight = .04) and the constant is 1.89. The multiple correlation of this equation is .56, which differs from zero at the .01 level.

Thus, the three best predictors of personnel file rating are the global psychological evaluation, and two scales of the CPI, dominance and sociability (dominance in a negative direction).

Supervisor Ratings

For each man in the study, two of his supervisors rated him on a five-point scale (poor to superior) for 35 characteristics which seemed indicative of desired police behavior. In addition, they gave him a general overall rating.

For purposes of analyses, the 35 items were divided into nine clusters. The nine clusters, and some representative items from each, were as follows:

1. *Use of authority:* "Ability to be firm when appropriate"; "Avoids being unnecessarily punitive with offenders".

2. *Initiative, responsibility:* "Ability to assume responsibility"; "Shows initiative."
3. *General competence and judgment:* "Ability to function under stress"; "Ability to make good decisions."
4. *Routine:* "Is prompt, observes time limits"; "Writes clear, concise reports."
5. *Self-control:* "Ability to avoid personal problems interfering with work"; "Can control his own feelings in handling his job."
6. *Public relations:* "Is courteous with the public"; Personal behavior reflects well on department."
7. *Empathy:* "Tries to understand the offender"; "Is courteous to offenders."
8. *Loyalty:* "Loyalty to the law enforcement profession"; "Loyalty to the Sheriff."
9. *Adaptable, cooperative:* "Ability to accept supervisions"; "Can grasp new concepts and ideas easily."

The average ratings of the two supervisors was taken as the criterion variable, and the data were analyzed in the same manner as for the personnel file, by means of multiple step-wise regressions.

The results of the regressions are presented in Table 2.

The equation is the same as that for personnel file, above, substituting 'criterion score,' for 'personnel file score.' In no case did expanding the equation beyond the first three steps produce a substantial increase in the multiple R.

The data on the supervisor ratings suffer from the fact that the correlation between the two independent supervisor's ratings was only .41. Considering this low index of agreement, it is surprising that the multiple R's usually manage to approach .50.

Despite this limitation, the data present an interesting pattern. The best predictors of supervisor ratings were the subscales of the California Psychological Inventory.

DISCUSSION

The data on which this research is based suffer from a substantial but unavoidable handicap: they figured into the actual hiring decisions made by the sheriff's department. Precisely how much weight was given them is impossible to determine. The results reported here in all probability would have been much stronger had extreme cases not been screened out at the time of the Oral Board and thus lost to the study. Considering this limitation, it is

Table 2 Supervisors' Ratings

Criterion	Variable #1 and Weight	Variable #2 and Weight	Variable #3 and Weight	Constant	Multiple R
Average Overall Rating	CPI Socialization .02	CPI Flexibility -.03	CPI Well Being .04	1.11	.41
Cluster 1 (Authority)	College -.24	Youngest child -.41	MMPI Manic .02	2.55	.50
Cluster 2 (Initiative, Responsibility)	CPI Flexibility -.05	MMPI Lie .02	CPI Responsibility .03	1.79	.48
Cluster 3 (Competence, Judgment	CPI Flexibility -.04	MMPI Lie .02	Psychological Global .13	2.49	.50
Cluster 4 (Routine)	CPI Flexibility -.04	CPI Wb .05	MMPI Hysteria -.01	2.24	.54
Cluster 5 (Self-Control)	CPI Flexibility -.04	Otis IQ -.02	Psychological Global .15	5.20	.49
Cluster 6 (Public Relations)	CPI Flexibility -.05	Psychological Global .17	CPI Well Being .04	1.93	.52
Cluster 7 (Empathy)	Otis IQ -.01	MMPI Manic .02	Youngest child -.36	3.51	.45
Cluster 8 (Loyalty)	College -.31	CPI Flexibility -.04	CPI Responsibility .02	3.22	.47
Cluster 9 (Adaptable, Cooperative)	CPI Flexibility -.04	CPI Well Being .05	Psychological Global .15	1.34	.48

somewhat surprising that the results came through as strongly as they did.

The conclusions one may draw from these data depend in large part upon one's choice of criteria. If selection of police applicants who stand a good chance of eventually being promoted is a prime concern, it would be best to focus on correlates of general intelligence, such as IQ, Civil Service score and educational level (IQ and Civil Service score, e.g., correlated .74). Conversely, applicants who later will be fired can be differentiated on more psychological variables (the psychologist's overall evaluation, the Rorschach, and two CPI scales, responsibility and socialization). In this study, the psychologist was strongly influenced by the Rorschach in assigning the global rating. This rating was essentially a clinical judgment. The best prediction of police performance, therefore, was a blending of clinical and psychometric data.

On the basis of the data presented in this study, one could insure a good personnel file by giving maximum consideration to the psychologist's overall evaluation of the applicant, along with two CPI scales, dominace and sociability.

The lack of agreement in the supervisors' ratings of police performance presents an interesting problem in its own right. A "good cop," it would seem, is in the eyes of the beholder. The evaluation depends more on who is doing the ratings than upon the behavior of the deputy in question. Despite the limitations placed on the data by the low inter-judge agreement, one might tentatively conclude that many of the scales of the CPI are potentially useful predictors of future evaluations.

The findings of this study are not without some paradoxes. Thus, the CPI "Flexibility" scale has a *negative* weight in predicting evaluations of competence, routine, self-control, public relations, adaptability and overall performance. The more flexible the individual scored at the time of application, the poorer he was evaluated by his supervisors later on. Before concluding that rigid people make the best policemen, one should examine the items which make up the scale. It would seem that the scale would be better labeled "tolerance for ambiguity". One man's "flexibility" may be another's "wishy-washyness." The nature of police work may be such that quick and firm decisions are frequently required, and philosophical suspension of judgment is not adaptive.

Also noteworthy is the finding that attendance at college negatively predicted loyalty and ability to deal with authority. If education breeds dissent, and assuming education to be a valued process, then perhaps police departments must reevaluate traditional notions of "loyalty." Evidently, one cannot have both educated and docile policemen at the same time.

Most surprising were the findings that the Responsibility and Socialization scales of the CPI were significantly *higher* for the group which was eventually fired than for those men who remained employed. The Responsibility scale is supposed to identify persons "of conscientious, responsible and dependable disposition and temperament" while Socialization is designed to indicate "the degree of social maturity, integrity, and rectitude which the individual has attained" (Gough, 1960, p 12). Clearly, these are not undesirable traits. While the fired group was higher on these two scales, it was significantly lower than some of the other groups on the overall psychological evaluation, the Rorschach, and the intelligence cluster. These seemingly contradictory findings defy explanation at this time, and should be replicated before they are taken into consideration in future screenings.

Among the more practical implications of this research is the fact that the California Psychological Inventory was clearly superior to the other major group-administered psychological test, the Minnesota Multiphasic Personality Inventory, as a predictive assessment device.

Also worthy of comment was the failure of the psychiatric interview to significantly predict any of the criterion events. This is consistent with the findings of other studies on the validity of the psychiatric interview in the prediction of job effectiveness (e.g., Fisher, Epstein and Harris, 1967; Harris, Fisher and Epstein, 1963). Blum (1960) found the psychiatric interview to correlate higher with Oral Board ratings than did the psychological report. This is not surprising since both are based on face-to-face interview data. The psychological evaluation samples a broader range of behavior potentials, a range which appears more predictive of future performance. It can be argued that psychiatric interviews of this nature cannot be evaluated solely in terms of predictive efficiency, since they are actually multipurpose devices (Ulrich and Trumbo, 1965). Among the ancillary goals of the psychiatric interview in a police screening situation might be rapport building with future consultees, dissemination of information about mental helath services, as well as more political considerations (it "looks good" to have applicants screened by a psychiatric interview). The data presented here might suggest that if these ancillary purposes are considered sufficient to justify the use of a psychiatric interview, then these purposes be made explicit and the interview be structured around rapport, education, etc., rather than being billed as a "screening" device.

It would appear that at the present time no screeing procedure *alone* can preselect "good" or "bad" law enforcement officers. Although men with certain characteristics can be identified by means of psychological tests, it is the law enforcement agency itself which must decide what kind of man it wants. Screening procedures can designate areas of concern and special talents to be developed. But if the agency is seeking to improve the quality of its personnel it must be alert to any opportunities to re-enforce the desired behaviors (especially by making them clear) and to use the available psychological data in supervising and guiding the new officers.

REFERENCES

Baehr, M., Furcon, J. and Froemel, E. *Psychological assessment of patrol-men's qualifications in relation to field performance.* Washington, D.C.: Office of Law Enforcement Assistance, U.S. Dept. of Justice, 1969.

Bard, M. and Berkowitz, B. Training police as specialists in family crisis intervention: A community psychology action program. *Community Mental Health Journal* 1967, 3 315-317.

Blum, R. *A study of deputy sheriff selection procedures.* Unpublished report, 1960.

Blum, R. (Ed.) *Police selection.* Springfield, Ill: Charles C. Thomas, 1964.

Cross, A. and Hammond, K. Social differences between 'successful' and 'unsuccessful' state highway patrolmen. *Public Personnel Review* 1951, 12, 159-161.

Federighi, E. Extended tables of the percentage points of student's t-distribution. *Journal American Statistical Association,* 1959, 54, 683-688.

Fisher, J., Epstein, L. and Harris, M. Validity of the psychiatric interview: Predicting the effectiveness of the first Peace Corps volunteers in Ghana. *Archives General Psychiatry.,* 1967, 17:744-750.

Friedman, M Community mental health education with police. In A. Bindman and A. Spiegel (Eds.) *Perspectives in community mental health.* Chicago: Aldine, 1969.

Gough, H. *Manual for the California Psychological Inventory.* Palo Alto: Consulting Psychologists Press, 1960.

Harris, M., Fisher, J. and Epstein, L. The reliability of the interview in psychiatric assessment for job placement. *Comprehensive Psychiatry,* 1963, 4, 19-28.

Johnson, D. and Gregory, R. Police – Community relations in the United States: A review of recent literature and projects. *Journal of Criminal Law, Criminology and Police Science,* 1971, 62, 94-103.

Levy, J. Summary of report on retrospective study of 5,000 peace officer personnel records. *The Police Yearbook,* 1966, pp 61-63.

Mann, P. Police responses to a course in psychology. *Crime and Delinquency,* 1970, 16, pp 403-408.

Mann, P. Establishing a mental health consultation program with a police department. *Community Mental Health Journal,* 1971, 7, 118-126.

McDonough, L. and Anderson, T. Consultation to courts and corrections. In H.R. Lamb, et al. (Eds.) *Handbook of community mental health practice.* San Francisco: Jossey-Bass, 1969.

Miller, R. *Simultaneous statistical inference.* New York: McGraw-Hill, 1966.

Mills, R. Use of diagnostic small groups in police recruit selection and training. *Journal of Criminal Law, Criminology, and Police Science.,* 1969, 60, 238-241.

Mills, R., McDevitt, R. and Tonkin, S. Situational tests in metropolitan police recruit selection. *Journal of Criminal Law, Criminology and Police Science.,* 1966, **57,** 99-106.

The President's Commission on Law Enforcement and the Administration of Justice, *Task Force Report: The Police.* Washington, U.S. Government Printing Office, 1967.

Rhodes, W. Regulation of human behavior: Dynamics and structure. In S. Golann and C. Eisdorfer (Eds.) *Handbook of community mental health.* New York: Appleton-Century-Crofts, 1972.

Shev, E. and Wright, J. The uses of psychiatric techniques in selecting and training police officers as part of their regular training. *Police,* May-June, 1971, pp. 13-16.

Smith, D. Police officer selection: A critical literature review. Paper read at the Western Psychological Association Convention, San Francisco, 1971.

Ulrich, L. and Trumbo, D. The selection interview since 1949. *Psychological Bulletin,* 1965, **63,** 100-116.

5

A Law Enforcement Training Program in a Mental Health Center Catchment Area*

EDWARD J. ROLDE, ELLSWORTH FERSCH, FRANCIS J. KELLY
SUSAN FRANK and MAURICE GUBERMAN

This paper describes a training program in the problems of children for police, probation, and parole officers from the catchment area of the Massachusetts Mental Health Center. This area has a population of approximately 200,000 and consists of parts of the city of Boston and the adjacent town of Brookline. It is in a central section of a large city and has a heterogeneous population. There is a complete spectrum of socioeconomic conditions and ethnic subcultures.

The 30 training program participants represented ten different law enforcement agencies and included officers from two police forces; probation officers from four municipal courts, a superior court, and a juvenile court; and parole officers from both the adult and juvenile system. For convenience, this group will be referred to as "law enforcement officers."

The program, which was managed by the Division of Legal Medicine, Community Mental Health Services, Massachusetts Mental Health Center, was designed to focus on two issues bearing on the development of a law enforcement training program by a community mental health center. The first issue is the difficult relationship that exists between many law enforcement agencies and other social service and community organizations. The second issue is the pressure on individuals to perform duties in the style of the agency or system of which they are members. This paper gives the background and overview of our experience.

*Reprinted from the *American Journal of Psychiatry*, 1973, **130,** 1002-1005, with permission. Copyright 1973, the American Psychiatric Association.

PAST PROBLEMS OF LAW ENFORCEMENT TRAINING PROGRAMS

Most law enforcement officers are given some training in the problems of children. The most common type of program is usually provided at the time of recruitment by a specific agency to its own staff. Arrangements made for individual officers to attend classes in academic institutions are increasingly common. Formal programs run for law enforcement agencies by outside groups are also common. Most often they are one of three types (1-9): didactic lectures or demonstrations, primarily for new recruits; sensitivity groups, most often led by a professional leader with law enforcement officers as group members: and training in special techniques for a subunit of the Agency (e.g., training of special family intervention teams). We are not aware of any combined inservice training programs for police, probation, and parole officers.

Our contacts with social service agencies, consulting firms, and law enforcement officials revealed a consistent opinion that training programs run by outside organizations for law enforcement personnel, especially those run by mental health organizations, were of little value. Most people felt, however, that there was a pressing need for programs providing contact between law enforcement and other disciplines. Many papers in the literature also reflect this concern (10,11).

In the past, training programs have faced a fundamental difficulty: ignorance, mutual disrespect, and absence of communication between lawmen and social service personnel working with the same clients. Many mental health workers believed that law officers as a group knew very little about behavior, both their clients' and their own. It was often in a patronizing and pejorative manner that mental health workers implied that they could teach law officers more about behavior and make them better at their jobs. Since a major part of the law officer's job involves understanding his "client's" behavior and controlling his own behavior in a professional manner, the mental health worker often appeared to be telling him that he did not know how to do his job.

A second common difficulty reported primarily by those involved in training programs is the relationship of the individual law officer to the system or agency of which he is a part. Those who felt they had overcome communication barriers and provided program participants with useful information often felt their work was undone because of the pressure on the individual officer to follow the behavior model of the agency. Several former faculty members of training programs said that their programs were useless: before individual officers could change their behavior, the law enforcement agency would have to change.

The problems of training for law enforcement officers are even further compounded by the diversity of the law enforcement system itself. There are major obstacles to the interaction and understanding of different components of the system. On the one hand, police, parole, and probation officers are often working in administrative isolation from and conceptual antagonism to one another. On the other hand, there are differences and barriers to cooperation between differing units of the same components. Differences in style among neighboring police departments are foremost among these.

CONCEPTUAL FOUNDATION OF THE PROGRAM

Our first premise was that the individuals who knew most about law enforcement work were the officers. This was especially true of our participants, most of whom had ten to 20 years of work experience in our geographic area. We believed that this group knew more than any other about the techniques and problems of handling a delinquent adolescent, for example. Consequently, we avoided telling the officer how to do his job; we felt that would be presumptuous and would most likely produce resistance and antagonism.

Our second premise was that a great deal of law enforcement work, especially that involving the maintenance of order, requires the officer to deal with community, family and individual problems (12-18). Consequently, we assumed that it would benefit law officers to hear how other agencies and professions approach the same problems. They might find some of these other approaches useful in their work and it might also give them a clearer perspective on what their clients experience in the community. Finally, they would be introduced to other agencies and their staff and would be able to contact them and work with them in the future.

Two features of the program were designed for maximum behavior change, not only in the officers' work routine, but in their organizations as well. The first was relevance. There were no "outside speakers." All guests were members of local agencies. They discussed their agency's policies and problems and were able to take back to their agency the reaction of the other participants. The second feature was the length of the training program. Participants had a chance to develop trust in the staff and each other over time and to become comfortable in the discussion meetings. There was an opportunity for them to think about the presentations and continue to react to them over a long period. The extended time also allowed us to continually adjust the program to the pace and interests of the officers.

MECHANICS OF THE PROGRAM

The group of 30 officers met every other week for about one year. They received a stipend roughly equal to their regular pay. Each session lasted two to three hours. The first half of each session consisted of a presentation by representatives of a guest agency; questions and discussion came from the group as a whole. The second part consisted of meetings in small groups, which included both officers and guest agency staff. The project staff helped the guest agency prepare the presentation and moderated the meeting and the smaller group discussions.

The program focused on youth and the development of delinquency. We emphasized both social and psychological points of view. We chose guest agencies and organized the presentations so that there would be a coherent and orderly sequence. At the same time, we tried to raise the interest level and enthusiasm of both the individual guests and the officers. We wanted lively and relevant discussions of definite points of view, rather than comprehensive reviews of subject matter. Invited guests included staff members of local universities and public school systems; local judges and public defenders; youth, family, and drug treatment agencies; funding organizations; and law enforcement agencies.

At the end of every fifth meeting or so, there was a review session in which there were no invited guests. The sessions were used to digest, review, and complete previous topics, to evaluate what had already happened, to plan future programs, and to consider suggestions from the participants for presentation to other community agencies.

EXPERIENCE WITH THE PROGRAM

Obtaining the cooperation of the participating agencies was a major task. Permission for members to participate was obtained from the ten different law enforcement organizations and numerous guest agencies. The full participation of the different groups in the sessions was one of the major intermediate goals and accomplishments of the program.

Although the law enforcement agencies agreed to participate, they expressed a good deal of skepticism about the value of the program. The skepticism was supported, in most cases, by what individual officers reported as bad experiences with past training programs and with social service and mental health professionals. At the first session, attendance varied among the different law enforcement groups. The one agency that did not offer a stipend to its staff was fully represented. The agency that had enrolled the largest number in the program, a police department, had only two men present at the first session. At the second session, all of its representatives were present. By the third session, additional men from that agency had asked to be included in the program. After the first two or three weeks, attendance at the sessions was close to complete for all the participating agencies.

PROGRAM SESSIONS

A sense of the structure and content of the program can best be conveyed by brief descriptions of several sessions.

The guests at one of the sessions were 30 grammar school principals, guidance counselors, and adjustment counselors from Brookline, Mass. The superintendent and staff of the department of education had expressed a great deal of interest in knowing more about the work of the law enforcement agencies and in working more closely with them. One of the guidance counselors raised the central issue confronting school personnel in cooperating with law officers. It was confidentiality, what they should do when a child comes to them and confides that he is breaking the law. The issue is complicated and raised many questions about the techniques used and roles assumed by school staff and law officers in their dealings with children.

During the second half of the session the participants broke into three smaller groups of about 20. There were equal numbers of school and law enforcement personnel in each. While the three discussions differed, a common theme appeared initially. The law enforcement officers tended to believe that the school staff were too lenient to be of help to children in many situations. The school personnel tended to believe that law enforcement officers would almost always be too severe. Soon both groups gave examples of how many wished to be more like the other. At the same time, both expressed fears of what would happen to their clients if the other group had its way. After the session both sides asked that we set up continuing sessions of this type in Brookline during the following years.

At another session, the guest speaker was the director of the state bureau that manages federal "safe streets" money. He discussed his bureau's policies and plans and mentioned in particular the problems it faces in funding programs for delinquent youth. The officers told him they had long felt that his agency had neglected to take advantage of their views and expertise and had never made it clear why certain decisions were made. The guest speaker explained the reasons for some controversial policies and asked the group's opinion on several issues that were under consideration at the time. The officers began to feel that they were being heard and some of the decisions were not reached as arbitrarily as they had thought, or that they at least understood the policies better. There was a noticeable increase in their morale and in their knowledge of program decisions and funding management.

Another of the meetings was held in the children's unit of the Massachusetts Mental Health Center. The law enforcement group met with several members of the staff including psychiatrists, psychologists, and social workers. The meeting began with a film on hyperactive children. After the film there was a presentation by one of the child psychiatrists and a general discussion of the film and presentation. The discussion centered on the way psychiatrists relate to children and on the hyperactive syndrome itself.

During the session and discussion period, the view each group held of the other began to emerge. The law enforcement officers felt that the mental health workers did not really know much about children who get into trouble with the law. They also felt that the doctors were not very warm in their dealings with children and tended to treat them as subjects rather than as persons. The mental health workers thought the officers were interested in law enforcement rather than people and felt that a law enforcement background did not prepare them for sophisticated concepts. This session was well received by most of the officers. They felt they had learned something useful about hyperactive children and gave this as an example of a subject the mental health workers knew something about and for which they had specific treatment methods that related directly to law enforcement work. Most important, however, was their feeling about a session with psychiatrists from the mental health center. Many commented on the doctors' willingness to listen to their points of view and said they felt much more comfortable about coming to the center when their work took them there.

RECEPTION OF THE PROGRAM

Several things indicated that the program was very favorably received by the law enforcement participants. The sessions themselves were enjoyable and the participants were enthusiastic. They often said they looked forward to the sessions and talked about them often with us and between themselves during the week. Attendance was very good throughout the duration of the program, even though the participants were busy and often had to make complicated arrangements to attend. Almost all the participants reported that the sessions were useful. This favorable response was made both in the discussion sessions and our formal evaluation interview and in subsequent reports to us.

Most important, there were numerous indications that the program changed the work behavior of the participants and influenced the practices of their agencies. Several instances were reported of improved working relationships between officers and agencies that had participated as guests in the program and between officers representing different departments or divisions within law enforcement agencies.

While this type of evidence does not constitute a controlled evaluation, it is still very encouraging. It is clear that we have learned a great deal about the problems and practices of law enforcment and have established relationships with individuals and organizations that would have been difficult to establish without the program. While the focus of the training was on changing the behavior of the officers, the learning process obviously worked both ways. In fact, the sessions were most often a very challenging and useful experience for the invited guests. We hope to focus on this aspect of the program more fully in a later paper.

REFERENCES

1. Bard, M., Berokowitz, B., Training police as specialists in family crisis intervention: A community psychology action program. *Community Mental Health J3*: 315-317, 1967.
2. Elkins, A.N., Papnek, G.O., Consultation with the police: An example of community psychiatry practice. *Am J Psychiatry* 123: 531-535, 1955.
3. Friedman, M.H., Community mental health education with police. *Ment Hyg* 49: 182-186, 1965.
4. Lipsitt, P., An experiment in police community relations: A small group approach. *Community Ment Health J5*: 172-179, 1969.
5. Matthews, R.A., Rowland, L.W.A., A manual for the police officer: How to recognize and handle abnormal people. New York, National Association for Mental Health, 1960.
6. Lonkes, G.A., How should we educate the police? *Journal of Criminal Law, Criminology, and Police Science 61*: 587-592, 1970.
7. Siegel, A.I., Federman, P., Schultz, D.G., *Professional police human relations training*. Springfield, Ill. Charles C. Thomas, 1963.
8. Sikes, N.P., Cleveland, S.E., Human relations trainig for police and community. *Am Psychol 23* 766-769, 1968.
9. Watson, N.A., Human relations training for police: A syllabus. Washington, D.C. International Association of Chiefs of Police, 1968.
10. Germann, A.C., Changing the police: The impossible dream. *Journal of Criminal Law, Criminology, and Police Science 62*: 416-421, 1971.
11. Taylor, E.M., McEachern, A.W. Needs and directions in probation training. *Federal Probation 30*: 18-24, 1966.

12. Barton, M. *The policeman in the community*. New York, Basic Books, 1965.
13. Bittner, E. Police discretion in emergency apprehension of mentally ill persons. *Social Problems* 14: 278-292, 1967.
14. Cummings, E., Edell, L., Cummings, I. Policeman as philosopher, guide, and friend. *Social Problems* 12: 276-286, 1965.
15. Liberman, R. Police as a community mental health resource. *Community Ment Health J* 5: 111-120, 1969.
16. MacNamara, J.H. Uncertainties in police work: The relevance of police recruits' background and training, in *The police: Six sociological essays*. Edited by Bordua, D.J. New York, John Wiley & Sons, 1967, pp 163-252.
17. President's Commission on Law Enforcement and Administration of Justice: Task Force Report: Police. Washington, D.C., U.S. Government Printing Office, 1967.
18. Wilson, J.Q. *Varieties of police behavior*. New York, Atheneum, 1970.

6

Training Police Recruits for Service
in the Urban Ghetto: A Social Worker's Approach *

JOHN J. HUGHES

Many Metropolitan police departments are attempting to recruit simultaneously from the total national and local minority-group communities in an effort to upgrade both the quality and the enlightenment of police services in cities with increasing proportions of black and other poor minorities.[1] At the same time they are seeking to diversify and improve police academy programs for training these disparate groups of recruits by introducing instructors drawn from other professions. This paper will describe and assess the recent experience of a social worker, the writer, in such a program in a large eastern city, and will sift it for whatever implications it may have for other cities, social workers, or police trainers.

BACKGROUND

The specific vehicle was a three-hour weekly course in the prevention and control of juvenile delinquency: a small part of the total police academy program, which consisted of thirteen weeks of classwork with a three-week break halfway through for on-the-job field training.

Before the spring of 1970, all the courses in the program were taught

*Reprinted from *Crime and Delinquency,* April 1972, **18,** 176-183, with permission of the National Council on Crime and Delinquency.

[1] Such recruitment follows recommendations made by the President's Commission on Law Enforcement and Administration of Justice. See the report of the Commission's Task Force on the Police, p. 123.

by police personnel attached to the academy. In 1970, a local university contracted with the police department to organize and offer the delinquency course. The writer was one of several social workers the university invited to serve as instructors, each one to lead a different recruit group. Since departmental recruiting was still under way at the time of the invitation, only the most generalized information about the recruits was available. Furthermore, the "crash" nature of the recruiting program and the newness of the university-police partnership made it difficult to draw up precise guidelines; instructors were encouraged to "stay loose" in their planning. As a result, each developed his own unique classroom experience.

The writer's group began training in May and finished in August. Classes were held at the police academy, an ancient and inadequate structure. The large classroom was equipped with the mobile desk-chairs typical of college classrooms, arranged in crowded rows ten deep. By the third week all the trainees wore the required uniform. Bells signaled the start and finish of classes and were meticulously observed by the trainees. The lecture was the teaching method almost exclusively used throughout the academy program. Recruits carefully addressed civilian instructors as "Sir." The general tone conveyed by the academy as a setting was one of inhibition.

THE POLICE RECRUITS

The recruits numbered forty-seven, including one woman; all were in their twenties. Two-thirds had completed their military service. All had a high school diploma or accredited equivalent; a handful had some college background. Twenty-six were white; twenty-one were black. Almost all of the black recruits resided in town, while almost all of the whites lived in nearby suburbs. Reflecting the national recruiting efforts of the department and the attractive starting salary, recruits hailed from eighteen states. Only thirteen of the forty-seven recruits, mostly black, had been local residents before they joined the force.

Two important inferences drawn from these group characteristics were to shape some of the course's directions: (1) most of the recruits were almost totally ignorant of the geography, culture, and services of the community they were to serve; (2) a large minority, though more knowledgeable about the community, was apt to share or be ambivalent about some of the community's views of the police system and its agents.

OBJECTIVES

All training programs should provide instruction on subjects that prepare recruits to exercise discretion properly, and to understand the community, the role of the police, and what the criminal justice system can and cannot do.[2]

Most of the recruits needed to learn something about the geography and the youth services of the city. Most had much to learn about the cultures and life-styles of its inhabitants, including the language. Some probably needed to confront their ambivalence about stepping from the culture of the ghetto into that of the police force. All needed to identify the components of their role in the prevention and control of delinquency and to develop their skills in fulfilling that role. These men were to be partrolmen, rather than juvenile officers; this fact dictated de-emphasis of specialized interviewing and referral skills — duties reserved for the juvenile officer — and recognition of offense rather than offender-oriented contact on the street rather than in the office. All could profit from exposure to the correctional system and to other systems that might serve youngsters with whom they would come into contact.

METHODS

The instructor's bias was toward participative learning, concrete and experience-based. The hunch that the instructional style should be colloquial and action-oriented proved correct after an early try-out. Accordingly, the instructional methods decided on were (1) role-playing, (2) small-group visits to agencies involved in the prevention and control of delinquency (and feedback sessions in class), (3) small-group discussions, (4) construction and presentation of a local ghetto glossary by recruits, (5) discussion of assigned interviews with experienced officers, (6) feedback from recruits during their three-week break for on-the-job training, (7) readings, and, of course, (8) instructor's lectures. Space permits only a brief discussion here of the major results of some of these approaches.

---

[2]President's Commission on Law Enforcement and Administration of Justice. *The Challenge of Crime in a Free Society*, Washington, D.C.: U.S. Government Printing Office, 1967, p. 112.

ROLE-PLAYS

Some of the role-plays were directed toward needs identified by the instructor; others were based on needs identified in recruits' field work and in their interviews with experienced officers. From the beginning the trainees made enthusiastic use of the role-plays, volunteering readily and participating freely.

The first role-play resulted in some spectacular dynamics. Six boisterous "teen-agers" confronted by two "officers" on a busy corner during a tense summer evening resisted the "officers" attempts to disperse and frisk them. Two of the black "youths" verbally assaulted the black "officers" as "Uncle Toms," accusing them of "trying to be the first black sergeant in the precinct." One "youth" refused to be frisked, and an "officer," intent on searching him, became increasingly and angrily determined to do so. The irresistible force finally met the immovable object as the "officer" slammed the "youth" against the portable blackboard to effect the search. The blackboard nearly broke the classroom door, as the instructor called a halt to the role-play and reassured an academy staff member who came rushing up to the classroom that nothing was the matter.

The class discussion that followed verged on pandemonium. Criticisms of the "officers' " behavior alternated with challenges to the validity of the "youths' " deportment, touching off scattered pockets of hot dispute all over the classroom. What finally cooled off the arguments was an observation by a recruit that, in the circumstances given, such police behavior would probably have started a riot. After a few moments of shocked silence, the discussion continued in a more sober and orderly fashion. The chief points centered on the possible reasons for the "teen-agers' " hostility to the officers, including group pressures, face-saving, etc., and the impersonal and direct approach of the officers.

During the week following the class, the role-play continued to be a source of lively, informal discussion among the recruits. In the next class, the situation was replayed by the same actors. A totally different pattern emerged: no dispersal, no frisk, a more casual approach with an emphasis on "rapping." The black "youths' " ambivalence toward black policemen took on the more subtle form of an effort to seduce them into a crap game. A major learning for the recruits was that, contrary to most of their earlier statements, good community relations might be important to law enforcement after all, offering access to local leadership and resources that could be helpful in cooling off situations of this type. Interestingly, the black recruits were not yet able to admit to ambivalence about their police role, despite the evidence of the role-plays. They ultimately did so later in the course, after such reaction was legitimated by the instructor's lectures and recruits' field visits.

Another role-play situation was the blocking of a street by anti-war demonstrators. The "students" sat on the floor and goaded the "officers," calling them "pigs" and throwing paper "rocks" at them. One such rock struck an "officer" and he responded angrily by trying to pull the offender out of the group. The "student" pulled back and the "officer" tumbled down among the group on the floor. Others went to his rescue and suffered the same fate. The role-play ended in a wrestling free-for-all, and once again a staff member ran up to see what was going on.

During a role-play on intervention in a family dispute, the "officers" failed to separate the disputants, permitted the argument to get out of hand, and wound up having to drag the "husband" off to the squad car and restrain the angry "wife" and "teen-age son."

Other role-plays included coping with a "sour cop" for a partner and understanding the importance of interracial cooperation within the department. The latter two were less directly concerned with skill acquisition than the others, having primarily cognitive objectives. A few recruits had encountered, during their on-the-job training experiences, veteran police officers of cynical mind, with extreme feelings of isolation and distrust of the public, including juveniles. The role-play was designed to help the recruits look at and work through some of their feelings about possible partnership with such an officer and to understand how he might affect their own attitude and work. The role-play on interracial cooperation was designed to help the recruits understand how the competition for intradepartmental rewards (including those built into the police academy program) might feed into racial polarity and obscure the importance of more cooperative relationships. As a result of the role-play the recuits went on to identify serveral problems common to all police officers which, in their opinion, were a source of lowered morale and merited their common attention.

The role-plays directed at skill acquisition were likely to result in physical violence of one form or another, at least initially, while those with more cognitive objectives were not. Some might conclude that the relative persistence of violent solutions reflects departmental norms of efficiency. Be that as it may, the role-plays effectively touched off spirited analysis of the police role, and the recruits' final evaluation of the course ranked the role-plays high as a source of learning.

VISITS TO AGENCIES DEALING WITH DELINQUENTS

Each recruit was asked to choose a team assignment to visit an agency dealing with preventive, control, or rehabilitative aspects of delinquency. The instructor designated the agencies with an eye to exposing the recruits to community services, particularly those into which their behavior as patrolmen might project juvenile offenders. Each recruit group had to report to the class and lead a general discussion on the agency and its services according to a flexible but comprehensive outline suggested by the instructor. Recruits were encouraged to talk, where possible, with recipients as well as staff, and to observe program services directly. All visits were carried out on the recruits' own time. Interestingly enough, despite the burden they placed on the recruits, these contacts were later adjudged by them the most valuable aspect of the course.

Trainees visited ten agencies, including the juvenile court, the detention center, a juvenile training school, a detached worker program, a halfway house, drug programs, economic development programs, ex-offender services, a youth correctional center, etc. Some of these programs were headed by community figures frequently identified as hostile to the police, and some recruits contemplated such visits with an anxiety that proved needless. Several group reports expressed surprise and admiration for the job being done by many ex-offenders. These reports touched off heated discussions among incredulous trainees.

Black recruits who had previously been reluctant to admit in class that some black citizens might resent their having joined the police force — a resentment unlikely to have come as a surprise to them — were confronted with open hostility at drug addicts' meetings. They reported, and white recruits corroborated, a special antagonism surpassing that directed at white officers.

At this report the trainees were finally able to discuss the bi-cultural "bind" of the ghetto-origin officer, pulled between community expectations of understanding and humaneness on the one hand and official and unofficial departmental standards of law-enforcing efficiency on the other.[3] In the instructor's judgment, black recruits had serious inner conflicts over this predicament, still far from resolved at the end of the course. Some felt that they had to be above suspicion of softness on crime in order to survive the probationary period, let alone to advance within the department. A local newspaper was currently running articles alleging departmental harassment of "militant" black officers, and these had a profound effect on the black recruits, a few of whom openly injected the issue into the classroom while most "played it cool." One black recruit who voiced strong feelings about departmental attitudes openly predicted that he would not survive his

---

[3]For example, see Egon Bittner, *The Functions of the Police in Modern Society,* Washington, D.C.: National Institute of Mental Health, 1970, p. 57: "Every officer knows that he will never receive a citation for avoiding a fight but only for prevailing in a fight at the risk of his own safety."

probationary year. The "cool" group avoided expressing their feelings in class but revealed their anxiety privately to the instructor in conversation and by presenting him with carefully clipped and underlined newspaper articles on the alleged harassment.

It may or may not be significant that of the nine recruits who left the group during the course of the training program for reasons never discussed with the instructor, seven were black.

The underlying tug-of-war for the black policeman's loyalties will probably continue to trouble the newly recruited black.[4] Most qualified black recruits will continue to find some way to live with the dilemma, and many will introduce into police service a necessary and salutary awareness of the strengths of the inner-city black community.

GHETTO GLOSSARY

The instructor asked three black recruits who were local residents to compile and present a glossary of ghetto terminology. They verbally presented a lengthy and repetitious lexicon heavily laden with sexual references. The out-of-towners found it enlightening (some shocking), but on the whole it was too disjointed and repetitious to be usefully assimilated. Such language skill is as vital in police work as in any cross-cultural endeavor. More orderly and systematic means (possibly borrowed from the language schools) such as short-term "immersion" should be adapted.

REPORTS FROM ON-THE-JOB TRAINING BREAK

The instructor sought to link classroom learning to the field experience by assigning responsibility in advance to three volunteers for providing the class with relevant feedback from their three-week break for on-the-job training (during which they were in the field with experienced officers). This linkage proved quite stimulating to the recruits — so much so that fully half the class offered feedback from their field experiences. Several reported being told by experienced officers to forget what they learn at the police academy.[5] One was jeered at as a "social worker" by his field instructor for

---

[4] As an illustration of this conflict Jerome Skolnick, "Why Cops Behave the Way They Do," in Simon Dinitz *et al., Deviance* New York: Oxford University Press, 1969, p. 46, cites the case of a CORE leader who left the police department during his training because he could not live with the seeming contradictions.

[5] Bittner, *op cit. supra* note 3, p. 60, claims this is the first thing the new policeman learns.

"rapping" with some youngsters. Another was told not to ask young people questions because "they all lie." Two investigated assaults by jueniles only to have the victims drop the charges. Most found young children friendly, teen-agers hostile. One had his pocket picked by a thirteen-year old. One worked with a partner who ordered demonstrators around "to show them who's boss." Several were shocked to find six-to eight-year-old children wandering around late at night. One had bottles thrown at him by young people shouting "pigs." One expressed horror at his first exposure to a public housing project — "those people just don't give a damn about their kids." (Response from a black recruit: "Black mothers been looking after white folks' children for years. That's pretty good loving.") Two or three had encountered bitter old-timers of the department, white and black, who had expressed total distrust of the public, the department, and even fellow officers.

It seems fair to say that their exposure to the field had effected something of a "reality shock," emphasizing the gap between the indoctrinative uniformity of the academy and the diverse discretion of held roles. For two full hours the recruits discussed their varied emotional reactions to the realities of patrol duty. Opinions and counter-opinions, buttressed or modified by field experience, flowed more freely than they had previously. Much of their feed-back ultimately found its way into role-plays, structured small-group discussions, and the instructor's lectures. Perhaps the greatest lessons of the field work aspect of the training program are the validity of linking it to a classroom process and the advisability of a more organized and less haphazard use of the training.

THE ROLE OF THE INSTRUCTOR

One of the surprising aspects of the trainees' evaluation was their relatively high evaluation of the "prof's lectures." It was surprising because such lectures not only were kept to a minimum but were usually directed at content that is supposed to antagonize policemen: the alleged conservatism of policemen,[6] the racially disproportionate application of the criminal justice system, the juvenile's view of the policeman (including issues of brutality and corruption), the culture gap between policemen and the poor, the deleterious effects of pretrial detention, etc.

But the instructor plays a much more diversified role than mere lecturing, particularly in a free-wheeling approach like the one described here.

[6]Skolnick, *supra* note 4, p. 46

Reaction to him depends on his ability to communicate in appropriate terms ("What's 'recidivism,' teach?") and to establish a climate of mutual respect. If some recruits had reservations about the instructor's attack on racist views of Negroes as subhumans, his equating of such views with calling policemen "pigs" may have put them in a new light. Though a "do-good social worker," the instructor sought to draw on his experiences with street gangs and other delinquent groups to communicate a realistic assessment of the problems they present and his real conviction about the importance of good police work in dealing with them. He further sought to express a sympathetic awareness of the degree to which the community has delegated many of its most difficult social problems to the police without adequate resources for referral. It should be of concern to social agencies that a nationally publicized police training program in family crisis intervention found them "unable or unwilling to provide flexible crisis services."[7] In many ways the police department is the biggest social agency in town, and the instructor did not hesitate to say so.

CONCLUSION

This paper has described one social worker's experience in training metropolitan police recruits. It suggests that as universities become more involved, social workers may have increasing opportunity to participate in such programs and that their participation may be both satisfying and helpful. Even in the less-than-ideal setting of the police academy, police recruits can be stimulated to examine their attitudes toward the humanity of their clients and to develop skills in peacekeeping rather than mere apprehension of offenders. Indeed, current recruiting patterns are creating a situation in which training programs need only release rather than supply much of the knowledge necessary for better police-community understanding.

Black recruits experience conflict when they join the force and resolve it in individual ways but primarily by "playing it cool" — i.e., meeting or seeming to meet the minimal demands of both the police and the community cultures. Most police recruits, to the extent that this group was typical, are not insensitive to the human needs of inner-city residents and are able to open themselves to experiences that address those needs. But there appear to be strong systemic forces toward the isolation of the policeman from the

---

[7]Morton Bard, *Training Police as Specialists in Family Crisis Intervention*, Washington, D.C.: Department of Justice, 1970, p.30.

community. Motorization and increasing centralization of operations have substantially taken the policeman off the beat and out of the neighborhood and have depersonalized the police function to a large extent. Official and unofficial departmental norms may offer inadequate support to integrative patrol behavior. These problems will need to be modified if good training is to result in the most effective work, but even then a major effort must be made to equip recruits to exercise wisely the discretion that inheres in their everyday role. That effort can be partly made by social workers who can help create and interpret flexible learning opportunities, particularly those rooted in an experiential base. Social workers close to the urban community would seem to be among the most likely candidates for such training roles.

7

The Role of Law Enforcement in the Helping System [*][1]

MORTON BARD

It is one of the ironies of social existence that the greatest progress often occurs at times of greatest social unrest. Indeed, it is the threat of violence that is frequently the most powerful force to promote change in the institutions of society. History attests to the fact that the most dramatic technological advances have occurred during periods when our nation was imperiled by war. There is little question that when "under the gun" we are able to marshal our resources, we can reappraise our priorities, and we can alter our institutions to enhance our survival as a social order.

Today threats of violence are legion — not so much from without as from within our society. Are we prepared to undertake critical appraisal of our institutions and alter them to insure survival? If the past is prologue, we will; there are signs that the necessary changes are taking place.

CHANGING ROLES OF LAW ENFORCEMENT
AND THE UNIVERSITY

Two institutions are in the forefront of social reappraisal: law enforcement and academe. It is hardly accidental that these two should be

[*]Reprinted from *Community Mental Health Journal*, 1971, 7, 151-160, with permission. Copyrighted by Behavioral Publications, New York, 1971.

[1]The project described herein was supported by OLEA Grant No. 157, U.S. Department of Justice. An earlier version of this paper was presented at the dedication of the Cumberland County Mental Health Center, Fayetteville, North Carolina, April 9, 1969, and was first published in the *North Carolina Journal of Mental Health,* Vol. IV, No. 3.

paired at this time in history. Both play critical roles with respect to the internal harmony of society: one primarily by thought, the other primarily by action; the one given to change, the other committed to the *status quo*. Unfortunately both have failed to adapt to rapidly changing conditions. The simplistic notion of the police as a repressive force in the defense of property is no more viable today than is the naive notion that the university is a medieval cloister given to abstract thought far removed from the realities of everyday life. As a consequence of adhering to outmoded functional concepts, both institutions find themselves increasingly remote from those they serve and decreasingly effective in fulfilling their primary missions (Bard, 1969).

Perhaps the key issue for both of these institutions lies in their failure to acknowledge present-day realities. Much of the university's prime function is regarded as irrelevant today. There seems to be less and less tolerance for abstract research exercises that fail to contribute to the world of real people. A similar charge of irrelevance is directed at law enforcement. There is increasingly less tolerance for police behavior patterned after the Hollywood-reinforced stereotype of the tight-lipped, gun-slinging frontier marshall.

There was a time when the myth of academic intellectual purity excluded practical application of knowledge in much the same way the law enforcement tended to reject all functions but those based on force. But each institution has had to confront its own myths. The university did so initially by incorporating elements of the practical in science and technology, creating schools of engineering and agriculture; later, medical colleges, schools of social work, and schools of education were added to the array of interests that could be said to serve the community without compromising the university's mission to extend the horizons of knowledge. The university accepted its responsibility in the preparation of society's professional helpers. Interestingly, save for rare exceptions the university ignored the education of one of the most direct helpers in society — the police. It is the thesis of this paper that our present national crisis makes it imperative that law enforcement be acknowledged as a participating profession in the helping system. To do so will mark the maturation of society toward progress and responsibility. There is no better barometer of the state of any society than the state of its law enforcement.

Recent changes in the helping system have created a particularly favorable climate for embracing the police as appropriate participants. Increasing population density, growing economic inequities, and even greater complexity and alienation have caused helping institutions to examine some of *their* myths. Selectivity in the delivery of services, organizational rigidity, educational limitations, and other givens of the "helping game" have become insupportable deficiencies. Agencies with long traditions of helping in particular ways have found their most hallowed methods under attack. The pressure for change has grown increasingly insistent. It is a never ceasing source of wonder that this kind of social unrest succeeds in bringing about the adaptive changes which, in the end, make for a better society.

The goals of the university, law enforcement, and the helping system can be said to intersect logically. Interrelating these three institutions in no way minimizes the primary law-enforcement function of the police. But there is ample evidence (Cumming, Cumming, and Edel, 1965; Epstein, 1962; McCann; McCloskey; Wilson, 1968) that in the United States between 80 and 90% of a policeman's daily activity in rural, suburban, and urban areas involved maintenance of order as distinct from law enforcement. As Wilson (1969) pointed out,

> The vast majority of police actions taken in response to citizen calls involve either providing a service (getting a cat out of a tree or taking a person to the hospital) or managing real or alleged conditions of disorder (quarreling families, public drunks, bothersome teenagers, noisy cars, tavern fights). Only a small fraction of these calls involve law enforcement such as checking on a prowler, catching a burglar in the act or preventing a street robbery.

Wilson's (1969) distinction between order maintenance and law enforcement is critical,

> The difference between order maintenance and law enforcement is not simply the difference between "little stuff" and "real crime." The distinction is fundamental to the police role, for the two functions involve quite dissimilar police actions and judgments. Order maintenance arises out of a dispute among citizens who accuse each other of being at fault; law enforcement arises out of the victimization of an innocent party by a person whose guilt must be proved ... Because an arrest cannot be made in most disorderly cases, the officer is expected to handle the situation by other means and on the spot, but the law gives him no guidance on how he is to do this; indeed, the law often denies him the right to do anything at all other than make an arrest ... Alone, unsupervised, with no policies to guide him and little sympathy from onlookers to support him, the officer must 'administer justice' at the curbstone.

ORDER-MAINTENANCE FUNCTION
OF THE POLICE

The helping system has virtually ignored the implications of "order maintenance." This is particularly striking in that the police of every community have been functioning as social and mental health agencies by virtue of their order-maintenance function. Instantly available 24 hours of each day (unlike other helpers, who operate between the hours of nine and five and not on weekends), they come when called (eliminating the frustrating delays of waiting lists and return visits) and *they do something* (unlike the typical verbal abstractions of the usual "planned intervention").

The "something" policemen "do," however, is the centrally crucial issue. The police establishment does not recognize order maintenance as "real" police work. Consistent with more pervasive social values, the police institution recognizes and rewards the quick draw on Main Street as the prototype of police excellence. It may be that acknowledgment of compassion and helping is regarded as threatening to the masculine mystique of law enforcement. Yet the basic occupational motivation for many police officers may be in opposition to this attitude. Many officers are primarily motivated by the desire to help others — a desirable attribute for beginners in any of the helping professions, it is not one usually attributed to policemen (Bard, 1969a):

> What happens to those policemen whose basic motivation is to help, to be the embodiment of the strong yet benign and giving father? Chances are they quickly get the message — they learn during the earliest months of service that the system does not reward "helpers," that those who "make it" do so by suppressing compassion and by adopting the masculine posture consistent with the establishment's expectations. Regrettably, this early learing is reinforced by a steady diet of real experiences with the most disordered and unpredictable elements in society. Confused and embittered, such policemen, if unable to work out compromise solutions (such as Youth Squad, Rescue Service, etc.), often become the most cynical transmitters of the traditional police mystique.

Institutional insensitivity to the order-maintenance function of police work has been costly. Recently, the FBI reported (1963) that 22 percent of policemen killed in the line of duty nationally were slain while intervening in disturbances such as family disputes. Estimates of time lost because of injuries sustained in the line of duty indicate that about 40 percent occur in the same way. Police myths notwithstanding, therefore, it would appear that the less glamorous and often helping functions of the police may be central in the institutions's operations more than has been suspected.

Indeed, this becomes even more striking when one compares society's investment in the helper most like the police officer — the physician. There are no other two professionals in the helping system whose identities and responsibilities approximate each other so closely. The physician is an authority with the power of life and death in situations that involve physical disorder. The policeman, on the other hand, is an authority with the power of life and death in situations of social disorder. And yet the average physician receives a minimum of 11,000 hours of training to prepare him for his role; the average policeman receives less than 200 hours of training to prepare him for his (Lipset, 1969).

SPECIALIZED POLICE TRAINING

There are undoubtedly many factors that contribute to the disparity in training. But in view of the escalation of social disorder, it is highly questionable that society can continue to ignore the extensive ramifications of the range of functions subsumed under the rubric of law enforcement. Perhaps the time has come for the kind of creative collaboration between law enforcement and the academic-professional communities which would maximize the potentials of the police as acknowledged members of the helping professions.

For a two-year period recently concluded, an experimental program operated that may serve as a model for demonstrating the potentials inherent in police helping-system collaboration. The program has shown that the mutual distrust of both institutions can be minimized while they cooperate to serve the community more effectively. What is more the collaboration permitted each agency to remain faithful to its own primary mission. For the police, enhancement of its law enforcement and order-maintenance mission; for the university the education of helping professionals (in this instance, clinical psychologists), research, and community service. Impetus for the program was derived from a number of sources: increasing crime rates, increasing violence and aggression, worsening police-community relations, and increasing social and professional pressure for innovation in preventive mental health.

The President's Commission on Law Enforcement and Administration of Justice commented on a phenomenon well known to every policeman (Wilson, 1969):

A great majority of the situations in which policemen intervene are not, or are not interpreted by the police to be, criminal situations in that they call for an arrest . . . A common kind of situation . . . is the matrimonial dispute, which police experts estimate consumes as much time as any other kind of situation.

The program to be described was designed to deal with this social reality. Crime statistics indicate that between 35 and 50 percent of all homicide victims in the United States are related to their killers and that in fewer than 20 percent of the cases are homicide victims and perpetrator complete strangers. It is apparent from these startling figures that family crisis intervention offers unlimited experimental and preventive prospects.

The psychological helping professions have become increasingly disenchanted with traditional methods of diagnosis and treatment. Not only are their methods found wanting in themselves, they seem to have lessening social impact as the demand for psychological services quickly outdistances man-power resources. Prevention appears to offer the greatest promise of relief. The project in police family crisis intervention embodies principles of at least three distinct tracks of mental health theory and research: 1) the training of the front-line mental health worker; 2) the role of the family in determining disordered behavior; and 3) preventive crisis intervention.

As Reiff and Riessman (1964) and Rioch (1963) have demonstrated, indigenous mental health aides can effectively extend the social impact of the highly trained professional. There appears little question that intelligent laymen can be trained to render effective mental health services under supervision. In such an approach the highly trained supervisor does little direct service but instead influences the functioning of those he supervises, thus extending the effects of his education and experience. It was proposed that a group of policemen be selected and trained to serve in the capacity of indigenous mental health personnel *in the course of their regular police duties.* This was based on the supported contention that policemen were already engaged in quasi-mental health roles and that specific training would simply enhance their effectiveness in doing what they were already doing.

A Model Research Program

A program was conceived that embodied crime prevention and preventive mental health principles, but, more important perhaps, it afforded a research framework within the psychological and social matrix of a living community — an opportunity to explore a variety of hypotheses regarding the natural history of aggression. Most important, perhaps, was the design of a model for the utilization of policemen as primary crisis intervention agents

(Bard and Berkowitz, 1967).

Briefly, 18 police officers were selected from among 45 volunteers. Because the community surrounding the campus (west Harlem) is largely black, the design called for the selection of nine white and nine black patrolmen who were to be paired interracially. No effort was made to induce participation except for the proffer of three college credits. Selection was based on evidence of motivation and aptitude for family crisis intervention and minimum of three years' experience as patrolman to insure sufficient skill in police work.

For the entire month following selection the men were released from all duties to engage in an intensive training program that included lectures, workshops, field trips, and a unique opportunity to "learn by doing." Three Family Crisis Laboratory Demonstrations involved the enactment of specially written plays by professional actors in which the patrolmen intervened in pairs. The value of the experience was to enable the men to see how different interventions could produce different outcomes. All the practice interventions were subjected to extensive critique and reviewed by all members of the unit. The intensive training also included human relations workshops which helped sensitize the men to their own values and attitudes about disrupted families.

The Family Crises Intervention Unit

After the month of intensive training, the Family Crisis Intervention Unit began its operational phase. For the subsequent two-year period, one radio car was designated for use by the unit and was dispatched on all complaints that could be predetermined as involving "family disturbance." A special duty chart permitted 24-hour-a-day coverage by men of the unit in a circumscribed experimental area of about 85,000 people.

The men continued their training by appearing on campus in groups of six for discussions with a professional group leader each week. In addition each man had an individual consultation with an advanced graduate student in clinical psychology who used the experience to enhance his own training as a mental health consultant.

In its 21 months of operation, the Family Crisis Unit engaged in 1375 interventions with 962 families. In addition the men of the unit performed all routine police duties on a par with the other men of their command. However, despite the high-hazard work involved in family crisis intervention, there was not a single injury sustained by any member of the unit. During the same period, three patrolmen not trained in family crisis intervention sustained injury while responding to family disturbances.

Although conclusions based on the method described will have to await final evaluation, preliminary findings can serve as a basis for speculation. For example, the remarkable absence of injury to a group of officers exposed in the extreme to dangerous and highly volatile aggressive situations strongly suggests the importance of the role played by the victim in the exacerbation of violence. Recently Sarbin (1967) characterized danger as connoting a *relationship,* pointing out that assaultive or violent behavior that leads to the designation *dangerous* "can be understood as the predictable outcome of certain antecedent and concurrent conditions . . . among these conditions are degradation procedures which transform a man's social identity."

Sarbin (1967) develops the notion that social identity is formed out of role relationships and that individuals who do not meet minimal social expectations may be classified as "brutes" or as "non persons," or, to put it another way, are deprived of their social identity. By the nature of his work a policeman is always ready to classify conduct as potentially dangerous. The officer's negative valuation of the other person in the power relationship may entail degrading behavior toward those he classifies as "non persons." Indeed, the officer may even be engaged in premature power display, thus further provoking the untrusted "non person" to behave as the expected "wild beast." In this connection the conclusion may be drawn that the dangerous person may, in large measure, be the outcome of the very institutions we have created to control him. It may be that the officers engaged in the project, because of their sensitivity training, avoided premature power displays and eschewed classifying people as "non persons" and hence avoided potentiating danger and violence directed at *them.*

Some Results of the Program

The project has many implications; space permits touching upon only a few. If there is a single most significant factor in its approach, it is that role-identity confusion in the officers was avoided. Throughout the project, every effort was made to avoid giving the men the notion that they were functioning in any way other than as police officers. Their professional identities were respected and preserved and, indeed, constantly reinforced. The members of the unit never lost sight of their primary objective: restoring and maintaining the peace. Their insight and training served to enhance their performance as policemen, yet this was in no way regarded as being inimical to the helping role.

This aspect of the experience was paramount, perhaps because it highlighted one of the greatest pitfalls in mental health community consultation. Frequently consultants succeed in confusing the role identity of their consultees. It is a central problem, for example, in educational consultation. Well-meaning consultation programs in the schools almost universally succeed in confusing the classroom teacher. Before very long, the teacher is not quite sure whether she is a teacher or whether she is a psychotherapist. It may be that pride and omniscience endow many consultants with a subtle form of proselytizing enthusiasm which only serves to confuse the consultee. Awareness of the problems of role-identity confusion must be regarded as a keystone in the mental health consultation process.

The validity of the concept of utilizing as mental health resources those individuals already in the psychological front lines needs no further emphasis here. What should be underscored, however, is the importance of identifying those in society who are in this front-line role. Mental health personnel typically move *in safe social subsystems.* The most popular is the educational subsystem; working through that institution is usually justified by the claim that the child is father to the man and as such represents the best of all preventive possibilities. Even though this may be true in part, it may not be the real reason for investing so much effort in the schools. A more subtle reason may be that the educational subsystem is more familiar, more comfortable, and hence *safer* for the mental health professional. The school establishment is well-traveled ground and requires little reorientation. Not so in other subsytems; the police establishment, for example, is a subsystem as remote from the world of mental health professionals as it is possible to be. And as such it is regarded as uncomfortable and, in a way, unsafe. There are many subsystems that offer unusual and creative opportunities for extending preventive mental health principles. They exist, however, outside of the safety of the schools and of the hospitals and the like; they exist in abundance elsewhere in the community. They represent the real challenge in preventive mental health, but it remains for us to search them out and use them effectively.

Aside from service potentials and fulfilling the objectives of prevention, such approaches open a wide range of research possibilities. The world of people as seen through the eyes of those unfamiliar subsystems can only enlarge and add dimension to our knowledge of human behavior. For example, as a result of the police family crisis intervention program, much will be learned about the social psychology of aggression — not in the context of the scientifically pure experimental laboratory, but in the pulsating, real-life laboratory that every community represents.

NEW STRUCTURING OF POLICE ORGANIZATIONS

The successful collaboration between a police department and a university has left both with capacities and insights they did not have before (Final Report, 1969). An exciting spin-off of the police family project is the promise it holds for a new structuring of police organizations. Typically, police departments follow the specialist model. Individual police officers are assigned to highly specialized tasks, for example, to traffic control, emergency services, community relations, youth detail, etc. The officer so assigned performs his specialized function to the exclusion of generalized law enforcement. But, unfortunately, that approach has had results with which specialists in other fields are only too familiar — psychiatrists, for example. The specialist officer is quickly regarded by his fellows as no longer a "real cop" and, following a fundamental biological principle, he is rejected as a foreign body. What is more, the public also views the behavior of the police specialist as not being typical of the police in general.

This project suggests the viability of the generalist-specialist model of police patrol (Bard, 1969c). It would entail utilizing the special talents and interests of each patrolman, while at the same time having each perform overall patrol duties. The unit operating as family crisis intervention specialists patroled like all other members of their command but were available within their precinct area whenever a family disturbance occurred. The same approach might be taken in relation to youth disorders, alcoholics, attempted suicides, or psychotics. It is too much to expect that every policeman should have specialized capacities in relation to the enormous range of human problems. It does make sense, however, to assume that a patrolman with special proclivities in managing a psychotic may not be so well suited to managing a group of unruly adolescents, or vice versa. What is more, the public is exposed to police whose behavior is consistent with special capacity and special training, thus vastly improving their impressions of the police. If the public attitude toward police is to improve, it will not be because of highly touted community relations gimmickry, but because policemen are handling their order-maintenance functions with skill, understanding, and compassion. If professionalism is to occur in law enforcement, it will be necessary to modify outmodes organizational structures that are no longer relevant in today's complex society.

The assumption of helping roles and responsibilities by law enforcement officers was completely unforeseen as recently as two decades ago. Even though it is not at all clear that these responsibilities should fall to the police, it is nevertheless a fact that they do. The helping system has failed to adapt to changing circumstances and in so doing has, by default, encouraged the assumption of helping roles by the police. This reality can be acknowledged, to the advantage of society, by organized efforts to bring the police into the helping system as coequal professionals.

REFERENCES

Bard, M. Family intervention police teams as a community mental health resource. *Journal of Criminal Law, Criminology and Police Science,* 1969(a), **60**, 247-250.

Bard, M. Extending psychology's impact through existing community institutions. *American Psychologist,* 1969(b), **24**, 610-612.

Bard, M. and Berkowitz, B. Training police as specialists in family crisis intervention: A community psychology action program. *Community Mental Health Journal,* 1967, **3**, 315-317.

Bard, M. Alternatives to traditional law enforcement. In E.F. Korten, S.W. Cook, and J.I. Lacy, (Eds.), *Psychology and the problems of society.* Washington, D.C.: American Psychological Association, 1970, 128-132.

Bard, M. *Training police as specialists in family crisis intervention.* Washington, D.C.: National Institute of Law Enforcement and Criminal Justice, U.S. Government Printing Office, 1970.

Cumming, E., Cumming I. and Edel L. Policeman as philosopher, guide and friend. *Social Problems,* 1965, **17**, 276-286.

Epstein, C. *Intergroup relations for police officers.* Baltimore, Md.: Williams and Wilkins, 1962.

FBI Law Enforcement Bulletin, January 1963, p. 27.

Lipset, S.M. Why cops hate liberals and vice versa. *Atlantic Monthly,* March 1969, 76-83.

McCann, R. Director, Chicago Police Department Training Division. Personal Communication.

McCloskey, C.C. Jr. Executive Director, Division of Police Administration Services, Office for Local Government, State of New York. Personal Communication.

Reiff, R. and Riessman, F. *The indigenous non-professional: A strategy of change in community action and community mental health programs.* New York: Behavioral Publications, Inc., 1965.

Rioch, M., Elkes C. and Flint, A.A. *Pilot project in training mental health counselors.* Washington, D.C.: U.S. Department of Health, Education and Welfare, Public Health Service Report No. 1254, 1965.

Sarbin, T. The dangerous individual: An outcome of social identity transformations. *British Journal of Criminology,* July 1967, 285-295.

Wilson, J.Q. *Varieties of police behavior.* Cambridge: Harvard University Press, 1968.

Wilson, J.Q. What makes a better policeman. *Atlantic Monthly,* March 1969, 129-135.

8
Training Police in Family Crisis Intervention *[1]

JAMES M. DRISCOLL, ROBERT G. MEYER and CHARLES F. SCHANIE

Why do police officers find themselves spending a significant proportion of their on-duty time dealing with families in conflict? On the surface, the reason is that no one else takes the responsibility for mediating family disputes. This *no one else* explanation is admittedly a superficial one as it stands, but becomes meaningful with reference to the fact that in less complex societies — or at least in some societies unlike current American society — family conflict is handled by the extended family or senior members of the kinship system. Parents, close relatives, kinship elders, or some other respected or legitimate insider mediates with authority, with the interest of the family and its immediate social extensions in mind.

In modern America, however, social mobility has placed most nuclear families in geographical settings distant from parents, relatives, or even neighbors who could be counted on to mediate a dispute fairly or to regulate

*Reprinted from *Journal of Applied Behavioral Science*, 1973, 9, 62-82, with permission of the NTL Institute for Applied Behavioral Science.

[1] This project was conducted under contract between the division of Police, City of Louisville and the University of Louisville. However, the opinions and conclusions stated in this article are those of the authors, and are not to be taken as those of the Louisville Division of Police. Projects such as this rely heavily on enthusiasm for effective social action on the part of many persons throughout the community. Those to whom a particular debt is owed are: the late David A. McCandless, former Dean of the University of Louisville's School of Police Administration; C.J. Hyde, former Chief of Police, George Burton, former Director of Safety, and Sgt. Bill Lamkin, Project Liaison Officer, all of the Louisville Division of Police; James P. Bloch and Stephen A. White. Training Assistants; J. Carleton Riddick, Simulation Supervisor; and Dr. Willard A. Mainord, who served as a group leader. Finally, special thanks are due Professor Morton Bard for his advice and guidance prior to the initiation of this project.

unacceptable behavior on the part of one or both marital partners. Consequently, when a nuclear family in such social isolation has exhausted its internal resources and methods for handling conflict, its members often have no place to turn but to public arbitration.

This isolation is aggravated by certain facts: the mental health system in most communities is not responsive to this type of problem, it is seldom avaiable 'round-the-clock on short notice, and many family conflicts involve violence. All this sets the problem squarely on the shoulders of the police.

The police are the only agents of society licensed to use counter-force against citizens prior to litigation (see Bittner, 1970). Since scores of family crises require the use of counter-force to prevent or offset violence, the problem of domestic trouble can legitimately be placed within their domain — at least in part. Ignoring the potential for violence in domestic disputes would be foolhardy: most homicides and assaults occur among family members or persons closely related to one another (Wolfgang, 1958; Federal Bureau of Investigation, 1970).

Additionally, since effective social control is dependent on the range of outcomes available to the controlling agent and his ability to use them, most will concede that the policeman is in an enviable position in this respect. It is also true that a police officer is a legally constituted authority of the entire community and, as such, possesses different stimulus properties than the mental health agent or the social worker. In his legitimately constituted role, a police officer may be perceived as a legitimate intervention agent more often than a mental health worker would be under the circumstances of most family crises. He is representative of the community as a whole, has that community's backing, and is powerful in terms of the action alternatives available to him. Disputants are therefore compelled to accept an officer's presence in the crisis as a sanctioned agent of society.

Most important, perhaps, is the fact that the police officer usually arrives at the point of crisis in family conflicts. Caplan and Grunebaum (1967) have noted that the turmoil in which crisis-plagued individuals find themselves often makes them particularly pliable. Characteristically, such persons realize that they have exhausted their repertoire of coping behavior and are no longer capable of handling the situation. They are therefore more susceptible to influence that might lead them to more adaptive behavior.

THE EFFECTIVENESS OF TRAINING

Unfortunately, the reasonable expectation that police responsibility for dealing with domestic trouble be met with some degree of competency is usually not satisfied. Few police officers have the behavioral science training necessary for an effective family crisis intervention. Bard (1970) has suggested recently, however, that such competency can be gained in a relatively short time within the context of an intensive and specialized training program; this possibility is certainly worth serious attention.

On the other hand, caution must be exercised, since several considerations suggest that training in family crisis intervention might not be accepted by police officers − and, if accepted, might not prove effective. Several major forces might militate against the development of a potential for effective handling of domestic trouble. For instance, most police systems currently reject family trouble as a legitimate aspect of policing, place low priority upon it, and fail to reward activities so directed. As a consequence, the begrudging police response to a family in conflict is usually either legalistic ("take a warrant, lady") or coercive ("if we have to come back again, we'll lock you all up"). Moreover, the educational level of most police forces is not particularly high, and there is a traditional distaste for service functions, along with an almost single-minded orientation toward crime control.

Evaluating the New York Project

Thus, prudence would dictate that evidence on the effectiveness of police training in crisis intervention be amassed before investing substantial money or manpower in such training. The initial project in family crisis training for police was designed and conducted in New York City by Dr. Morton Bard (1970). Unfortunately, it provides, at best, equivocal support for the efficacy of such training. However, serious problems in the study, stemming from Bard's evaluation strategy, appear primarily responsible for the failure to obtain convincing evidence in favor of the training program. Since the goal of our project was a different evaluation strategy, we present here a brief review of the New York project.

The New York project focused on six evaluative criteria, with expectations for each as to the direction of change. It was hypothesized that, in comparison with a control precinct, in a demonstration precinct of trained patrolmen: 1) the number of family disturbance complaints would decrease; 2) the number of repeat interventions for trained officers would decrease (as a function of problem resolution); 3) homicides would be reduced; 4) homicides among family members would decrease; 5) assaults would decrease; and 6) injuries to policemen would be reduced.

Disturbingly, results on four of these six criteria in the evaluation of the New York project were *opposite* to expectation. There were three times more disturbance complaints in the demonstration precinct than in the control precinct; more repeat cases; an increase of three and one-half per cent in the number of homicides in the control precinct; and an increase in family homicides in the demonstration precinct as compared with no change in the control. Fortunately, fewer assaults were found in the demonstration precinct than the control precinct; and no trained officer was injured, while two members of the regular force in the demonstration precinct and one officer in the control precinct sustained injuries in family disputes.

All in all, the results of the New York project permit little confidence to be placed in the type of training devised by Bard to help police officers deal effectively with family disturbances. Had the number of family disturbance calls been fewer, and had homicides decreased in the demonstration precinct, the logic of the experimental design would have permitted the conclusion that the project was responsible for these positive effects. But since family disturbance calls increased and homicides were greater in the demonstration precinct than in the control, the conclusion that the project was responsible for these negative effects is equally valid.

The only recourse from this conclusion is the existence of confounding variables extraneous to the experimental design. Bard (1970) argues that differences in reporting between the Family Crisis Intervention Unit (FCIU) officers and untrained control officers account for the differences found in the number of disturbance complaints and the number of repeat interventions. This is perhaps an acceptable explanation (knowing the aversion of most police officers to completing written reports). As an explanation of the greater number of domestic trouble calls in the demonstration precinct, Bard (1970) also suggests that ". . . the availability of a more effective police service in this connection may have resulted in greater and more effective community utilization of the FCIU."

It is somewhat more difficult to explain the increases in both general and family homicides found in the New York project, and Bard's (1970) conclusion that ". . . the operation of the FCIU failed to effect any change in overall homicide incidence in the demonstration area" is patently erroneous, given the logic of the design of the evaluation, within which an increase in homicides must be considered a probable effect of the experimental treatment. Furthermore, in the case of homicide statistics, differential reporting cannot be suggested as a plausible external confounding factor, since homicide statistics were collected independently of the project, in the usual manner of the New York City Police Department. Thus, either the effects must be accepted as due to the project or a reasonable argument must be made that it is extremely unlikely that such effects could emerge from the project and that other extraneous factors were responsible for them.

Using crime statistics in evaluation. One possible extraneous consideration is that the New York project was run during the summer of 1967 − a time of notable black unrest. The increase in homicides *may* have been a reflection of heightened tensions in the black community. The difference between the demonstration and the control precinct, then, might be more a function of the unfortunate fact that the demonstration precinct was almost totally black and the control precinct largely Puerto Rican. There is no evidence to support this argument, however, and it rests on a chain of possible intervening variables too long to warrant its casual acceptance.

This set of design problems, however, did prevent the sort of direct and unconfounded evaluation deserved by a training program as creative and promising as that devised by Bard. While the reduction of crime incidence is obviously a worthy goal, the problems inherent in the use of crime statistics as indices of success of a police training project invite near-certain failure. Two major problems encountered by Bard seem to have been differential reporting and the operation of variables extraneous to the project that may have been much more powerful than the effects of the project itself. Relatedly, there is usually considerable cross-district variation in crime statistics, which make them unreliable for assessment of all but very large projects.

An Alternative Evaluation Approach: Louisville

The Louisville project was accordingly conducted to evaluate the Bard model of crisis intervention training for police by using an evaluation strategy that focused directly on the efficacy of the intervention. In this manner, the problems associated with crime statistics can be avoided and evaluation can be made directly at the point of program impact, the most probable locus of unconfounded effects — the crisis situation itself.

Using psychosocial criteria. If training is effective in helping officers conduct efficient and effective family crisis interventions, several consequences pertaining to the intervention itself should ensue. In general, citizens could be expected to respond to police intervention more favorably along several psychosocial dimensions. In particular, it was predicted that citizens dealt with by trained officers would report higher levels of rapport between themselves and the officers, a greater involvement on the part of the officer, a greater level of success in working with the problem, more satisfaction with the way the situation was handled, an increased regard for police, and a greater acceptance of police in similar circumstances.

Trained officers could be expected to report changes along several dimensions related to their experience in interventions: an increased understanding of the problems with which they are dealing; an increase in the acceptance of them by citizens; a greater receptivity to their suggestions; a decrease in the necessity for force; an increase in their effectiveness in dealing with domestic trouble; and an overall favorability toward the new techniques and the training program.

Each of these conceptual dimensions was operationalized by a question put to either citizens or participating officers. Results for questions put to citizens were analyzed for statistically significant differences between responses of citizens dealt with by trained and untrained officers. Results for questions put to officers were dealt with descriptively as self-reported differences between experiences before and after training.

THE LOUISVILLE TRAINING MODEL

The Bard training model was followed as closely as possible, given local conditions, such as the makeup of the training staff and orientation of available expert contributors.

Theory

One major difference produced by these local conditions was in the theoretical underpinnings of the project. Although the training schedules of the New York and Louisville projects (see Bard, 1970; Driscoll, Meyer, and Schanie, 1971) appear very similar, the explanatory concepts behind topics presented and the procedures employed were quite different. The New York project contained elements suggestive of sensitivity training, and relied to some extent on psychodynamic concepts for its theoretical base. An explicit effort to change the police officers as persons, both dispositionally and affectively, was made, and a good deal of attention was paid to self-examination and awareness. Intervention procedures were based to a considerable extent on assumptions about personal and interpersonal dynamics underlying the crisis situation.

In contrast, the theoretical basis of the Louisville project was that of contemporary experimental social psychology, combined with a behavior modification approach to intervention. Within social psychology, basic social learning and imitation principles were used for the understanding of behavior and of its etiology, while exchange theory (Thibaut and Kelley, 1959) provided the context for analyzing interpersonal relations. Behavior modification principles (Wolpe, Salter, and Reyna, 1964) were used largely as the basis for intervention techniques and actions directed at a solution to problems encountered.

One immediately obvious benefit of the theoretical orientation of the

Louisville project was that the release from demands on the police officers to achieve personal change yielded an immediate gain in rapport. When the officers saw that they were not to be tested, probed, or submitted to criticism for personal attitudes, beliefs, or values, they soon accepted the staff and approached training with some measure of trust and enthusiasm. Philosophically, the orientation was one in which educators and police officers were mutually involved in changing policing techniques; officers brought their expertise in police matters, and training staff offered their expertise as educators and behavior scientists.

Throughout the course of training, the emphasis on intervention skills and techniques emerged as the dominant concern. The training philosophy became, in the main: provide the techniques, provide an opportunity for their practice under conditions of diminishing supervision, and count on their application in the field.

Selection

Police officers were recruited by superiors within the Louisville Division of Police, who provided an initial group of 13 volunteers. Each of these men was interviewed, and 12 were judged acceptable for the project.

The extent to which the police officers in the Louisville project were selected is an important issue, since it forms a potential point of comparison with the New York project, which used highly selected men. Accordingly, some basic data on crisis unit officers were compared with data from a nominal group formed by a random selection of 12 patrolmen from the Louisville force. Men of the crisis unit were on the average 33 years of age, some 4.4 years younger than the average of the nominal group, and had 5.6 years less experience on the force.[2] However, if crisis unit officers and officers of the nominal group are ordered by age, 8 of the 12 men of the crisis unit can be paired with a nominal group counterpart within three years of age, either younger or older. Nearly the same holds true for date-joined-the-force; half of the men from the crisis unit and nominal group can be paired in experience within one year. In contrast, Bard (1970) decided to limit the New York project to volunteers ". . . with at least three years, but no more than 10 years, of service." Eighteen men were selected from 42 volunteers in the New York project. At the very least, a comparison of selection procedures

---

[2] Comparison of selected with unselected officers on attitudinal and value dimensions was precluded by the decision not to test officers. This decision was made within the context of the philosophy of thy project, which stressed that officers were not to be treated as subjects but as equals engaged in the joint enterprise (with the academic staff) of developing techniques and skills in family crisis intervention.

suggests that officers in the Louisville project were less subject to volunteer bias and somewhat more representative of policemen in general. However, some selection obviously operated on the Louisville sample, and whatever conclusions are made possible by our results hold strictly and only for policemen selected in a comparable manner.

In the formation of teams, the staff policy to involve police officers in decisions about the program led to the officers' rejection of the staff's proposed sociometric techniques in favor of choosing partner assignments for themselves. This wish was stated strongly and with unanimity, and was accepted by the training staff. Officers were thus left free to work out their own partnerships and to report them to the staff at the end of the day. No complaints were made to the staff and no partners separated before the end of the evaluation.

Training

Intensive training consisted of five to seven hours of activities each weekday for a five-week period.

Presentations, readings, and films. Presentations with discussions were intended to provide officers with information basic to the understanding of problems in family crisis and with the background needed for application of the techniques to be taught. Officers received presentations on the role of the police in family disputes, new concepts of police work, causes of behavior, effects of early experience, changing behavior, children in families, family structure and interactions, and alcohol and drug abuse (see Bard, 1970; Driscoll, Meyer, and Schanie, 1971).

Contributors were told of the intent of the program and left free to direct their comments in any way they, as experts, felt was most appropriate.

Review, extension, and integration of the above material took place in discussions after each presentation, in training groups, in morning feedback sessions, and in informal contact between officers and staff. Readings and films were used to supplement and extend the presentations, while simultaneously providing the implicit support gained through the use of multiple media.

Field trips. Two agency field trips were arranged to take place at opportune times in the intensive training program, with an eye toward impressing upon the officers the importance of community agencies. At this time, a condensed listing of referral agencies and a supply of referral slips were given officers; these were to be carried with them at all times when on duty.

Simulations. In changing long-standing practices, such as those used over the years by police officers in handling family trouble, lecture techniques can be anticipated to have only limited impact. Most psychologists would agree that to consolidate such learning the person must actually execute the new behavior and find it successful. For this general reason, and because of Bard's strong recommendation, simulated family crisis interventions were included as a major aspect of the training programs. In contrast to the format of the New York project, which provided partially written scripts, a decision to work with groups of actors for new, more creative simulations was made.

A week or so before each simulation, the project staff worked with actors to decide upon the main story line in terms of the requirements of good stage production and systematic psychology. These sessions resulted most often in a significant extension of the initial plan, given input from the actors and ideas generated by them while they played out the basic scene. (A basic scene was played out prior to each "intervention" as a sort of warm-up.) This scene changed a little each time it was played, since a script was never used, but its main themes remained essentially the same. However, once the team of officers arrived, scenes took unpredictable turns, since actors were instructed again and again to respond to the officers from the viewpoint of the role being played.

More simulations were included in the Louisville project than were used previously. In the New York project, each team of officers was involved in one simulated intervention and observed other teams six times. Three different plays were seen: the one in which each officer intervened and two in which other officers intervened. In the Louisville project, each officer intervened in three simulations and observed, on the average, 17 others, involving three different plays. Each team of officers handled each simulation, then went behind a one-way mirror to observe their colleagues handling the same situation. Officers were scheduled so that they did not observe before they "intervened."

The last two simulations represented an innovation; officers in the project helped devise simulations for their colleagues. In retrospect this seems to be an excellent practice and is strongly recommended.

Feedback sessions: Conference with actors and video replay. Following the format of the New York project, feedback sessions were provided. On the day after the simulation, selected actors were asked to meet with policemen and to comment on their reactions to the officers. Another innovation was a videotape replay of each intervention. Replay was controlled by the trainer, who replayed segments so that officers, actors, and psychologist-trainers could comment on whatever occurred that could be used for learning purposes.

Simulations, supplemented by actor conferences and videotape feedback (in particular), proved, we believe, to be the most effective and stimulating aspect of the entire intensive training program.

Field interventions and reports. In addition to videotape feedback, the Louisville project was also able to add field interventions to the basic design of the New York project. These were possible because the Louisville Division of Police has the enlightened policy that qualified persons interested in seeing police work can, with proper arrangements, ride in patrol cars with beat officers. Under this provision, field interventions were made by each team of police officers in the company of a staff member. On these interventions, teams were permitted to roam freely and to answer family dispute calls. Each team answered at least one call and several answered two in the one evening. On the following day, the staff member worked with the officers, who later reported on their field interventions to the entire unit.

Reports on field interventions proved valuable in two ways: they provided an opportunity for officers to convince one another that they could make effective crisis interventions in the field under actual conditions, and provided a format for the training groups in the operational phase of the project.

Training groups. Training groups were the main source of flexibility, informal discussion, and opportunity to deal with feelings, uncertainties, and other personal matters in the program. Two permanent training groups operated throughout the course of the intensive training program, each with the same six officers, graduate assistant, and group leader. As might be expected, each group performed somewhat different functions for the persons in them. Following training, groups were kept intact with the same graduate assistant and membership. Groups met once every two weeks for the first two months of the operational phase of the project and once a month thereafter. The purposes of the groups during the operational phase of the project was multifold, but the major amount of time was spent in what might best be called case conferences.

Field Operation and Evaluation Procedure

As indicated earlier, assessment of the effectiveness of crisis intervention training for police in terms of crime statistics seem the obvious evaluation technique. However, crime statistics have many shortcomings which make them inappropriate for evaluation of a project such as this. The two most serious are their sizable natural variation within samples no larger than police districts and their susceptibility to extraneous influence. For this reason as well as others, evaluation efforts were directed to the effectiveness of the crisis interventions themselves.

The option of evaluating at the point of the crisis intervention, though perhaps not as immediately compelling as a focus on crime statistics, is not an intrinsically undesirable one: most persons, we believe, would agree that direct demonstration of effective crisis intervention by police would be a most significant step. To this end, a structured Client Telephone Questionnaire was designed to assess the reaction of citizens to several dimensions of an effective crisis intervention and to compare the effectiveness of trained with untrained officers. In addition to the Client Telephone Questionnaire, an effort was made to gauge the reactions of the participating officers to the novel intervention procedures with an Officer Participant Questionnaire.

Late in July of 1970, following the completion of the five weeks of intervention training, formal operation of the six 2-man crisis teams was initiated. Trained officers were given regular assignments, consistent with the understanding that training in family crisis intervention was intended not to produce police specialists but to make the general patrolman more adept at a task he was already performing as a general patrolman. Two of the six teams were assigned to each of the three 8-hour shifts, so that at any given time of the day there were two crisis intervention teams on duty in the eight-beat district. This arrangement was maintained from late July through December of 1970 to allow for the data collection. During this period, radio dispatchers assigned domestic trouble calls in any part of the district to trained intervention teams whenever possible.

When this was not possible (as when crisis officers were busy with regular beat duties), the call was assigned to another patrol in the district manned by two untrained officers. This provided an asystematic assignment of domestic cases to trained and untrained officers for subsequent evaluation follow-up in the form of the Client Telephone Questionnaire.

Over the data collection period, 421 domestic trouble runs were made in the third district by all officers, and of these runs, 129, or 31 percent, were made by trained officers (who constituted 25 percent of the officer teams on duty).[3]

The Client Telephone Questionnaire. Six evaluative questions were included on the Client Telephone Questionnaire, each designed to assess a particular dimension relevant to the effectiveness of the intervention. These dimensions were:

---

[3] Comparison of arrest rates and other crime statistics for trained and untrained officers was not made because of the problems associated with such indices discussed in the introduction to this paper.

Rapport
Question 1: How friendly would you say the officers were? Would you say that:
A.   They were friendly like a stranger in the street.
B.   They were friendly like a neighbor.
C.   They were friendly like a big brother or sister.

Involvement
Question 2: How hard do you think the officers tried to help you with the problem that brought them? Would you say that:
A.   They tried very hard to help.
B.   They tried a little to help, but not much.
C.   They didn't try to help at all.

Perceived Success
Question 3: How helpful did you feel the policemen were in settling your problem? Would you say that:
A.   They were very helpful.
B.   They were a little helpful, but not much.
C.   They were not helpful at all.

Satisfaction
Question 4: How happy were you with the way the policemen handled the situation? Would you say that:
A.   You were happy with the way they handled the situation.
B.   You think they handled it okay.
C.   You were unhappy with the way they handled it.

Regard
Question 5: Did the way these police officers acted in your home change your opinion of police?
YES   NO
If yes, do you think:
More of the police?   Less of the police?

Acceptance
Question 6: Now that the police have visited your home, would you be more likely, less likely, or about as likely as before to call them back if you needed them?
A.   More likely to call them.
B.   Less likely to call them.
C.   About as likely as before.

Three questions not related directly to the impact of the intervention but of use in other ways were posed: one as to whether a referral was made, a second on whether the agency was visited, and a third asking if the police had made a previous visit for a similar problem.

A procedure of interviewing the first adult of the household arriving at the phone was deliberately adopted over a theoretically more desirable equal-sex sampling procedure. This was done out of concern for its potential for exacerbating conflict in the home (by perhaps implying to the spouse who happened to answer the phone that the other's opinion was preferred). Three householders seen by the untrained group and one seen by the trained group admitted at this point in the interview that the police had been to their home but refused to talk to the interviewer. After elimination of these cases, the number of completed interviews with householders seen by the untrained and trained groups was 26 and 29, respectively.

One question which might be reasonably posed is the extent to which the asystematic (but not random) sampling procedure and the necessity of telephone contact produced like samples for the two groups. One available indicator of similarity was average family income. Average family incomes for the census tracts into which the households fell were determined from the 1960 United States Census. The median, mode, and mean of these incomes were then computed for each group. Median and mode for both samples were exactly equal at a value of $7,052. The mean for the households seen by the untrained group was $6,689; for those seen by the trained group, $6,625, or $64.00 less. On this basis the groups appear comparable.

The Officer Participant Questionnaire. The 12 participating officers were mailed the Officer Participant Questionnaire four months after formal operation of the crisis intervention units began, with instructions to return it anonymously. Five items on this questionnaire concerned the officer's perception of the amount of change on several dimensions indicative of his handling of domestic trouble calls after, as compared with before, training. The issue of participant overall favorability toward the program was examined by a sixth question. All questions were stated in a form allowing for both positive or negative change. Most questions were followed by a seven-point scale with a center position labeled *no change,* the extreme left position labeled *a great deal . . .* or *much more . . .* , and the extreme right position labeled *much less* or *a great deal less. . .*

The six dimensions assessed and their respective questions were:

Understanding
Question 1: How much better or worse do you feel you understand the nature of family crisis as a result of your training?

Acceptance
Question 2: How much more or less welcome is your presence in the homes of disputants as a result of your training?

Receptivity
Question 3: How much more or less receptive do the disputants seem to be to what you have to say in family crisis interventions as a result of your training?

Force Reduction
Question 4: How much more or less force have you found necessary to employ in handling family crises as a result of your training?

Effectiveness
Question 5: How much more or less effective are you in handling family crises as a result of your training?

Overall Favorability
Question 6: What type of recommendation would you give a fellow officer if he asked for your opinion concerning whether or not he should participate in a crisis intervention training of this sort?

Results and Discussion

Either the Client Telephone Questionnaire or the Officer Participant Questionnaire alone would have provided rather tenuous support for crisis intervention training of police officers. However, the two questionnaires complement one another and offer cross-validation of their findings. Their results will be discussed together.

The results from both evaluation instruments provide reasonable support for the proposition that trained policemen managed to resolve the immediate conflict in the crisis situation more adequately than did untrained policemen (see Table 1). The Officer Participant Questionnaire showed strong changes in the direction of improved understanding of interpersonal conflict (q. 1), plus enhanced acceptance of officers by clients (q. 2), greater receptivity to suggestions (q.3), less need of force (q. 4), and increased overall effectiveness (q. 5). The Client Telephone Questionnaire showed statistically significant effects in trained officers' rapport with clients (q. 1), perceived involvement in the problem with accompanying efforts to help (q. 2), overall satisfaction with the intervention (q. 4), and increased regard for the police (q. 5).

Table 1 Frequencies of Choice of Response Categories on the Client
Telephone Questionnaire and Officer Participant Questionnaire

Client Telephone Questionnaire

Question	Trained (N = 29)			Untrained (N = 26)			Sig.*
	Neg.	Neut.	Pos.	Neg.	Neut.	Pos.	
1. Rapport	1	17	11	8	17	1	$p < .01$
2. Involvement	1	5	23	3	11	12	$p < .05$
3. Perceived Success	5	6	18	3	10	13	n.s.
4. Satisfaction	1	5	23	3	14	9	$p < .01$
5. Regard		19	10		25	1	$p < .02$
6. Acceptance	3	11	15		14	12	n.s.

Officer Participant Questionnaire (N = 12)

Question and Scale Positions	Negative or Negative Change			Neutral or No Change			Positive or Positive Change
	1	2	3	4	5	6	7
1 Understanding					1		11
2. Acceptance				1	2	5	4
3. Receptivity				1	1	6	4
4. Force Reduction				2	1	5	4
5. Effectiveness					1	2	9
6. Overall Favorability					1		11

*By chi-square analysis. Low-frequency categories collapsed where necessary and possible.

Any one specific effect listed here might easily be questioned, but the consensus that is apparent between officers and clients on the different dimensions involved in dealing with family crisis argues persuasively that trained officers injected themselves into the crisis situation more satisfactorily and managed a de-escalation of the conflict more effectively than did untrained officers.

The above findings recommend crisis intervention training generally, with results in the change in use of force (q. 4, officers) and opinion of police (q. 5, clients) perhaps of particular interest to police administrators. Police administrators might, however, be even more inclined to consider the results for question 6 of the Officer Participant Questionnaire, which showed that most trained officers, four months into the operational phase of the project, reported that they would strongly recommend the training to a colleague.

Two questions from the Client Telephone Questionnaire failed to show statistically significant differences and thus leave two issues largely undetermined: question 3, "How helpful do you feel the policemen were in settling your problem?" and question 6, which asked about the likelihood of calling the police again. Apparently, question 3 suffers from an unfortunate choice of words; the intention of the question was to ask about the resolution of the immediate crisis, but the term, "your problem," appears to direct attention to long-standing difficulties. In this light, it is not too surprising to find that trained officers failed to out-perform their colleagues, since the problems with which they were dealing were, for the most part, notably intransigent (half the cases with which officers dealt were repeaters); i.e., the police had previously been to the home for similar reasons. If it is accepted that question 3 inappropriately directed attention to the solution of more severe problems than the policemen could be expected to deal with in the 20 or 30 minutes usual for an intervention, then the satisfaction question, which showed results favorable to trained officers, stands alone as the best indicator of success in resolving the immediate crisis.

COMPARISON OF FINDINGS: LOUISVILLE AND NEW YORK

The issue of long-term problem resolution and aid is not completely unanswered, however, since officers were able to make referrals to agencies which provide help with such problems. Of the 21 referrals made by trained officers in the Louisville project, three persons (14 per cent) reported that they went to an agency. Unfortunately, frequencies are too low here to rely heavily on this estimate of referral rate; this is one shortcoming of the current evaluation in its focus on crisis interventions rather than on outcomes. However, the New York project was outcome-directed; and on several issues, such as referral rates, the New York and Louisville projects particularly complement one another. Of the 719 families referred to a social agency in New York, it could be verified that 69 (9.6 percent) took advantage of the referral and contacted the agency. Though the referral rate for both projects is quite low (it appears to lie somewhere within 10 to 14 percent), it is obvious that some persons received help who would otherwise have remained unaided.[4]

A second area of complementarity of findings between the New York and Louisville projects is the issue of call-backs and increased utilization of

---

[4] Referral rates for untrained policemen are unavailable. Such rates were not obtained because of the relative certainty that they are at or near zero, except for referrals to family court.

police in domestic disturbances. Here, the New York finding that FCIU officers made more repeat calls combines with the positive findings from the Louisville project (such as greater regard for and satisfaction with the police) to make it at least likely that the program enhances the police function in a community by affecting variables one would expect to be positively associated with the voluntary use of police in family quarrels. Thus, the failure to obtain significant differences on the call-back question (q. 6 of the Client Telephone Questionnaire) in the Louisville project appears to be out of line with both actual call-back data obtained by Bard and with the implication of reports by citizens of increased satisfaction with the police obtained in this present evaluation. Many reasons (such as the unwillingness of people to admit the possibility of calling police again for a similar problem) might be advanced for the failure of question 6 to show the expected results, but none can be substantiated from available data. Thus, the actual call-back results of the New York study should be taken as the best indicator of willingness to recall trained police, with the possible realization that people might not be willing to state such a possibility before the fact.

A third area of comparison between the New York and Louisville projects concerns the issue of force and violence. In the New York project, no FCIU officer was injured, while three untrained patrolmen in the area were injured on domestic trouble calls. These frequencies are too small for statistical tests, so additional support is desirable. Such support seems to be provided by the officers' reports in the Louisville project that they required less force in handling domestic conflicts after training than before. Thus a benefit of crisis intervention training appears to be that it provides officers alternatives to force, which in turn reduce their own liability to injury.

The final comparative point is that results of the Louisville project make it somewhat less likely that the increases in homicides found in the New York project were due to the application of crisis intervention techniques in domestic trouble situations. If trained policemen were inadvertently exacerbating domestic conflict, negative consequences might be understood. If, on the other hand, trained policemen are responded to positively by citizens, as shown in the evaluation of the Louisville project, it is unlikely that they are contributing to conflict, or to increases in violence.

Thus, results from the Louisville project's evaluation showing effects such as increased friendliness, satisfaction, and appreciation of the officers favor the argument that whatever the cause of the increased incidence of assaults and homicides in the New York project, it is unlikely that FCIU officers contributed to conflict and violence through their crisis interventions. Interventions which produce high levels of positive psychosocial reaction are unlikely to leave a residual for violence.

ADAPTATIONS FOR FUTURE TRAINING

These comparisons assume that the differences between the two programs are not so substantial as to preclude meaningful comparison. Such differences can also serve as a source of information relative to future applications, and to answering the general question about any program: is it transferable—can others apply the same procedures and expect comparable outcomes?

The success of the Louisville project, modeled after the New York project, argues that crisis intervention training for police can be generally applied. Indeed, the program appears to be robust, since it can tolerate a number of significant deviations from the initial plan. Some deviations made successfully in the Louisville project are instructive:

1.   Police personnel in the New York project were highly selected, whereas in the Louisville project little selection beyond the recruitment by superiors was possible. Given the success of the Louisville project, it follows that highly selected police officers are not a prerequisite, and the program can be applied to larger groups without major revision based on the qualities of the police personnel.

2.   The theoretical point of view of the New York project was generally anlytic, compared to the more behaviorally oriented Louisville staff. At the least, such differences in theoretical orientation do not seem crucial to the success of the project.

3.   The Louisville project placed considerably more emphasis on simulations, on videotaping, and on field intervention practice. There is no way to know from the data available whether this difference, combined with the theoretical difference, accounted for success.

4.   The target population in the New York project was almost exclusively black, while in the Louisville project the target population was over 90 per cent white. These differences seemed unimportant in the training, save for requiring a few special presentations on special aspects of the target population. Whether they influenced project success is not known.

Many other differences can probably be tolerated in any new application of crisis intervention training for police. However, some problems encountered in the present project point to a few areas where laxness may seriously restrict the effectiveness of the program. One of these areas is the support of immediate superiors. Support for the Louisville program came from the top command of the Police Department, and the officers in the program soon became advocates of crisis training. However, command personnel at the level of sergeant, lieutenant, and captain proved indifferent, at best, and hostile, at worst. The New York FCIU officers were subject to ridicule at times from untrained officers, which was felt as particularly harsh in the absence of active support from immediate superiors. However, the most serious obstacle was pressure from sergeants against investing time and effort in domestic cases. Bard (1970) avoided many of these problems by a program of conferences with all personnel indirectly involved with the project. This procedure is strongly to be recommended. However, we even more strongly recommend a procedure in which an autonomous subsystem is selected, and everyone within that subsystem (say, a precinct) receives the training program. This, in effect, isolates the trained personnel from counter-influences from the larger organization.

Another shortcoming shared by the New York and Louisville projects was inadequacy of the service agency liaison. In both projects, for instance, agencies proved indifferent to the extent that agency referrals could not be traced. This is a particularly insidious problem. Surface cooperation is often easily obtained from colleagues working in agencies, but the day-to-day demands upon staff in these agencies seem so pressing that they invariably neglect their participation in the project. Closer liaison with social agencies is one answer, but an established Crisis Center with an adequate referral and follow-up service is strongly recommended.

Given the precautions stated above, there appears to be reasonable assurance that the Bard model of crisis intervention training, with some adaptation, can produce more satisfactory and effective family crisis interventions by police officers.

REFERENCES

Bard, M. Training police as specialists in family crisis intervention. Washington, D.C.: U.S. Government Printing Office, 1970.

Bittner, E. The functions of the police in modern society. Public Health Service Pub. No. 2059. Washington, D.C.: U.S. Government Printing Office, 1970.

Caplan, G., and Grunebaum, H. Perspectives on primary prevention: A review. *Archives of General Psychiatry*, 1967, **17**, 331-346.

Driscoll, J.M., Meyer, R.G. and Schanie, C.F. Police training in family crisis intervention. Louisville, Ky.: University of Louisville, 1971.

Federal Bureau of Investigation. *Uniform Crime Reports—1969.* Washington, D.C.: GPO, 1970.

Thibaut, J. and Kelley, H. *The social psychology of groups.* New York: Wiley, 1959.

Wolfgang, M. *Patterns of criminal homicide.* Philadelphia: University of Pennsylvania Press, 1958.

Wolpe, J., Salter, A. and Reyna, L. *The conditioning therapies.* New York: Holt, Rinehart & Winston, 1964.

9
Diversion from the Juvenile Justice System and the Prevention of Delinquency *[1]

ARNOLD BINDER, JOHN MONAHAN and MARTHA NEWKIRK

About four million youths in the United States come into contact with law enforcement agencies every year. Half of these contacts result in arrests, and half of those arrested are referred to the juvenile court (Gemignani, 1973). Of the approximately one million juveniles referred to the court, about 50 percent are handled informally by court staff, about 40 percent are formally adjudicated and placed on supervised release, and the remaining 10 percent or about 100,000 juveniles, are placed in a custodial institution (Gemignani, 1971). Extending such figures over lives, it has been estimated that between 20 percent (Blumstein, 1967) and 35 percent (Wolfgang, Figlio and Sellin, 1972) of the male population can expect to have a police record before the age of 18.

The sheer magnitude of juvenile problems in this country, documented by the above data, belies the notion that the juvenile court can serve as an effective agent of delinquency prevention, as its designers had originally envisioned. Moreover, the juvenile court has not been conspicuously successful in changing the behavior of those juveniles it has processed (Ferster and Courtless, 1972) and there is substantial reason to believe that the labeling and stigmatization associated with the formal juvenile justice process may actually exacerbate delinquent behavior (Lemert, 1971; Cressey and McDermott, 1973).

These and other criticisms of the juvenile court has coalesced into two questions of public policy:

*This chapter was written especially for this book.

[1] The preparation of these materials was financially aided through a Federal grant from the Law Enforcement Assistance Administration and the California Office of Criminal Justice Planning under the Omnibus Crime Control and Safe Streets Act of 1968, as amended. The opinions, findings, and conclusions in this publication are those of the authors and are not necessarily those of the Law Enforcement Assistance Administration or the California Office of Criminal Justice Planning.

OCJP reserves a royalty-free, non-exclusive and irrevocable license to reproduce, publish and use these materials, and to authorize others to do so.

1. whether some of the actions of children and parents now subject to definition as delinquency or unfitness should not be conceived as nonproblematical and either ignored or written off simply as part of the inevitable, every day problems of living and growing up;

2. whether many of the problems now considered as delinquent or preludes to delinquency should not be defined as family, educational or welfare problems, and diverted away from the juvenile court into other community agencies (Lemert, 1971, p. 15).

This paper deals with the latter policy issue — diversion from the juvenile justice system. The fact that diversion *from* the juvenile court is becoming an increasingly recognized need contrasts with the original intent of the juvenile justice system — that youths be diverted *to* the juvenile court from the adult criminal court (Nejelski, 1973). Rather than a strange anomaly, perhaps that shift represents a cyclic pattern characteristic of many social phenomena. For example, it was deemed desirable during the nineteenth century to remove the mentally ill from communities, and so, many state asylums were built to house them. But the community mental health movement of recent years has led to the closing of the state hospitals and the return of the mentally disordered to the communities. A similar pattern may be seen in the current "paraprofessional movement", which represents a return to what was the practice before it became *de rigueur* for human service practitioners to have such advanced degrees as the M.S.W., M.D., or Ph. D.

Diverting youth from the juvenile justice system to more appropriate and, hopefully, more effective and less stigmatizing alternatives received a major endorsement from the President's Commission on Law Enforcement and Administration of Justice (1967), recently reaffirmed by the National Commission on Criminal Justice Standards and Goals (1973). These commissions recommended the creation of Youth Service Bureaus to act as central coordinating units for all community services for young people, and to focus on attracting diversionary referrals (Norman, 1972). Currently over 150 Youth Service Bureaus are in operation in the United States, and the goal of the Federal Youth Development and Delinquency Prevention Administration is to reduce referrals to juvenile court by 25 percent between 1972 and 1977 (Gemignani, 1973).

The approach employed in the present project (Binder, Green and Newkirk, 1973) is distinguished by a close collaboration with law enforcement personnel, since "police should become the chief source of referrals to diversion agencies because that's where most official processing starts" (Lemert, 1971, p. 94); and by the use of a staff thoroughly trained in the principles of community mental health and administratively independent of the police. "Early offenders" are the target group of interest. As such, the program aims at early identification and intervention, or the secondary prevention of delinquency.

HISTORY OF THE PROJECT

The Youth Service Program began in January 1972 after a local police captain[1] approached one of us (A.B.) and expressed his concern that the juvenile justice system was not providing service to juveniles until they had established an extensive police record. His emphasis was less on the effectiveness of the juvenile justice system than on the general ineffectiveness of society in channeling early behavior patterns in a positive direction. A youth could commit many offenses before being apprehended by the police. The police would often wait until the third arrest before referring the youth to the probation department, who, in turn, would wait until several offenses had been committed before petitioning the youth to the juvenile court. By the time any service was provided, stable behavior patterns appeared to have formed.

The Youth Service Program originally operated as part of the field study courses of the Program in Social Ecology. Social Ecology is a new interdisciplinary program at the University of California, Irvine, concerned with the application of behavioral science knowledge to contemporary social problems (Binder, 1972). Two undergraduate students spent 10 hours a week on the Program. Since September, 1973, the Youth Service Program has been funded by a grant from the California Council on Criminal Justice. This funding allows for a paid staff of three — a coordinator and two full time counselors. All three are recent Social Ecology B.A. graduates. Supervision is provided by a Director and Associate Director, who are both on the faculty at the University (and have Ph.D.s in Clinical Psychology). Six field study students are also serving in the Program for 10 hours per week each.

THE PROGRAM

All referrals to the Youth Service Program are made by the police. The police contact may be originally initiated by the parents requesting police help in child rearing, a juvenile requesting aid for family problems, or it may stem from a juvenile code violation. Referral criteria include: (a) juvenile under 18 years old; (b) no more than three previous arrests; (c) the current arrest (if there is one) cannot be for a hard drug offense; (d) willingness of the

---

[1] Captain Robert Green of the Costa Mesa (California) Police Department.

parents and juvenile to participate in the program without coercion; (e) willingness of the police to take no further action on the case after referral.

Upon referral to the Program and acceptance into the treatment group (see Evaluation Design, below), a staff member sets an appointment to see the entire family together, if at all possible. At the initial meeting the program is described and the family's problems assessed. The family may, of course, choose to discontinue service after the initial meeting. But if service seems appropriate to family and staff, the family is seen for between four and eight weekly sessions, at which time referral for long-term treatment may be made if necessary.

The modes of intervention used in the program are derived both from the extensive pilot project and from a review of the current literature on behavior change techniques. An effort is made to avoid, on the one hand, the extreme of relying completely on unspecified "clinical judgment" in determining the course of intervention and also to avoid, on the other hand, dogmatically adhering to one narrow treatment model and forcing cases to conform to the model. Four modes of intervention were developed. While some overlap undoubtedly exists among them, the four modes have proven a useful guide to the conduct of the program. The modes of intervention are:

1. *Contingency contracting.* Contingency contracting is a form of bargaining or negotiating demands which appears to have special relevance to the families of "pre-delinquents". Defined by Stuart (1971) as "a means of scheduling the exchange of positive reinforcements between two or more persons", contingency contracting makes explicit the expectations of every member in the family. A frequently encountered situation in problem families is one in which the parents want their child to do something that he is not doing (e.g., make his bed), and the child wants his parents to do something that they are not doing (e.g., permitting him to watch a certain TV show). A "contract" could be set up where the child gets to watch the TV show contingent upon making his bed.

2. *Parent-child communication.* Therapists from several orientations (e.g., Haley, 1971; Alexander and Parsons, 1973) have stressed the importance of communication patterns in analyzing and resolving problem families. Patterson and Reid (1970) have demonstrated the lack of reciprocity which often exists in family interactions. Strenuous efforts are made during the interviews to foster clear and responsive communication from one family member to another (e.g., avoidance of lengthy monologues).

3. *Coping Skills.* At times, explicitly educating the parents or juvenile concerning a problem area is undertaken. Parents ignorant of the rudiments of child rearing techniques might be instructed in the method of Patterson and Guillon (1968). Juveniles might be provided with sex education where it

is obvious that their misconceptions might have serious consequences for them. The mutual idiosyncracies of people might be highlighted with emphasis that avoidance of confrontation may be more easily accomplished than change of the idiosyncracies.

4. *Community Involvement.* The program functions as a "service broker" in making maximum use of existing community support systems. A thorough survey of existing community resources is made and each resource is analyzed in terms of it appropriateness for referral. Where no resource exists for a given need, an attempt is made to create the resource. For example, the Program created a Big Brother/Big Sister group of college student volunteers to aid in providing service to boys and girls in need of an appropriate role model. In addition, all counselors work closely with school personnel in the development of potential modes of environmental change.

EVALUATION DESIGN

From the outset it was recognized that only a sophisticated and stringent evaluation of the program could advance knowledge in the field of delinquency diversion. It was decided that a randomized control group design with pre- and post- measures, was both feasible and appropriate. Data from the police, parents, juveniles and staff, in addition to recidivism measures, are routinely collected.

The evaluation procedures take the following form: (1) the referring officer supplies a minimal amount of background information on the case and assesses the probability that the juvenile will have subsequent police contact; (2) the staff consults a random number table which assigns a minimum of 20 percent of the cases to a no-treatment control group and 80 percent to treatment — the proportion to control goes up if the number of referrals exceeds staff capability, but the procedure of randomized assignment continues; (3) at the first interview, a structured assessment of the family's problem areas is undertaken and various information release forms are signed; (4) at the conclusion of service, an evaluation form is given to the juvenile and parents and one is completed by the staff member; measures of problem improvement and attitude change are sought; (5) six months after referral a follow-up telephone evaluation is used with families of both the treatment and control groups; a record check is made of juveniles and school records are checked for truancy and disciplinary problems; (6) a similar follow-up using both evaluation forms and record checks is performed one year after referral; (7) police attitudes toward the project are assessed by means of a periodically administered questionnaire.

PRELIMINARY RESULTS

Data are available from the evaluation form distributed to juveniles and their parents at the time of their termination from the program. Between October 1, 1973 and January 31, 1974, 83 cases had been terminated with the youths ranging in age from six to 17. Both the parents and juveniles were asked "Has the problem which led to your referral changed since you began the program?" A five-point rating scale, ranging from "much worse" (1) to "much improved" (5) was supplied. Both parents and juveniles had a mean score of 4.5, midway between "somewhat improved" and "much improved".

To the question "Would you recommend this program to other parents in a similar situation?", 100 percent of the parents responded "Yes." When asked "Would you recommend this program to a friend in a similar situation?", 93 percent of the juveniles also answered affirmatively.

A large majority of both parents and juveniles reported that progress had been made in their communicating better as a family, in changing each other's behavior by making agreements, in dealing with everyday problems, in handling serious problems in the parent-child relationship, and in improving the juveniles' relationships outside the family.

Some anecdotal evidence of program impact can be gleaned from the spontaneous comments about the program written on the evaluation forms. One youth wrote: "I liked the way I could talk so easily with the two of you. I feel that if it hadn't been for you I would have kept silent and all of my problems would never be solved." Another remarked: "The only part that I personally dislike is having to expire my relationship with Cathy Brody (a staff counselor). I have had a very rewarding time and I have benefited very much." Testimonials from parents were equally positive: "At this trying time, it was a comfort to me to have a confidential and constructively critical individual to talk to." Another parent commented: "I feel the program was responsible for a better communication between us and our son and also helped our son to evaluate some of his actions and what he wanted out of life. I am very thankful the program was available."

ETHICAL ISSUES

One cannot mount an intervention program on the border of mental health and criminal justice without confronting numerous ethical quandries. The staff of the Youth Service Program has spent a great deal of time working through such issues and formulating explicit positions. The most relevant concepts are:

Voluntary nature of the Program

While the decision to refer is made solely by the police, once referral has been made to the Program, the police agree to forego further processing, even if the family declines the referral or drops out of treatment. This is in keeping with the recommendation of the National Commission on Criminal Justice Goals and Standards (1973) that "youths should not be forced to choose between bureau referral and further justice system processing".

This issue has been easier to resolve among the personnel of the Program than in the larger context that includes the police. Clearly, the orientation of many police officers has been in a more coercive direction and it was not easy for them to accept the voluntary arrangement. Discussion of the wisdom of the arrangement has recurred at several of our regular meetings with juvenile officers, and, it seems certain, will recur in the future.

While the decision has been full accepted that there will be no further police action if service is declined, one obviously cannot control every phrasing, intonation or other form of implied coercion in the structuring of the police officers who make the referrals. Each Program staff counselor, therefore, points out the voluntary nature of the program during the initial interview.

Provision of a control group

Denying a proven service to some individuals solely for the "sake of science" is a practice which society has recently and justly begun to question. In the field trails for the Salk poliomyelitis vaccine, for example, the one million children used as controls and not given the vaccine had triple the rate of paralytic polio as the vaccinated children, and all the cases of fatal polio occurred among the controls (Meier, 1957).

When one does not have substantial reason to believe that a service is actually beneficial, society is rightly more tolerant of controlled experimentation. Indeed, it is becoming increasingly accepted and even legislated that those who would offer the public a supposed boon are obligated to verify empirically the beneficial nature of their service. It is this mandate for accountability to both consumers and funding sources which motivates the present evaluation.

It is clear that the beneficial effects of youth service bureaus or programs are far from established. Moreover, the consequences of the failure to provide service would, at worst, be far less catastrophic than in the case of experimentation on physical diseases (e.g., the polio experiment). Finally and most importantly, it was clear to us from the pilot project that we would not be able to service all police referrals because of our relatively small staff. This latter restriction means that placing some cases into a control group at the time of referral results in no less total service being provided than if we stopped accepting referrals when our service capacity was reached.

While no service is rendered by our staff to those in the control group, the police officers are, of course, free to provide whatever service or referral they would have provided to these juveniles were the Youth Service Program not in existence.

On the basis of staff size and expected referral numbers, we established that 80 percent of referred families would be assigned to treatment group and 20 percent to control group. Assignment is accomplished by a table of random numbers. If, moreover, referral numbers exceed expectations sufficiently, the random assignment table has provision to allow increase in the proportionate assignment to control group. This procedure results in no increased deprivation since we are assigning to controls approximately that percentage of referrals that exceeds the staff's capacity to service. And we have in the process accomplished the substantial advantage of allowing for a systematic and experimental analysis of the effects of the program.

Avoidance of "labeling "

A recurrent sociological criticism of programs aimed at the prevention or treatment of juvenile delinquency has been that such programs may label nondelinquent youths as delinquents. This label may become internalized, with the result that "agencies of social control may exacerbate or perpetuate the very problems they seek to ameliorate" (Lemert, 1971, p. 13). While there has been much recent critique of labeling theory (Davis, 1972) and some data to suggest that its effects may not be as severe as had been feared (Berleman, Seaberg and Steinburn, 1972), the staff of the YSP has been extremely sensitive to the issue of labeling. The voluntary nature of the program is stressed to the youth and his parents, as is the fact that the staff are not police agents. Great care is taken to avoid substituting the label "sick" for the label "bad". When it is clear that the locus of the problem resides in the parents rather than in the juvenile, the intervention effort is focused on the parents, and the youth may not be seen at all (beyond the initial interview) except as a last resort to help him or her cope with an impossible family situation. The short-term nature of the program (four to eight weeks) also inhibits labeling and dependency.

Lemert (1971) notes that programs of juvenile diversion have most often failed for two reasons: (1) alienating police officers, who are led to believe that the program is usurping their authority, and (2) alienating the community, which is led to believe that the program is "soft" on delinquents. Bearing this warning in mind, we have made strenuous efforts to maintain good relations with all levels of the police and community. Police officers are given immediate feedback on every case they refer and kept up to date on the progress of the Program (within the limits set by confidentiality). A prestigious community Board of Directors has been of considerable help in forming policy and overseeing the Program.[2] Publicity concerning the program in local newspapers as well as the *Los Angeles Times*, in addition to a local half-hour television program on the Youth Service Program, has been abundant and very favorable.

CONCLUSIONS

Preliminary data indicate that the Youth Service Program may be a fruitful approach to the prevention of delinquency. We are painfully cognizant that many in the past have had their hopes for delinquency prevention shattered by the findings of controlled experimentation, and we await further data with guarded optimism.

[2] The Board includes Captain Robert Green of the Costa Mesa (California) Police Department, Captain Harold Mays of the Huntington Beach (California) Police Department, Mr. Arthur McKenzie, former Chief of Police and City Manager for the city of Costa Mesa and Rev. Thomas W. Overton, Senior Minister of the First Christian Church, Huntington Beach.

REFERENCES

Alexander, J. and Parsons, B. Short-term behavioral intervention with delinquent families: Impact on family process and recidivism. *Journal of Abnormal Psychology*, 1973, **81**, 219-225.

Berleman, W., Seaberg, J. and Steinburn, T. The delinquency prevention experiment of the Seattle Atlantic Street Center: A final evaluation. *The Social Service Review*, 1972, **46**, 323-346.

Binder, A. A new context for psychology: Social ecology. *American Psychologist*, 1972, **27**, 903-908.

Binder, A., Green, R. and Newkirk, M. University-police cooperative approach to juvenile diversion: Evaluating its applicability and effectiveness. *Journal of Criminal Justice*, 1973, **1**, 255-258.

Blumstein, A. Systems analysis and the criminal justice system. *The Annals of the American Academy of Political and Social Science*, 1967, **374**, 92-100.

Cressey, D. and McDermott, R. *Diversion from the juvenile justice system.* Ann Arbor, Michigan: National Assessment of Juvenile Corrections, 1973.

Davis, N. Labeling theory in deviance research: A critique and reconsideration. *Sociological Quarterly,* 1972, **13**, 447-474.

Ferster, E. and Courtless, T. Post-disposition treatment and recidivism in the juvenile court: Toward justice for all. *Journal of Family Law,* 1972, **11**, 683-709.

Gemignani, R. Congressional briefing to the Subcommittee to Investigate Juvenile Delinquency of the Senate Committee on the Judiciary. January, 1971.

Gemignani, R. Diversion of juvenile offenders from the juvenile justice system. In U.S. Department of Justice, *New approaches to diversion and treatment of juvenile offenders.* Washington, D.C.: U.S. Government Printing Office, 1973, pp. 8-38.

Haley, J. *Changing families: A family therapy reader.* New York: Grune and Stratton, 1971.

Lemert, E. *Instead of court: Diversion in juvenile justice.* Chevy Chase, Maryland: Monograph Series of the National Institute of Mental Health, Center for Studies of Crime and Delinquency, 1971.

Meier, P. Safety testing of poliomyelitis vaccine. *Science,* 1957, **125**, 1067-1071.

National Commission on Criminal Justice Standards and Goals, *A national strategy to reduce crime.* Washington, D.C.: U.S. Government Printing Office, 1973.

Nejelski, P. Diversion of juvenile offenders in the criminal justice system: in U.S. Department of Justice, *New approaches to diversion and treatment of juvenile offenders.* Washington, D.C.: U.S. Government Printing Office, 1973, pp. 83-92.

Norman, S. *The youth service bureau: A key to delinquency prevention.* Paramus, New Jersey: National Council on Crime and Delinquency, 1972.

Patterson, G. and Guillon, M. *Living with children: New methods for parents and teachers.* Champaign, Illinois: Research Press, 1968.

Patterson, G. and Reid, J. Reciprocity and Coercion: Two facets of social systems. In C. Neuringer and J. Michael (Eds.), *Behavior modification in clinical psychology.* New York: Appleton-Century-Crofts, 1970.

President's Commission on Law Enforcement and the Administration of Justice. *The challenge of crime in free society.* Washington, D.C.: U.S. Government Printing Office, 1967.

Stuart, R. Behavioral contracting within the families of delinquents. *Journal of Behavior Therapy and Experimental Psychiatry,* 1971, **2**, 1-11.

Wolfgang, M., Figlio, R. and Sellin, T. *Delinquency in a birth cohort.* Chicago: University of Chicago Press, 1972.

10
Law Enforcement, the Judiciary, and Mental Health: A Growing Partnership *

ALLAN BEIGEL

During the past few years, an important focus of mental health agencies has been the development of partnerships with the law enforcement and judicial systems. All three systems deal with behavior that society has defined as deviant, and that is the principle that brings them together. Because of the vague and shifting definition of deviancy, sometimes only a fine line separates individuals who are referred to the mental health system from those referred to the law enforcement and judicial systems. Thus it is important for planners and administrators in the three areas to consider what target populations and services are appropriate for cooperative efforts.

Until recently, in many communities, deviant behavior was often called first to the attention of law enforcement agencies, whether or not it involved breaking a law. Consequently, mentally ill individuals were held in local jails until they could be sent to mental institutions. Although that now occurs less often because of the development of community mental health programs and changes in commitment laws, many localities are still struggling to clarify the relationships between the mental health, law enforcement, and judicial systems.

For example, it is still a common practice in many communities for individuals to contact law enforcement or judicial officials rather than the mental health agency when they wish to obtain a psychiatric examination for someone they think is in emotional distress. In Pima County, Arizona, that issue was the critical focal point from which cooperative relationships began.

*Reprinted from *Hospital & Community Psychiatry,* September 1973, **24**, 605-609, with permission. Copyright 1973, the American Psychiatric Association.

Before 1970 anyone in the county who wished to obtain such an examination could go to the courthouse, get the order for detention, sign it, and return it to the judge for signature. The judge would then forward it to the local law enforcement agency, which would pick up the individual. Thus each year hundreds of persons were detained in local hospitals for psychiatric examination without any professional prescreening. If patients' rights were to be protected and appropriate services delivered, it was imperative that the procedures be changed.

Discussions about the kinds of behaviors each system should deal with made it easier for law enforcement and jucicial agencies to transfer those responsibilities to the mental health system. The separate roles of the three systems were recognized: law enforcement as the keeper of the peace, the judiciary as the interpreter of the law and guardian of individual rights, and mental health agencies as providers of evaluation and care to those acting aberrantly because of emotional problems.

As a result, now when someone appears at the county courthouse requesting a petition for a psychiatric examination, he is referred to the walk-in clinic of the local mental health center to discuss the situation. If he and the mental health professional who evaluates the situation cannot agree on an appropriate course of action, he may still sign a petition. However, the judge has the final responsibility for authorizing an inpatient examination. If the mental health professional feels that the request for detention is not appropriate, he may forward his recommendations to the judge along with the petition. Not only do mental health professionals have earlier and primary responsibility for the diagnosis and evaluation of emotional problems, but also the judiciary is relieved of responsibilities for which it ahs not been trained.

The law enforcement system has also changed some of its procedures as a result of the cooperative relationships. Until recently, when law enforcement officers were confronted by behavior for which an individual could not be arrested, they usually took him to the county hospital and signed an order detaining him on the psychiatric unit. By doing so, they removed him from his environment, protected others from the effects of his deviant behavior, and were able to respond to the demands of those who had called them. However, the procedure was nothing more than a quasi-arrest. It provided even less protection of the individual's rights than if he had been taken to jail and booked for a crime.

In discussions with law enforcement officials, we found the procedure was followed partly out of the belief that if someone was taken into custody, an officer could be accused of illegal detention unless the individual was booked either into the local jail for violation of a law, or, if no law had been broken, into the county hospital as emotionally disturbed. With advice from the local judiciary, we pointed out that if an officer had wrongly detained someone, he could not be absolved of responsibility by placing the individual on the psychiatric unit.

The ruling helped steer law enforcement officials to a more appropriate means of handling deviant behavior that did not violate the law. Currently, if an officer encounters an individual whom he believes to be emotionally disturbed, he takes him to the local mental health agency, where the final decision about treatment is made by mental health professionals. This arrangement, which presents no more problems in operation than the previous unsatisfactory one, demonstrates what can be accomplished through discussion and clarification of issues.

In our community it was also a common practice to hold hearings for people who were legally detained in the county hospital, even if the doctor had determined that continued hospitalization was not indicated. Thus such patients were often forced to remain in the hospital for several days until the hearing took place. That complicated any efforts to begin out-patient treatment.

Consequently it was necessary to further clarify the responsibilities of judicial and mental health agencies. Once it was agreed that medical considerations had priority in this situation, the judges assented to the right of the physician to discharge the patient without a formal hearing. However, the physician must first inform the judge, who authorizes the release of the patient by dismissing the petition. A way is being sought to carry the process one step further and rewrite the order of detention so that the doctor can dismiss it without judicial consent.

BENEFITS OF CLARIFICATION

Clarification of such issues has implications for community acceptance of the mental health system. When the responsibilities of the three systems were confused, the mental health system was overshadowed by a pervasive legal aura that negatively affected the attitudes of those who needed help for emotional problems. They were unwilling to enter the system for fear that their deviant behavior would be labeled a violation of the law.

I would suggest that in some communities the reluctance to disclose emotional difficulties by seeking help is not solely a result of a fear of the stigma of mental illness, but also a manifestation of very real concern that there will be an accompanying stigma of criminal behavior. In our community, when the functions of the three systems were clarified, many who appeared for treatment commented that they had been reluctant to do so in the past because of the fear that they would be placed in the county hospital, brought before the judge, and "sentenced" to the state hospital.

Such clarification can also lead to expanded partnerships between agencies. For example, through a grant from the Law Enforcement Assistance Administration, the judicial and mental health systems have developed a court clinic. It provides diagnosis, evaluation, and short-term treatment of prisoners seen after conviction, before sentencing, or after probation is granted. This kind of partnership can have an impact on recidivism because it creates linkages through which an individual can be transferred to the mental health system. That facilitates continued treatment of deviant behavior that does not violate the law.

Recognition that jail personnel must often deal with such behavior has led to the development of a training program for them. It was designed to help them be more effective in handling manipulative, depressed, and suicidal behavior in prisoners. It also prepared them to be diagnostic aides who could bring to the attention of mental health professionals those prisoners who required treatment. Volunteers are now being trained under an LEAA grant to help provide evaluation and consultation.

Our counseling program for victims of sexual attack is another example of how cooperative efforts can benefit people whose needs transcend a single system. Law enforcement officers who question the victims give careful attention to their emotional reactions to the attack. If they seem to need counseling and supportive therapy, they are referred to health and mental health professionals who, along with the officers, function as part of a team.

FLOW OF FUNDS

When considering the flow of funds between the mental health system and other human service systems, it is important to recognize that while all are having funding problems, the mental health system is still the low man on the totem pole. Although that may not be reflected by the actual dollars available to the mental health system, it is still the "new game in town" and therefore receives a lower priority when it attempts to obtain financial support from other systems in return for the services it can provide. Other human-service systems have been visible to the public longer than the mental health system and have built up a bigger constituency in most communities. Furthermore, flow of funds from other agencies will also depend on the relevance of services to target populations and community attitudes toward those services.

Each of those factors has important implications for the flow of funds. Agencies may be more willing to purchase direct services, such as patient care, because they are visible and can yeld tangible results. They are often less willing to contract for indirect services, such as consultation and education. In any case, the mental health agency that approaches other agencies and says, "This is what we have to offer; what will you pay for it?" may find itself quickly rebuffed. The rejection may result solely from the factors already mentioned, disguised by the statement "We have no money."

Even so, mental health agencies must keep their services available and accessible to other agencies. It may be more realistic for them to adopt the philosophy that they must prove their worth before either expecting or demanding that other agencies channel dollars to them. Thus services must be directed at target populations that are already of legitimate concern to other service systems. Our own experience provides some examples.

Originally it was the courts who paid physicians and psychiatrists to examine those who had been placed in the county hospital on detention orders. The physicians were reimbursed on a fee-for-service basis from court funds budgeted specifically for that purpose each year. Those funds were the only county funds available for mental health services. When the new partnerships were being developed, it was agreed that the money should be turned over to the mental health system. The physicians who had been providing the services were asked to continue to do so under contract.

In their negotiations to obtain the funds, mental health officials argued that all they wanted was access to money that was currently being spent on mental health services, and the freedom to spend it in the way that was most appropriate without dictation from either the courts or law enforcement agencies. Authorization problems were minimized because no new funds were being requested, and those available had already been earmarked for providing mental health services.

The budgetary shift, along with the other changes in the service relationships between the systems, resulted in a decrease in the number of hearings, the time required of law enforcement and judicial officials, and the number of referrals to the state hospital. The mental health system was then able to go to the county, which had provided the original funds to the courts, and request increased funding based on documented effectiveness of the program.

Alcoholics were another target population of mutual interest. Community studies had documented to law enforcement and judicial authorities that their handling of public inebriates showed excessive costs in manpower and no demonstrable effectiveness. Thus those officials worked with mental health agencies to develop a pilot project to examine the impact of treatment services on public inebriates. The project was funded primarily by the local community and the state. After it ended, the mental health system was able to obtain additional funds to continue the program.[1]

---

[1] A. Beigel, "Planning for the Development of Comprehensive Community Alcoholism Services," *Texas Journal of Alcoholism*, Vol. 4, Winter 1972-73, pp. 17-42.

Shared staffing arrangements are another means of obtaining funds for mental health. For example, the personnel in the court clinic were supported financially by both the judicial and the mental health systems.

New projects that develop through cooperative planning and funding appear more likely to achieve financial viability than those that begin as isolated projects of a particular service system, even though the services overlap into other areas. Partnerships also open up possible funding resources not normally available to mental health agencies, such as LEAA grants. Similarly, funds available to the mental health system can be used to support mental-health-related projects in other human-service areas.

EXCHANGING INFORMATION

The advent of a more open delivery system for mental health services has already involved a number of professionals in the treatment of patients. Thus the issues of information-sharing and confidentiality have become more complicated than when the treatment relationship included only the doctor and his patient. The issues are even more complex when professionals from the law enforcement and judiciary systems are also involved.

Strict guidelines that go beyond the doctrine of informed consent must be established on how information obtained in one system may be shared with another. In all likelihood, the mental health system should restrict its role to being a friend of the court and keeping the treatment relationship outside the adversary process.

We are often faced with the problem of the patient who seeks help with an emotional problem while facing trial or sentencing. In this situation, it is even more important for all staff to have clear guidelines that have been agreed to by all systems. As a critical first step, other professionals should be educated in the principles of confidentiality followed in the mental health system. Mental health professionals should also be informed about those followed in the courts and law enforcement systems. This educational process is important, since other service systems do not define confidentiality in the same way as mental health agencies. Therefore, when partnerships are formed, the initial consultation and education process should include a series of inservice training programs about how information should be handled between the various systems.

Second, mental health records should clearly identify patients who are involved with other systems, particularly law enforcement agencies and the courts. That will alert mental health professionals to limit the abount of information placed in the records. Some mental health agencies have attempted to get around the problem by maintaining a dual record system.

One, which contains relatively few details about the patient's condition, is available to other agencies, while a second with more detailed information is not made available. However, dual systems should be discouraged because they require extra work and unnecessary secretiveness. A single record-keeping system can work when professionals understand the importance of confidentiality and the principles of appropriate information-sharing with other human-service systems.

Third, before any information is released, it is important that the patient be told the nature of the information requested. If the mental health agency cannot contact the patient, then only limited information should be provided until the other system has specified in writing the questions it wants answered. Too often agencies request release of all information without specifying what is actually needed.

In our program, we provide psychological and psychiatric consultation to residents of the jail who have emotional problems. To avoid becoming involved in the adversary process, we require that requests for consultation come from officials at the jail. Similar requests from prosecuting or defense attorneys must be routed through the courts. When the client is seen at the jail, information gathered there is not included in the jail records. That protects the client from prejudicing himself. The protected consultation arrangement was worked out through mutual agreement between the parties involved. It has helped bring more immediate professional attention to jail residents in need of such support.

Another instance in which the flow of information is carefully limited is in requests from the court to perform examinations of an individual's competency to stand trial. We believe such examinations are an appropriate function of the mental health system because they are not directly part of the adversary process. Although the law protects an individual from having information gathered in a competency proceeding used against him at his trial, both we and judicial officials recognize that this legal protection is not guaranteed.

Reports are therefore carefully phrased and the information provided is carefully limited to the issue of competency. That helps protect the client from the release of inappropriate information that has no bearing on his competency to stand trial. On the other hand, we do not participate in examinations related to pleas of insanity because they are directly a part of the adversary process.

Another important aspect of the flow of information between human-service systems is the extensive use of computers. Computer technology has revolutionized information-gathering in all human-service systems. Although information-gathering in all human-service systems. Although information-gathering in all human-service systems. Although information-gathering by computer can have benefits for research, data sought by one service system, such as mental health, may not be applicable in another system. Therefore, careful negotiation is required between the different systems before computerized information is exchanged. That is necessary not only to protect confidentiality, but also to maximize the potential for beneficial information-sharing.

USE OF PERSONNEL

The expansion of partnerships between mental health and other human-service systems has created a growing need for new training programs that will make mental health professionals more acceptable to other workers. It may be hypothesized that mental health professionals have difficulty in working with other human-service systems in direct proportion to the distance they perceive between their system and the other one. Although this distance will vary among mental health professionals, the principle is useful in devising training programs. Such programs should stress knowledge of both systems by personnel on both sides.

Contributing to the issue of perceived distance is the professional jargon found in every system. If representatives of the various systems are to communicate clearly with one another, a common language, free of jargon, must be developed. Simply educating professionals in the jargon of the various systems is not enough; a more basic level of communication that all can respond to is needed. In that regard, it is useful to consider once again the bond that unites the various systems: human behavior. Development of a common language should therefore proceed from the common experiences that all such workers share.

Role definition is another critical factor in preparing individuals to move easily between systems. People who are particularly suited to working within multiple service systems are those who have a more flexible view of their role, one that guards against rigid adherence to the concepts and goals of one system. But just as all law enforcement officers are not amenable to training to handle family disturbances, not all mental health professionals can be trained to fill consultative roles to law enforcement agencies. We must begin to identify the personality characteristics that enable professionals to work effectively with other systems.

At the same time, we must examine the effects of attempts to alter a professional's role definition so that he is more competent to work with other systems. For example, when we trained jail personnel in behavioral observation so they could serve as diagnostic aides, many of the more cooperative men quickly faced the possibility of ostracism by their more resistive co-workers. Similarly, the mental health professional who becomes competent in working with other human services may be ostracized by colleagues who hold a more traditional view of their role. They may see the new interservice role as an abrogation of traditional responsibility and a deviation from their sanctioned function.

Notwithstanding those important issues, there are still many innovative ways in which personnel can be used in partnerships. For example, most law enforcement agencies are now including courses on principles of behavior in their training programs. That presents an opportunity for a mental health professional to participate in the training process. However, he must approach the task from the point of view of law enforcement and adjust his training methods to conform with that system.

The potential roles of the paraprofessional and the volunteer and their relationship to these expanding partnerships are also being examined. In each system, appropriately trained paraprofessionals and volunteers can play an important adjunctive role. However, without proper training they will be neither accepted nor considered competent. We must not assume either that they can make important contributions to mental health, law enforcement, and judicial services simply because they are not professionals, or conversely that by training them we will diminish their effectiveness. Paraprofessionals and volunteers should be incorporated as partners in the staffing pattern of the human-service system in which they are involved.

The success of expanded partnerships between human-service systems will depend on the ability of workers to move freely and effectively between them. Suitable people must be selected and appropriately trained, or such cooperative relationships are doomed to failure.

11
Bail Reform as an Example of a
Community Psychology Intervention in
the Criminal Justice System *[1]

MICHAEL T. NIETZEL and JERALD T. DADE

While the relatively new disciplines of community mental health, social psychiatry, and community psychology remain distinguishable (Cook, 1970), they also share several important principles. One of the most important principles is an attempt at system level as opposed to individual interventions. Briefly, this position holds that many of man's problems in living are the result of negative influence exerted by important social institutions. If problems are seen in this light, the most efficient approach to society's "mental health" is through changing existing institutions or creating alternatives rather than attempting ameliorative interventions with individuals. Cooperative day care centers and private "free schools" are but two examples of recently attempted alternative institutions.

Mental health professionals for some time have been involved in the criminal justice system. Examiniations of present professional functions have shown that a wide range of possibly more valuable services are being ignored (Nietzel and Moss, 1972). Indeed, the interests of psychologist have broadened recently to include such preventive legal services as training the police as family crisis-intervention specialists (Bard, 1969).

The defects and deficiencies of the bail system have been matters of concern to the legal professional since the 1920's (Freed and Wald, 1964; Goldfarb, 1965; Morse and Beattie, 1932). The major dissatisfactions expressed

*Reprinted from the *American Journal of Community Psychology*, 1973, 1, 238-247, with permission. Copyrighted by V.H. Winston and Sons, Inc., Washington, D.C.
[1]Gratitude is expressed to Dr. Julian Rappaport for his direction in the preparation of this report.

have centered on three general areas. First, the present administration of bail is often inconsistent with the specific goals defined by the history and theory of bail. Second, the financial or property-owning requirements necessarily discriminate against certain groups of people. Third, the financial condition of the accused is an inappropriate criterion for determining the probability that accused will return to court when required.

Perhaps more serious than problems in the use and determination of bail are the effects of pretrial detention, whether because bail has been denied or because the defendant has been unable to meet financial requirements. The consequences of pretrial detention are numerous and constitute several obstacles to equal justice, particularly for the indigent (Ares, Rankin and Sturz, 1963; Foote, 1965; Foote, Markel and Wooley, 1954; Rankin, 1964). Unconvicted defendants are subject to the identical physical and psychological punishments experienced by convicted criminals. Detention often results in a person's losing his job, thus further jeopardizing his already precarious financial situation. As a result, the innocent members of his family may also suffer the burden of his imprisonment. Perhaps most crucial are the restrictions placed on his participation in the preparation of his defense. Free, uncensored communication with the outside is frequently denied, and confidential interviews with counsel are difficult, if not impossible, in most American jails. There is no opportunity for the enlistment of character witnesses in his behalf. He is unable to accumulate any type of pretrial work record that might suggest probation as a suspended sentence if convicted. Finally, the physical signs of imprisonment are likely to be prejudicial to the detained at future court appearances. Several studies indicate that after all other factors have been held constant, a person who is living in the community at the time of his trial has a better chance of acquittal or of receiving a suspended sentence or probation if convicted than has a person who is being detained at the time of adjudication (Ares et al., 1963; Foote, 1965; Foote et al., 1954; Rankin, 1964).

As well as being discriminatory, high money bail is not a valid criterion for judging which persons are "good risks" for appearance at their court dates. The success of numerous bail projects has not only rectified some of the legal inequities which typically plague the poor, but has led to a basic reevaluation of the bail system in its entirety. Faith in the deterrence value of money forfeiture involved in standard bail is rapidly decreasing as a result of these investigations and related experiences. The crucial factors involved in compelling appearance in court may have very little to do with the threat of money loss. Foote et al. (1954) concluded that "the real deterrent force against nonappearance in commercial bail is the threat of apprehension."

The American bail system is faced with the reconciliation of two separate and often conflicting demands. On the one hand is the moral and legal preference that the accused by free prior to any determination of guilt. On the other hand there is society's justifiable demand that the defendant will appear at court whenever required. As has been described, the traditional means of resolution of these demands has been soundly criticized. Recently, in response to such criticism, attempts have been made to develop alternative methods of assuring the accused's presence at trial.

The Manhattan Bail Project (Ares et al., 1963) was the first recent attempt to change bail procedures so as to eliminate (or at least lessen) the hardships faced by the indigent. The project workers conducted a quick interview with the accused prior to the setting of his bail by the arraigning magistrate. This inquiry assessed factors thought to be related to the probability that a defendant would appear for his trial — the defendant's roots in the community, residence factors, employment status, contact with friends and relatives, past arrest record. The information supplied by the defendant was verified through telephone or field contact with relatives or friends of the accused. Objective point values were assigned to the degree to which a given person satisfied the above criteria. If the person met some minimum number of total points set on the above areas, the magistrate was given a recommendation by the interviewer to release the accused without money or property bail (often termed ROR or release on own recognizance). The findings indicated that in the pretrial situation the rate of ROR "jumping" may actually be less than failure to appear under traditional bail procedures. Of the 10,000 defendants who were interviewed, approximately 3,500 were recommended for ROR. Of the defendants released on their own recognizance, only 1.6 percent failed to appear for their trial; of those released on bail bond, 3 percent failed to appear (Goldfarb, 1965).

The importance of the Manhattan Project is that it not only demonstrated that a large number of defendants could be released safely without money bail, but also led to similar projects in many major jurisdictions. A recent survey estimates there have been over 100 similar projects in the United States to date (Wice and Simon, 1970). Almost every major urban center in the country has developed a program patterned after the Manhattan experience. Many innovative variations have also been introduced, one of the most important being the use of a wide range of professionals and volunteers to gather information from defendants, verify it, and present it to magistrates (Goldfarb, 1965; Kennedy, 1968; McCarthy, 1965; Scott, 1966; Smith, 1965).

At its beginning, the Manhattan Project excluded several types of offenders from consideration. Defendants charged with homicide, assault on a police officer, rape, and narcotics offenses were among those not considered. Gradually, most projects (including Manhattan) have come to consider all defendants (Scott, 1966). Along with the liberalization of types of offenders considered has come a relaxation in the requirements for a ROR release. Many projects no longer employ strictly objective bases for recommendation decisions.

The success and acceptance of these programs have been unequivocal. Repeatedly, they have demonstrated that nonfinancial release of the accused is as effective as traditional money bail in assuring the appearance of the accused at court (Wice and Simon, 1970).

The present program introduced to the Champaign County (Illinois) Court system a demonstration bail project based on the Manhattan Project's procedures. The procedures were not limited to indigents or misdemeanants, but were extended to all defendants. Comparison of preproject, project, and postproject data was used in testing the following hypotheses:

(1)   More ROR would be employed during the project than either before or after.
(2)   ROR is a feasible form of pretrial release.
(3)   ROR would be significantly associated with subsequent rates of conviction and sentence if convicted.

The project in addition to providing a service to the local judicial system, serves as an example of a new role for psychologists in the legal system as well as a training device for both graduate and undergraduate students who normally have little contact with the population served. Finally, the project is one example of a research contribution that behavioral scientists can make in the evaluation of social system change.

METHOD

Staff

The staff consisted of two advanced graduate students in clinical psychology at the University of Illinois under the supervision of a clinical psychologist. Eight undergraduate psychology majors at the University of Illinois served as assistants.

Subjects

Interviews were conducted with 80 persons charged with a violation of the criminal code of the State of Illinois, including serious moving traffic violations. There were 73 males (91.3%) and 7 females (8.7%). Ages ranged from 17 to 66 years with a mean age of 24.7 years. The defendants were both black (37.5%) and white (62.5%). Of the total population, 51.3 percent had been arrested previously and 30 percent had at least one prior conviction. Although formal assessment of socioeconomic class was impossible, the majority of defendants appeared to be of lower or lower middle class background.

Procedure

The interviewers investigated five basic factors considered essential in determining a "good risk" for ROR: prior record, family ties, employment, residence, and time in area. Each defendant was interviewed individually for approximately 15 minutes by one of the graduate students. The defendant was told that the purpose of the interview was to aid in obtaining his release by recognizance bond and that any information supplied would be used only for that purpose. Defendants were further instructed not to discuss the present charge with the investigator. The interview was summarized in a questionnaire, which was given to an assistant for verification and scoring. A score of 5 points was needed for a recommendation of ROR; the possible range of points was from −2 to 12. Points were based on a set of objective criteria that quantified the questionnaire information. Verification of the information was made by telephone, in person if family or friends were present, or by field investigation. In most cases verification could be completed in 10 minutes. After the information was verified as to its truthfulness, a prepared summary was given to the presiding magistrate. This summary consisted of the sheet on which the criteria were listed with the particular scores for each defendant recorded under the proper category. It was usually the case that this written summary was not given to the magistrate in those cases in which a recommendation could not be made. In such cases it was simply stated that a recommendation could not be made at that time. In cases where a recommendation for recognizance was made, a brief oral presentation of the data was also made to the magistrate. The recommendation summary was given to the State's Attorney and defense counsel (if any) whenever possible. Previous to his appearance before the magistrate, the defendant was always advised as to the interviewer's decision to make or not to make a recommendation.

The project was in effect for 1 month, beginning on May 4, 1971, and ending on June 7, 1971.

RESULTS

An analysis was made of the first 400 criminal dockets occurring during January-April 1971 in the Champaign County Circuit Court. Of the 400 cases, 231 (57.8%) had completed adjudication at the time of analysis. These cases constituted the preproject data against which project and postproject data were compared. The first 100 cases completed immediately following the project served as the postproject data.

Project Defendants

Of the 80 defendants interviewed during the 1-month period, recommendations for release on recognizance were made in 63 cases, and of these 63 recommendations, 43 defendants were granted release on their own recognizance.

Comparison of the "recommended" defendants with regard to racial composition, age, or prior arrest reveals the following figures:

(1) Of the defendants recommended and receiving ROR, 34.9 percent were black and 65.1 percent were white. Of the defendants recommended but not receiving ROR, 40 percent were black and 60 percent were white.

(2) The mean age of ROR defendants were 25.6 years. Of those not receiving ROR, the mean age was 23.5 years.

(3) Of the ROR defendants, 43.2 percent had at least one previous arrest while 65 percent of the non-ROR defendants had at least one previous arrest ($X^2 = 2.63$; 1 $df; p < .20$).

Differences in Rates of ROR

A comparison of rates of release on recognizance among the preproject, postproject, and project groups reveals that ROR was granted to 34.2 percent of preproject defendants, 55 percent of project defendants, and 38 percent of postproject defendants ($X^2 = 10.88$; 2 $df; p < .01$).

Differences in Reappearance ("Jumps") among Defendants

Of those defendants released on recognizance, the "jump" or failure to reappear rate was lowest among those defendants released during the project (2.3%) as compared with preproject (10.1%) and postproject (15.8%)

($X^2 = 4.50$; 2 *df; p* < 20). For defendants released on some type of financial bond, the failure to reappear rate was 6.6 percent (preproject), 13.9% (project), and 1.6 percent (postproject).

Difference in Disposition and Sentence

At the time of this report, 68.8% of the cases in the project has reached a final outcome. Combining these completed cases with preproject and postproject cases, the percentage of defendants receiving an outcome of "dismissed" or "not guilty" among defendants receiving ROR does not differ significantly ($X^2 = .02$) from that of defendants released on financial bond or detained before their final disposition. Of the defendants found guilty before, after, and during the project, however, those defendants released on recognizance received a lesser percentage of jail or prison sentences (10.4%) than did those defendants in the "other arraignment decisions" category (26.6%) ($X^2 = 6.5$; 1 *df;p* $< .02$). The latter category included other types of arraignment decision. Specifically, this group was composed of people released on 10 percent cash deposited, property, surety, or cash bond (73.9%); those pleading guilty at their first appearance (6.9%); those having their charges dismissed immediately (2.5%); and those not able to pay any type of bond and remanded to the custody of the sheriff and not released before their final court decision (16.7%).

DISCUSSION

During the operation of the project, a significantly greater number of defendants were released on recognizance than either before or after the project. The percentages of recognizance bonds for both preproject and postproject defendants were already considerably higher than the average (27%) for several cities (Des Moines, St. Louis, San Francisco, Tulsa, and Columbus) already using bail reform procedures (Wice and Simon, 1970). The present data indicate, however, that an even greater percentage of defendants could be released on recognizance with the introduction of a systematic information-gathering procedure. Not only was such a procedure administratively feasible, it also provided information that allowed the magistrate to make release decisions on the basis of factors other than past record or present charge. At the minimum, such information facilitates more careful bail setting. Maximally, the information is necessary to support the expanded use of recognizance release. The present study confirms the notion that financial deterrents to flight are unnecessary in most cases. Not only do financial requirements discriminate against the indigent defendant, they seem to serve no defensible function for those defendants who can afford bail. A substantial percentage of the defendants released on recognizance during the project could have afforded the 10 percent deposit on bail bonds required in Illinois.

These results have importance beyond the specific court involved. Criticisms of the bail system and attempts at its reform have focused on court practices in large metropolitan areas. Bail practices in smaller jurisdictions (the 1970 census of Champaign County showed a population of 162,107) offer certain similarities and contrasts, two of which appear especially important in the present case. First, detention of an accused pending his trial is as much a problem in the smaller jurisdiction as in major urban centers. Second, smaller districts have certain administrative characteristics that greatly facilitate the expanded use of ROR. Careful, confidential interviews are much more feasible when 5-10 defendants are to be interviewed rather than 50-100. Problems stemming from continual, excessive demands made on the judicial machinery are minimal in comparison to larger districts. Furthermore, and perhaps more important, the judge is quite often acquainted to some degree with the defendant before him.

One important result meriting further consideration is the fact that the failure-to-appear rate of defendants released on recognizance was lower during the project than either before or after the project. While the difference is not statistically significant ($p<.20$), perhaps as a result of the attenuated sample size during the project, it is of sufficient magnitude to be of interest to a court concerned with the safe pretrial release of its defendants.

Assuming for the moment that some aspect of the project was responsible for the lower rate of recognizance "jumping" among project defendants, one can propose at least two possible explanations. First, it may be that the additional information provided by the prearraignment interview results in the selection of those defendants most likely to reappear when required. An alternative explanation is that it is not so much the information supplied by the interview, but the interview encounter itself, that is important in determining the return of the defendant to court. Several factors could be operative here, including the fact-to-face commitment made between defendant and interviewer, the emphasis placed on the possible penalties associated with a failure to reappear, or a feeling of indebtedness or trust that motivates reappearance. A final explanation, of course, is that these influences combine in some way to provide for the more reliable use of ROR.

The present study did not reveal a significant relationship between ROR and the frequency of "guilty" and "dismissed" or "acquitted" outcomes. The type of release, however, is significantly associated with the type of sentence received. Convicted defendants released on recognizance received a significantly lower ($p<.02$) incidence of prison or jail sentences than did those defendants either released by some other means or detained previous to a final decision or pleading guilty at their first appearance. Possible factors underlying the association between detention at time of trial and final sentence have been discussed elsewhere (Wald, 1964). In the present case, recognizance defendants are being compared with a group the majority of which were not detained prior to a final decision, but were released on some type of bond. One may hypothesize that the conditions of recognizance bond approximate the conditions of probation to a degree that allows a judge or probation office to make some prediction as to how well convicted defendant would do on probation. It is possible that the financial aspects of other types of bonds render them less of a representative test of the probation period.

Of course, alternative hypotheses relating recognizance release to severity of present charge, past record, or apparent weight of the evidence could account for the fact that recognizance defendants receive less severe sentences. Case-by-case examination of project defendants, however, resulted in substantial agreements with Wald's conclusion (1964) that the much greater likelihood of a defendant receiving a prison sentence if he spent his pretrial period in detention could not be accounted for by differences in the backgrounds of defendants detained as compared with those released on bail.

The ultimate importance of the present program can be realized only if its procedures are incorporated permanently into the criminal justice system. It can be seen from the postproject data that the use of ROR returned to its preproject level. It appears that the project itself was unable to induce lasting changes in court practices. Presently, plans are being made for the utilization of the part-time help available to the public defender's office as the means by which the program can be institutionalized. Examples of this strategy have already proven successful in other jurisdictions (Freed and Wald, 1964).

Within the criminal justice system, bail reform has been proven to be both desirable and attainable. The present project has demonstrated the necessity and feasibility of bail reform in a jurisdiction quite distinct in many ways from those inwhich bail reform has traditionally been attempted. It has provided evidence that in the future the professional resources of behavioral science can be applied to a much broader range of problems within the criminal justice system than has been the case.

REFERENCES

Ares, C., Rankin, A. and Sturz, H. The Manhattan Bail Project: An interim report on the use of pre-trial parole. *New York University Law Review*, 1963, **38**, 67-95.

Bard, M. Family intervention police teams as a community mental health resource. *Journal of Criminal Law, Criminology, and Police Science*, 1969, **60**, 247-250.

Cook P. (Ed.) *Community psychology and community mental health.* San Francisco: Holden-Day, 1970.

Foote, C. The coming constitutional crisis in bail. *University of Pennsylvania Law Review*, 1954, **102**, 1031-1079.

Freed, D. and Wald, P. *Bail in the United States: 1964.* U.S. Department of Justice. Washington, D.C.: U.S. Government Printing Office, 1964.

Goldfarb, R. *Ransom: A critique of the American bail system.* New York: Harper & Row, 1965.

Kennedy, P. VISTA volunteers bring about successful bail reform in Baltimore. *American Bar Association Journal*, 1968, **54**, 1093-1096.

McCarthy, D. Practical results of bail reform. *Federal Probation*, 1965, **29**, 10-14.

Morse, W. and Beattie, R. Survey of the administration of criminal justice in Oregon. *Oregon Law Review*, 1932, **11**, Supplement.

Nietzel, M.T. and Moss, C. The psychologist in the criminal justice system. *Professional Psychology*, 1972, **3**(3), 259-270.

Rankin, A. The effects of pre-trial detention. *New York University Law Review*, 1964, **39**, 642-646.

Scott, R. Bail factfinding project at San Francisco. *Federal Probation*, 1966, **30**, 39-43.

Smith, R. A new approach to the bail practice. *Federal Probation*, 1965, **29**, 3-6.

Wald, P. Pre-trial detention and ultimate freedom: A statistical study. *New York University Law Review*, 1964, **39**, 631-655.

Wice, R. and Simon, R. Pre-trial release, a survey of alternative practices. *Federal Probation*, 1970, **34**, 60-63.

12
Participant Observation and Attempted Mental Health Consultation in a Public Defender Agency *

MARC F. ABRAMSON

While I was a fourth-year psychiatric fellow in a community mental health training program, I had the opportunity to be a participant observer and to attempt mental health consultation in a public defender agency in a large city in the western United States. Rather than discuss the specific problems of participant observation or mental health consultation technique as they evolved in this experience, I shall describe some general aspects of the public defender's role and show how these may pose obstacles to a mental health consultant attempting to relate to a public defender agency.

Although the observations were made primarily in a public defender agency, many of the obstacles to mental health consultation apply generally to the defense attorney's role, whether he is a public defender, legal aid defender, privately retained defense counsel, or assigned or appointed defense counsel.

AMBIGUITIES OF PLEA BARGAINING

One problem of the public defender's role is that much of it is underground. In legal theory the defense attorney is a diligent adversary who does everything legally possible to get his client acquitted. Unless the public prosecutor can be convinced to dismiss all the charges, the only way to obtain acquittal is by trial. Trials, however, especially jury trials, are extremely time

*Reprinted from *American Journal of Psychiatry*, 1971, **127**, 964-969, with permission. Copyright 1971, the American Psychiatric Association.

consuming. If every criminal defendant demanded a full jury trial the courts would be hopelessly clogged. To avoid this, criminal defendants are encouraged to plead guilty to expedite their processing through the courts.

At least 90 percent of all criminal prosecutions are disposed of by a negotiated guilty plea (1, p. 128). But what kind of inducements can or should be offered to encourage guilty pleas? Should the judge know of the negotiations between defense and prosecution, and to what extent should he be limited in his sentencing discretion by the negotiated "deal"? Should the judge participate in the negotiations, oversee them from a distance, or remain totally aloof? If he participates, what happens if the negotiations fail and the case goes to trial? These concerns are still being debated by legalists.

In commenting on negotiated guilty pleas, the President's Commission on Law Enforcement and the Administration of Justice said:

> It would be a serious mistake . . . to assume that the guilty plea is no more than a means of disposing of criminal cases at minimal cost. It relieves both the defendant and the prosecution of the inevitable risks and uncertainties of trail. It imports a degree of certainty and flexibility into a rigid, yet frequently erratic system. The guilty plea is used to mitigate the harshness of mandatory sentencing provisions and to fix a punishment that more accurately reflects the specific circumstances of the case than otherwise would be possible under inadequate penal codes. It is frequently called upon to serve important law enforcement needs by agreements through which leniency is exchanged for information, assistance, and testimony about other serious offenders (1, p.135).

The President's Commission also pointed out:

> . . . the facts in most cases are not in dispute. The suspect either clearly did or clearly did not do what he is accused of having done. In these cases a trial, which is a careful and expensive procedure for determining disputed facts, should not be needed (1, p.130).

In jurisdictions with responsible police departments and public prosecutors, the presumption of innocence is a matter of "due process" rhetoric rather than actual probability. Truly improper charges are usually weeded out in screening processes by the police and the public prosecutor's office. One major function of the public defender is to spot those improper charges that do slip through the screening procedures on the law enforcement side and to provide pressure to maintain the quality of those screening procedures.

To withstand appelate court examination in the event of subsequent appeal, a guilty plea should be factual; it should be made by a defendant who has been informed of and understands all the possible alternatives; and it should be fully consented to without apparent inducement. Although the practice of bargaining for a guilty plea is ubiquitous, there is always the concern that a defendant will be persuaded to sacrifice some of his due process rights by unfair inducements to a guilty plea. Therefore, to preserve the appearance of due process and to guard the trial transcript against appelate reversal, the defendant almost always denies in open court that there have been any inducements — such as a promise of sentence leniency — to plead guilty. Usually he even denies that there have been negotiations at all (1, p. 130).

In this confused, subvisible context of plea bargaining the public defender functions as a kind of agent-mediator-broker for his client. Some public defenders take pride in being efficient and settling nearly all their cases with negotiated guilty pleas. These attorneys are often highly regarded, and their success in negotiating pleas is predicated on high prestige with legal colleagues and the ability to convince defendant clients that they are getting "the best possible deal."

To convince a defendant client to accept a deal is sometimes a complex process. The public defender informs his client about the progress of negotiations with the prosecutor and often delicately encourages the defendant to accept the bargain and plead guilty. This procedure often involves a subtle collection of mixed messages. An attorney will sometimes coax a guilty plea while denying that he is doing so.

Private defense counsel also participate in plea bargaining but do not have to be so delicate in suggesting a guilty plea. If the defendant does not like this advice, he can theoretically hire new counsel. The indigent defendant, however, cannot so easily discharge his public defender, whose advice to plead guilty must be more subtle. This does not imply that public defenders give their clients poor legal representation. In fact, some observers (2) feel that a public defender generally gives legal representation and gets deals at least as good as those of the private counsel. Also, the public defenders must maintain a certain degree of credibility for reasonable legal representation in the eyes of their clientele.

CONTRASTS WITH MENTAL HEALTH STYLE
OF INTERACTING WITH CLIENTS

The legal determination of guilt usually focuses attention on a defendant's discrete physical behaviors and presumed mental state during a short period of time. A man can be killed in a fight that was started and completed in 30 seconds. Who hit or threatened whom first, and what was the defendant thinking or feeling during that brief period? Were there witnesses? What did they see? Will they be available to testify? Will their versions conflict? These are the issues that concern the defense counsel. His interviews with his client focus on these issues; his adversary role is to create as much uncertainty as possible about the relevant events. I have observed a skilled public defender interview a defendant and convert what began as a simple, straight forward narrative into a dazzling sea of confusion. Sometimes even the defendant was amazed by this transformation.

In contrast, the mental health worker probably has had experience in psychotherapy, in which the goal is to create clarity about events in the patient's life. There would usually be consensus on what recent events had occurred, even if their underlying psychological causes were initially obscure. In evaluating a case, the mental health worker might accept a version of events based on all the available data acceptable by common-sense criteria, even if these data would be inadmissable in court because of technicalities of the rules of evidence. The mental health worker may assume the very events the defense counsel is trying to disprove.

The mental health worker's understanding of the case is in great part historical; his formulation usually relies considerably on past events in the patient's life. Past events in the defendant's life may be legally irrelevant to the adjudication of guilt or innocence.

In short, the mental health worker and the defense attorney have quite different ways of thinking about people and problems. Except for the mental status examination, the former's usual approach is historical, while the latter's is intensely cross-sectional in time. The mental health worker often assumes the accuracy of the best available description of behavior given him, and then attempts to understand and explain that behavior psychologically. Defense counsel often tries to creat confusion about what behavior actually occurred.

The interviewing style of most mental health workers is open ended. Questions are designed to elicit emotionally meaningful material. The interview flows in a direction determined by the patient's emotional needs. The interviewer permits and even encourages digressions and topic changes if he feels the new directions are toward a more open expression of the client's feelings.

In contrast, a public defender often perceives such an interview as meandering and directionless. Often pressed for time while interviewing a defendant, he wants only information strictly relevant to legal defense strategies.

Occasionally I have attempted to interview a client jointly with a public defender in an effort to acquaint him with some aspects of psychiatric interviewing technique. However, it soon became apparent that we had different goals in our interviewing styles, and the effort was abandoned. Another factor may have been involved here. Most defendants appeared with a great array of social and psychological problems. Often a public defender would feel unable to deal with a defendant's catalog of troubles. If the client started to discuss personal or intimate problems the public defender cut him off. Dealing with such material can be personally stressful to the interviewer. In addition, there was a common fear among the public defenders that discussion of such problems might lead to an embarrassing emotional display, such as rising anger or tears. There was the fear that once the floodgates were open the emotional torrent might be hard to stop. The public defenders were thus reluctant to open a Pandora's box of troubles they felt incompetent to deal with. Excessive sympathetic listening to a defendant was often disparaged as mere "handholding."

Often a group of defendants was interviewed together in a holding cell adjacent to the municipal court where minor cases were heard and serious (felony) cases bound over for superior court. This group interview was an effort to handle efficiently the tremendous number of defendants the public defenders had to deal with. But it discouraged intimate or sustained discussion of problems between the public defender and his client. The defendant was forced to be brief and to adhere to the legally relevant points in this public setting.

Different groups of public defenders handled the municipal and the superior courts. If a defendant were bound over to superior court after a preliminary hearing on a felony charge, a new public defender would take over this case in the higher court. This practice discouraged sustained emotional dependence on a single public defender.

Unless appeals were contemplated, the public defenders usually felt their roles were terminated when the charges were disposed of, either by dismissal, acquittal, or adjudication of guilt. They were often reluctant to talk with clients after disposal of the charges. If the defendant was judged guilty, his fate was then up to the judge, usually with the assistance of the probation department for a pre-sentence evaluation. If there was an acquittal, the public defenders often knew or suspected that their clients had actually committed the offense as charged. In this circumstance, many of the public defenders were reluctant to talk with their former clients. There was a common feeling that it would be childishly moralistic to try to make a referral to a social agency or to point out to the client that he had been "lucky to get off this time" but still needed some kind of help. Both the public defenders and their offender clients seemed to share a certain cynicism about the workings of the machinery of criminal justice. These attorneys generally did not think it would be helpful to try to reduce their clients' cynicism about the law by explaining the due process theories that had permitted their acquittals.

CRIME CONTROL, DUE PROCESS, AND SICKNESS

Herbert L. Packer, a Stanford law professor, proposes two models of the criminal justice system. As described by Blumberg,

> The first he calls a "crime control model." This version of criminal justice presumes the guilt of the accused and operates with assembly line speed and efficiency to process large numbers of defendants. The crime control model balances the interests of the individual and society, and individual interests must often give way. The other system is the "due process model." Here the system of criminal justice is a legalistic obstacle course to serve the needs and rights of individual defendants (3).

Some of the public defenders I observed were torn at times between the two models. Their professional roles in the adversary process demanded allegiance to the due process model. Their citizen roles, on the other hand, made them concerned with public safety. Sometimes they were appropriately frightened of offenders whom they had gotten acquitted or who had otherwise "walked out the door."

Sometimes a latent discontent with the limited adversary defense role was revealed. However, open espousal of the "crime control" model was not common. Some of the public defenders seemed to seek a third model as a compromise between the due process and the crime control models. This was the "sickness" model, which they used to soften the conflict between a dangerous offender's apparent desire for freedom and the state's need to isolate him from society. If this offender could be classified as mentally ill, he could then be isolated from society in a therapeutic institution where he would be "treated" and rehabilitated.

THE PUBLIC DEFENDER'S COMFORT IN HIS ROLE

Most of the public defenders seemed comfortable in their professional roles. Legal training had convinced them of the ultimate utility of the adversary process, and that process required someone to play the defense role. They seemed relatively inured to what an outsider with no legal training might have perceived as unbearable role conflicts.

Yet there were some complaints. They complained of overwork. Many were concerned that the large number of cases would prevent them from doing a professional, craftsmanlike job. They were particularly conscious of professionalism when a case actually went to trial. Some of the public defenders would assist a defendant who wanted to handle his own defense. Others would not, on the grounds that it would be impossible to do a truly professional job under those circumstances. Even though they generally wanted to avoid discussion of very personal material, they were often quite conscious of the psychologically powerful role they played for their clients. Often an indigent defendant's only perceived ally in the criminal justice system was his public defender, and some of these attorneys were anxious to create and protect a relationship of trust with their clients.

They had varied opinions about how far to push the adversary role. Some public defenders admitted that they occasionally encouraged a defendant to lie to aid his case. Others felt that their status as paid public servants prevented their extending the adversary role to that extent. Some expressed frustration at being lied to by clients and felt that privately retained defense council got more truthful stories from clients. One frustration was the frequent ingratitude of clients. This was particularly true when a client did not appreciate a deal a public defender had gotten for him, while the latter felt that the deal had been a particularly good one in the plea bargaining market. They recognized that nonlawyers were occasionally unsympathetic to their work. For example, some of the public defenders were hurt that nonlawyer personnel in the law enforcement and correctional fields were sometimes hostile when they "walked out" a dangerous offender because of some due process technicality.

Despite the attorneys' apparent subjective comfort in harmonizing the conflicting demands of the public defender role, it appeared to me that the resultant role conceptions were quite personal and varied. Each public defender might be willing to discuss his operating philosophies with trusted colleagues, but an open discussion of these conflicts with the entire agency staff seemed impossible. Previous trainee mental health consultants to the agency had reported that open discussion of different operating philosophies in group consultation sessions had often led to protracted argument among the staff attorneys. There was no open discussion of what minimal degree of role consensus would be necessary for adequate agency functioning. Once an attorney had worked out an operating philosophy for himself he did not seem to want it tampered with.

Another hazard to the attempted mental health consultation was my interest in the legal process. Vicarious participation in the adversary combat was exhilarating and seductive. While discussing a case with a public defender, I was sometimes caught up in the excitement of trying to map out defense strategy. I usually returned to the realization that I was there to try to provide mental health consultation to the agency, but sometimes not until one of the attorneys had reminded me that I was starting to "think like a lawyer."

CONCLUSIONS

It was not clear from my experience that discussion with a mental health consultant could help any public defender who was having difficulty in harmonizing the conflicting demands of his role. In fact it sometimes appeared that mental health consultation in such a situation might disrupt an individual attorney's previously workable conception of his role.

On the other hand, it must be admitted that my relationship with the agency was short-lived, limited as it was by the one-year duration of my fellowship with the community mental health training program. Possibly a more open-ended relationship with the agency would have resulted in my being sufficiently trusted and knowledgeable to help some of the public defenders harmonize their conflicting role demands.

It is more likely, however, that a public defender agency is not receptive to a mental health consultant, especially if he tries to adhere to an indirect service model. If a mental health consultant wishes to function in some part of the criminal justice system, his time might better be spent with police, judges, or probation officers, instead of with attorneys playing stylized, ritualized adversary prosecution or defense roles.

An exception might be the situation in which a defense attorney has a sustained, supportive relationship with a mentally ill defendant on trial[4]. The prosecutor probably has more actual discretion that the defense attorney, whose strategies are generally limited to responses to the prosecutor's decisions before conviction. Thus, prosecuting attorneys might be a better target for mental health consultation, although they probably would be less receptive than defense attorneys because the prosecutor's allegiance is more toward punishment and the protection of the public interest as he sees it than to the rehabilitation of the individual offender.

Another factor possibly limiting the feasibility of mental health consultation with public defenders was their circumscribed relationship with their own clients. The public defenders in this agency seemed little involved with the postconviction disposition of their clients. This lack of involvement was even more true in the event of acquittal, and many defendants who are personally troubled or socially troublesome may be acquitted for a variety of reasons.

Some public defender agencies (5-7) are experimenting with rehabilitative planning as part of the defense attorney role. If this potential activity becomes more common, public defender agencies may become more receptive to mental health consultation. It must also be noted that there is a real paucity of community resources to help offenders. Were these increased, the enlarged number of dispositional possibilities for offenders would make all workers dealing with offenders in the criminal justice system more receptive to mental health consultation.

REFERENCES

President's Commission on Law Enforcement and Administration of Justice: The Challenge of Crime in a Free Society. Washington, D.C. US Government Printing Office, 1967.

Oaks, D.H. and Lehman, W. Lawyers for the poor. Trans*action* 4(8):25-29, 1967.

Blumberg, A.S. *Criminal justice*. Chicago: Quadrangle Books, 1967, p 7.

Balcanoff, E.F. and McGarry, A.L. Amicus curiae: The role of the psychiatrist in pretrial examinations. *Amer J Psychiat* 126:342-347, 1969.

Cayton, C.E. Relationship of the probation officer and the defense attorney after Gault. *Federal Probation* 34:8-13, 1970.

Dash, S., Medalie, R.J. and Rhoden, E.L. Jr. Demonstrating rehabilitative planning as a defense strategy. *Cornell Law Review* 54:408-436, 1969.

Portman, S. The defense lawyer's new role in the sentencing process. *Federal Probation* 34:3-8, 1970.

REFERENCES

[text faded and illegible]

Part III
Treatment—Intervening in the Offender's Behavior

Rehabilitation has been steadily gaining on punishment as the primary objective of the correctional system (Kittrie, 1971). Karl Menninger asks rhetorically, "Do I believe there is an effective treatment for offenders and that they *can* be changed?" He answers: "most certainly and definitely I do" (1969, p. 261). Ramsey Clark states that "we know corrections can rehabilitate" (1971, p. 233).

Fortunately, the past decade has seen a move from "the period of the promise of treatment" to "the period of treatment program evaluation" (Kassebaum, Ward and Wilner, 1971). Unfortunately, it has been a sobering experience.

Bailey's (1966) review of 100 outcome studies of correctional treatment concluded that "the evidence of the effectiveness of correctional treatment is inconsistent, contradictory, and of questionable validity". Robison and Smith (1971) analyzed many large-scale studies of the California Department of Corrections and found that "there is no evidence to support any programs claim to superior rehabilitative efficacy". The most recent and exhaustive review of the effectiveness of treatment programs in a correctional context located 231 studies in the literature which met minimal standards of scientific methodology (including 27 studies on the effectiveness of psychotherapy). Martinson (1972), the reviewer, stated: "On the whole, the evidence from the survey indicated that the present array of correctional treatments has no appreciable effect — positive or negative — on the rates of recidivism of convicted offenders" (see also Jew, Clanon and Mattocks, 1972).

Kassebaum, Ward and Wilner (1971), whose controlled study of group counseling in California prisons showed no benefit to the program, make a cogent assessment of the literature:

> The most fundamental requirement for further research on the effectiveness of prison and parole programs would seem to us to be a frank recognition that psychological treatment programs involve assumptions about the causes of crime, the informal and formal organization of the prison and parole, and the nature of the postrelease experience, all of which may be quite unrealistic when applied to actual existing conditions (p. 320).

It seems clear that the rehabilitation procedures of the future must be radically different from the strategies of the past. The selections in this part were chosen to reflect new orientations which hold potential for breaking out of the morass of negative results. Scharf, Kohlberg and Hickey (Chapter 13) begin this section by presenting a unique perspective on psychological intervention in a prison. They describe an attempt to create a "just prison" utilizing Kohlberg's theory of moral development.

Wenk and Moos (Chapter 14) provide community mental health personnel with a new and potentially useful tool for the assessment and modification of prison settings (cf. Katkin, 1972; Musante and Gallemore, 1973). Their Correctional Institution's Environment Scale (CIES) may provide a link between the growing field of environmental psychology (e.g. Craik, 1973; Ittelson, Proshansky, Rivlin and Winkel, 1974) and the practice of community mental health. Perhaps it will be possible to link certain psychosocial climates with positive impact on various classes of offenders, and then design institutions to maximize these climates. Elsewhere, Moos (1973; Moos and Insel, 1974; Wenk and Moos, 1972) presents more extensive discussions of this promising methodology.

While the previous selections concerned prisons, Klapmuts (Chapter 15) provides an in-depth review of community alternatives to the total institutionalization of offenders. Reintegration of the offender into the community is her goal. She notes that community corrections need not be demonstrated to be *superior* to prisons in terms of reducing recidivism in order to be implemented. As long as community alternatives are *no less effective* than prisons in deterring crime, economic and humanitarian considerations support their adoption (see also Fixen, Phillips and Wolf, 1973; Lamb and Goertzel, 1974). The most radical shift from institutional placement to community corrections has occurred recently in Massachusetts. Preliminary data suggest that the move has been a substantially successful one (Ohlin, Coates and Miller, 1974).

Finally, Alexander and Parsons (Chapter 16) describe and evaluate a short term intervention program for delinquent families, based on an ingenious combination of social learning and interpersonal communication theories. Their rigorous evaluation at both the process and outcome levels could serve as a model for other intervention programs in this field.

REFERENCES

Bailey, W. Correctional treatment: An analysis of one hundred correctional outcome studies. *Journal of Criminal Law, Criminology, and Police Science,* 1966, **57**, 153-160.

Clark, R. *Crime in America.* New York: Simon and Schuster, 1970.

Craik, K. Environmental psychology. *Annual Review of Psychology,* 1973, **24**, 403-422.

Fixen, D., Phillips, E. and Wolf, M. Achievement Place: Experiments in self government with pre-delinquents. *Journal of Applied Behavior Analysis,* 1973, **6**, 31-47.

Ittelson, W., Proshansky, H., Rivlin, L. and Winkel, G. *Introduction to environmental psychology.* New York: Holt, Rinehart and Winston, 1974.

Jew, C., Clanon, T. and Mattocks, A. The effectiveness of group psychotherapy in a correctional institution. *American Journal of Psychiatry,* 1972, **129**, 602-605.

Kassebaum, G., Ward, D. and Wilbur, D. *Prison treatment and parole survival.* New York: Wiley, 1971.

Katkin, E. Psychological consultation in a maximum security prison: A case history and some comments. In S. Golann and C. Eisdorfer (Eds.), *Handbook of community mental health.* New York: Appleton-Century-Crofts, 1972, pp. 641-658.

Kittrie, N. *The right to be different.* Baltimore: Johns Hopkins University Press, 1971.

Lamb, H.R. and Goertzel, V. Ellsworth House: A community alternative to jail. *American Journal of Psychiatry,* 1974, **131**, 64-68.

Martinson, R. Can corrections correct? *The New Republic,* April 8, 1972, 13-15.

Menninger, K. *The crime of punishment.* New York: Viking, 1969.

Moos, R. Conceptualizations of human environments. *American Psychologist,* 1973, **28**, 652-665.

Moos, R. and Insel, P. *Issues in social ecology.* Palo Alto: National Press Books, 1974.

Musante, G. and Gallemore, J. Utilization of a staff development group in prison consultation. *Community Mental Health Journal,* 1973, **9**, 224-232.

Ohlin, L., Coates, R. and Miller, A. Radical correctional reform: A case study of the Massachusetts Youth Correctional System. *Harvard Educational Review*, Winter 1974, in press.

Robison, J. and Smith, G. The effectiveness of correctional programs. *Crime and Delinquency*, January 1971, 67-80.

Wenk, E. and Moos, R. Prison environments: The social ecology of correctional institutions. *Crime and Delinquency Literature*, December 1972, 591-621.

13
Ideology and Correctional Intervention: The Creation of a Just Prison Community *

PETER SCHARF, LAWRENCE KOHLBERG, and JOSEPH HICKEY

In recent years, there have been a number of efforts to use psychological theory to reconstruct the prison environment to facilitate the rehabilitation of the offender. While at least since the pioneering days of Slavson in the nineteen thirties (1945), psychologists have worked individually and in groups with inmates, the idea that psychology can intentionally reorder the social structure of the prison is a relatively new concept. Working from a range of psychological theories, this notion of psychological intervention in the prison has given evidence of coming of age.

It must be pointed out that this wave of reform has not, to date, provided many examples of success in terms of meaningfully reducing inmate recidivism. Some conceptually impressive, well-planned interventions (Warren 1969; Jessness 1969, 1972, 1974; Empy, 1971) have failed to show the hoped-for results in terms of effects on inmate lives. As well, a number of organizational studies (Sykes, 1958; Cressy, 1961; Studt, 1969) indicate that there is perhaps an endemic tension between what might be called the task of maintaining order in the prison and the task of rehabilitation. Inevitably those responsible for rehabilitating the inmate and those responsible for keeping him in custody conflict, with the result being that many programs instituted within prisons have been both ineffective as well as short-lived.

Several critics have argued that any efforts at such psychological intervention are both doomed to failure and, in a sense, merely legitimating what they regard as an unjust, corrupt prison edifice. Mitford (1973) and Ryan (1971) each argue that only through reordering the broad opportunity

*This chapter was written especially for this volume.

structure of society and ultimately "tearing down the prisons" can the current system of dealing with offenders be altered. They also suggest that the fact of coercive incarceration ultimately conflicts with the goal of rehabilitation and that efforts to reorient the prison are beset by unresolvable contradictions. Even some prison officials within the system have taken this position. Jerome Miller, former commissioner of the Division of Youth Services in Massachusetts, for example, in a period of three years has demolished the youth prison system in Massachusetts. Similarly, the recently published report of the National Advisory Commission on Criminal Justice Standards and Goals (1973) offers both that "the myth of rehabilitation is both bankrupt and misleading.

In spite of these binds, the authors of this chapter wish to offer a model of psychological intervention they believe is morally and psychologically adequate in a way that earlier attempts were not. Most earlier efforts at psychological intervention have been oriented towards two broad schools of psychological theory: First, the psychoanalytic school emanating from the followers of Freud; and second, the tradition focusing on social learning and behavioral change. The neo-Freudian tradition assumes that delinquent behavior is caused by neurosis akin to nondelinquent neurotic disorders. The approach assumes that the offender suffers from a personality disorder which should be treated from what might be called a "medical" model (i.e., the criminal is "sick" and should be treated as one who is suffering from something akin to a medical infirmity). Practitioners such as Slavson (1945), Friedlander (1960) and Frazier (1972) offer that the goal of institutional treatment should be to provide a climate offering interpersonal trust, and opportunity for the offender to interact with clinically trained correctional personnel. The notion put forth is that through a process of active therapeutic interaction within the setting, the offender gains insight into the "causes" of his delinquency and through active support is able to reverse his criminal course.

A second wave of reform begins with the behavioral tradition in animal and human psychology — the tradition from Hull to Skinner and the social learning theorists (Bandura, 1969). This view holds that criminal behaviors are learned through mechanisms similar to "normal" social behaviors. Rather than seeing him as "sick" (as do the psychoanalytic theorists), they see him as having been rewarded and conditioned in the "wrong" kinds of social behaviors. For example, the inmate has been rewarded by peers and possibly parents and teachers for stealing cars, rather than for holding a job and being punctual. The therapeutic strategy focuses on teaching "socially acceptable" behaviors and extinguishing "unacceptable" behaviors. Staff, through contracts and a token system, attemp to reward inmates for behaviors which approximate "appropriate" "street" behaviors. For example, inmates are given points transferable to an early release and privileges within the institution for acting in ways defined as acceptable (e.g., going to school, finishing job assignments, etc.).

While both psychoanalytic and behavioral traditions have made inroads into modifying the overt horrors of the custody prison (*cf.* Cressy, 1960), they have failed in our view in two key respects. First, they have not demonstrated that they are capable of meaningfully altering the behavior of criminals outside of the institution. Second, neither approach has developed an ethical philosophy vis a vis the inmate which is at once philosophically justifiable and is accepted as being just by the inmate.

A large number of studies document the first point. Many of the most conceptually promising of recent efforts at correctional treatment have failed to produce meaningful (and often even significant) results in terms of reducing inmate recidivism. Such sophisticated efforts as those instituted by the Center for Differential Treatment (Warren, 1969) or efforts by the California Youth Authority to implement institutional psychotherapy or behavior modification programs have not been met with significant results in terms of reducing inmate recidivism. (Jessness, 1969, 1972, 1974).

In addition to failing to produce programs which may be judged psychologically efficacious, psychology has failed to develop treatment modalities which provide agreeable bases of justice for the inmate. Several critics such as Szasz (1963) and Mitford (1973) have criticized what might be called the "Catch-22" moral logic of correctional treatment programs. Inmates in this view (a view we generally share) are subjected to a mode of justice which is both arbitrary and often transparently unfair. Decisions in the prisons are made through reference to psychological rather than ethical principles. For example, a counselor will decide to have an inmate placed in punitive segregation, not because he is in danger of violating the rights of others, but "in order to teach him to deal with his aggression". In several psychotherapy treatment programs parole and furlough decisions are made solely through psychologists making judgements about the inner "motives" of the inmate, rather than by making a rational decision involving a conflict of claims between the inmates' rights and those of the community. In the social learning programs we find a second type of moral incongruity. Generally, in these programs the goals of treatment are defined by the authorities' definition of conventionally acceptable behavior. Inmates are released when they demonstrate through their behavior that they will conform to societal norms. This definition ignores the issue of both the justice of such norms as well as the inmates perception of their moral rightness. This problem is especially acute in the case of politicized, highly intelligent inmates. Does a radical inmate, for example, find the goal of his conformity to the laws of the State a legitimate ethical goal?

Thus, we argue that in both psychotherapeutic as well as behavioral learning programs there is offered what Weber referred to as a form of "Kadi" justice (the nonrational proclamations of the Moslem village wiseman). We argue this both by reference to the ethical structure of the psychological judgments imposed in correctional treatment settings, and by looking at inmates' perceptions of justice in such programs.

In a study conducted by the first author (Scharf, 1973), we found that inmates in both psychoanalytic and behavior modification prisons often rejected the moral logic implied in each of the therapeutic ideologies. For example, an inmate in the prison based on the principles of transactional analysis offered:

> That they are just trying to brainwash you into being a middle American dude. The staff and all are liberal, but they are just trying to get you to conform, not smoke marijuana and stuff.

Similarly, in a behavior modification prison an inmate suggested:

> The idea is to make you like a pigeon. This stuff was started with retarded kids. They take your values and try to make you act like they want. It's like bribery and stuff.

In each case, it is clear that the basic moral orientation of the program is rejected by the inmate involved. This pattern, we found, held true for most inmates in the behavior modification prison and the most mature inmates in the insight therapy prison. In the behavior modification prison, roughly 60 percent of the inmates interviewed were scored as rejecting the basic mode of justice in the prison. A similar, though less dramatic pattern was found in the insight therapy, T.A. prison (Scharf, 1973).

Given these findings, we set out to use a psychological orientation which avoided some of the pitfalls of both the psychotherapeutic and social learning psychological models. Using a model of development conceptualized and empirically validated by Kohlberg (1969) over a period of 18 years, we sought to apply what we saw as a third psychological tradition — that of Dewey (1933), Mead (1934) and Piaget (1969) to the problems of corrections. This tradition (see Langer, 1969) offers that instead of focusing upon specific inner conflicts or behavioral patterns, psychologists interested in human growth should focus upon broad organizing structures of experience as their basic unit of psychological intervention. Following Piaget, it reports that there is an invariant sequence of stages which organize both the individuals' perception of physical reality as well as his conception of relationships with social others and the institutions of society.

Kohlberg's stages in the moral domain offer the most fully elaborated and empirically validated of these schemes of social development. Kohlberg argues that moral development may be conceptualized in terms of 6 stages. Each higher stage offers a moral perspective which is more adequate, logical and rational, in that it considers in a more coherent manner, conflicts of moral claims among individuals. In a variety of social and cultural situations, individuals have been found to move through the stages in the same order, though the rate of development and final stage achieved varies depending upon the types of social experiences offered the individual.

Studies in this area (Kohlberg, 1969) indicate certain specific conditions associated with rapid and complete moral development. One condition involves the experience of moral conflict in such a manner that there is group support for resolution of such conflict and tension. A second postulate offers that moral change is associated with active role taking and participation in the political and justice process of the setting. Finally, we have found that moral change occurs when individuals accept the social setting's atmosphere as being legitimate and positive as understood at the person's state of moral maturity.

The Moral Stages are given in Table 1.

This psychological orientation, we hoped, would be more appropriate to corrections than the psychotherapeutic or social learning interventions had proved to be. We believed that our concern with broad structures of experience would encourage inmates to develop life plans and life orientations which would be reflected in such life adjustment measures as recidivism. As well, we hoped that our concern with moral values and our position that morality should be defined in terms of universal principles, rather than specific social norms, would lead to a mode of justice within the institutions which would be just and would be perceived as just by inmates and staff involved.

Our efforts in the correctional field began rather modestly. For a period of a year, we ran moral discussion groups with inmates in a traditional custody prison. Where we were able to induce small changes in moral reasoning. (Hickey, 1971), we felt that both our ability to change inmates' thinking and our ability to change inmate lives was limited by the nature and structure of the institution. Specifically, we observed and documented (Scharf, 1971).

1. The custody prison denies the inmate simple procedural justice. He is told when to eat, sleep or work. He often has no appeal to constitutional rights or civil liberties. Discipline hearings lasted, on the average, only three minutes. Punishments tended to be automatic: generally, four to 30 days in the *Box*. This punishment meant that the inmate was stripped of his clothes, fed an inadequate diet,

Table 1 Classification of Moral Judgment into Levels and Stages
of Development

Levels	Basis of Moral Judgment	Stages of Development
I	Moral value resides in external, quasi-physical happenings, in bad acts, or in quasi-physical needs rather than in persons and standards.	Stage 1: Obedience and punishment orientation. Egocentric deference to superior power or prestige, or a troubleavoiding set. Objective responsibility. Stage 2: Naively egoistic orientation. Right action is that instrumentally satisfying the self's needs and occasionally others'. Awareness of relativism of value to each actor's needs and perspective. Naive egalitarianism and orientation to exchange and reciprocity.
II	Moral value resides in performing good or right roles, in maintaining the conventional order and the expectancies of others.	Stage 3: Good-boy orientation. Orientation to approval and to pleasing and helping others. Conformity to stereotypical images of majority or natural role behavior, and judgment by intentions. Stage 4: Authority and social-order maintaining orientation. Orientation bo "doing duty" and to showing respect for authority and maintaining the given social order for its own sake. Regard for earned expectations of others.
III	Moral value resides in conformity by the self to shared or shareable standards, rights or duties.	Stage 5: Contractual legalistic orientation. Recognition of an arbitrary element or starting point in rules or expectations for the sake of agreement. Duty defined in terms of contract, general avoidance of violation of the will or rights of others, and majority will and welfare. Stage 6: Conscience or principle orientation. Orientation not only to actually ordained social rules, but to principles of choice involving appeal to logical universality and consistency. Orientation to conscience as a directing agent and to mutual respect and trust.

placed in a dark windowless cell and given nothing to read but the
Bible and the *Reader's Digest*.

2. Inmates perceived the prison world as operating at primitive
levels. Inmates were seen as *ripping-off* and *ratting out* their friends.
They were viewed as living in a Hobbesian "war of all against all"
with no norms or standards to regulate the violence between inmate

and inmate. Authority and rules were typically perceived as the Stage One imposition of punitive force. The authority of the guard lay simply in his power to throw inmates in the *Box*.

3. The effect of the traditional prison is to stifle higher stage moral thinking. Inmates remain fixated in terms of their moral thinking through denial of the types of experiences likely to change moral thinking. Specifically, the prison strove to suppress intellectual and moral conflict, block inmate participation in the justice process and was perceived by inmates below their own stage of reasoning.

Given these observations, we conceptualized an institutional intervention program which had a number of goals, related both to our theoretical framework and to our observations in the custody prison. Specifically, we offered that a correctional psychological atmosphere could be constructed which would:

1. Be objectively just in terms of both the formal procedures and substantive justice offered the inmate. Inmates and staff would jointly arrive at a definition of the rules and work to maintain them.

2. Be designed so that the types of experiences which were related to moral growth might be present in the correctional community. We hoped in this respect to create a climate which would be perceived above the inmate's own stage, which would force him to participate in the justice process of the community and which would force him into active conflict with and dialogue with other inmates.

3. Provide a context for inmates giving active support to one another in terms of their developing and maintaining positive life plans upon release. It would hope that the sense of community we thought could be created in a prison context could be maintained in the "streets".

Given these goals, we sought to find an institution in which a basic structural shift in the prison structure would be possible. After a number of negotiations, the Connecticut Corrections Department suggested that such a project might be possible in the Niantic State Farm for Women. There were a number of conditions which made the project seem propitious. The administration was generally encouraging from the outset. Staff seemed unusually oriented towards finding a "better way" of working with the inmates. In addition, the farm was decentralized into a number of small living units

(20-30 inmates), each of which could function in an administratively autonomous manner. Though relationships between inmates and staff were tense when we arrived (Summer, 1971, when the Attica takeover occurred), there was a beginning willingness among staff, inmates and administrative groups to work together in defining a more equitable basis for running the prison.

As an initial step, we proposed a "constitutional" meeting with inmates and staff in which the groups could air differences and, most importantly, begin to explore possible bases for a new program in the institution. Though both inmates and staff expressed a reluctance to attend the "convention" at the first meeting, nearly the entire inmate population and many of the staff appeared.

The initial sessions were marked by suspicion between inmates and staff, and a gap in terms of moral perspective. In one session, there was a debate about whether there should be a rule against stealing all property or just inmate property. The inmates argued in seemingly Stage Two categories that they would "rip-off" institutional property with few qualms. The prison matrons, on the other hand, argued, using Stage Four notions, that "stealing was absolutely wrong" and that there had to be a hard and fast rule against all theft:

> Brenda (staff): How about stealing from the institution and not another woman?
> Barbara (inmate): Good for them.
> Alice (inmate): I guess it's how the individual feels.
> Brenda (staff): Isn't stealing wrong no matter who it is from?
> Barbara (inmate): The State of Connecticut is rich and the taxpayers are paying for it, so why not steal when you are at work?
> Alice (inmate): A couple of gallons of ice cream was stolen out of the kitchen. Do you really think the girls stole it? The staff takes a lot of stuff out of the kitchen.
> Linda (staff): The girls stole it. It was found in their room.
> Pat (inmate): If we got some decent food we wouldn't have to steal from the central kitchen.
> Brenda (staff): But any way you look at it, stealing is stealing.
> Judy (staff): I feel the same way. This is theft, and theft is theft.

After a number of months of such conflict, there evolved a definition of a program and common rules which were acceptable to most of the staff and inmates. The inmates would control discipline within the cottage through community meetings, and would receive many privileges which had not existed previously on the farm. Inmates agreed to make some accommodation with staff and also agreed to try to settle grievances and conflicts within the cottage.

The structure of the program primarily involved a concept of group decision-making. Within the cottage, there were two major decision-making forums: small groups and community meetings.

The small groups discussed personal issues effecting members of the cottage. Inmates brought up problems they had faced in their communities, or in the streets. They might also "run a beef" they might have with another inmate. The number of participants enable the groups to develop a mini-culture of their own with a greater intimacy than possible at the large community meetings.

The community meetings were the central political forum of the cottage. The entire group would decide joint disciplinary action to be taken against particular members (either inmates or staff). It would also determine important policy issues for the cottage. Common topics included the resolution of conflicts between inmates, dealing with violations to institutional or cottage rules, and attempts to influence prison policies and restrictions. In each type of action, the critical element involved giving inmates actual control over the particular decision to be made. In no case, even one dealing with a serious incident such as contraband or assault, was the cottage community meeting decision overruled by the prison administration.

The key to the success of the program involves inmates actively identifying with and maintaining the rules of the cottage. Initially, inmates found it impossible to discipline other inmates. One inmate said bluntly in one of the first meetings, "I'll do anything you like in this program. I'll talk in groups. The only thing I won't do is lock or rat out one of my sisters."

After a long series of meetings in which inmates successfully "covered-up" for other inmates who had committed minor offenses, the women began to see that if they didn't maintain the rules, the cottage would plunge toward anarchy and the project fail. The crisis came in a meeting in which an inmate named Melinda announced that if anyone brought up her name, she would "stomp their heads in with her stomp boot". After a long hush, the same woman who had announced that she would not punish another inmate stood up and said:

> Melinda, if we let you go around saying you gonna stomp people, we are gonna lose all respect for this house, the cottage and ouselves. We are going to punish you not to hurt you, but to keep respect.

This meeting marked the beginning of inmates actively identifying with the cottage self-government system. Increasingly, they trusted staff within the house and, reciprocally, staff began to feel confident that the inmates would deal fairly with conflicts which occurred within the cottage. We hoped that this process of their becoming actively involved in resolving conflicts and maintaining a social community would result in both moral and personal growth among the inmates.

Judged from a number of perspectives, the group process created in Niantic seems promising. Inmates, seen both in terms of qualitative and quantitative analysis, were judged to perceive the project positively. Seventy-two percent of inmates interviewed were judged as accepting the basic justice assumptions of the project. One inmate, somewhat characteristically, offered:

> In the model cottage I found something I never thought I would find: concern and love. People treat you like a human being, not like an inmate or a number. They care for you here and treat you with respect. This is different from any other prison I heard of . . .

The project also demonstrated that redesigning the moral atmosphere of the cottage had an apparent effect upon inmate moral reasoning. Inmates in the project changed an average of one-quarter of a moral stage over a six-month experimental period. The change was especially dramatic among the younger inmates in the project (i.e., those under 24 years old). These inmates changed an average of roughly 4/10ths of a moral stage. This result was consistent with Kohlberg's observations (1969) that moral judgment tends to stabilize in the mid-twenties. Typically, the change among inmates was from stage two to stage three. Those inmates who made a full stage transition were found to have the cognitive prerequisites for the next stage of moral thinking. The results compared favorably with an earlier intervention using moral discussion groups in a traditional custody prison (Hickey, 1971). Among the younger inmates the change was more than twice as great in the Model Cottage intervention than in the experiment using moral discussion groups in an unchanged prison setting (17/100ths of a moral stage – discussion groups alone – vs. 39/100ths of a stage in the Model Cottage). These results, where tentative, seemed to argue that an intentionally designed moral climate along with discussion groups had a more powerful effect upon moral thinking than would running moral discussion groups in an unchanged prison environment.

The recidivism results allow us to be cautiously optimistic. A preliminary recidivism count after a mean of one year indicated that only five of 33 inmates had returned to prison, four of the recidivists being parole violators (i.e., only one of the inmates commited a new felony). In summer 1974, a formal recidivism study will be conducted (matched with a comparable control group) to ascertain the true two-year recidivism rate. However, our preliminary results compare so favorably with statewide norms for female felons (16 percent compared with 35 percent) that we are confident that the program has made an impact upon the lives of the offenders involved. Life-interviews with women reveal that the vast majority are leading productive lives. Several are working, having meaningful relationships with others and their families, and are generally quite happy. One woman who had had a record of 10 arrests over a seven year period now is an administrator of an antidelinquency project. Several others who had had nearly perpetual confrontations with the law prior to their experience with the project are now leading clearly drug-free and crime-free lives.

The program, too, has undergone a dramatic evolution. The cottage at Niantic is now supplemented by a Community Correctional Alternative in New Haven. The inmates of the Niantic project wrote the first rules, created the program goals and were the first subjects for the new facility. The New Haven project, now a year old (founded June 1973) offers a dramatically different alternative to the traditional prison experience. The women live in the hub of New Haven, work during the week, and are involved in a range of community activities and experiences. The experience in the institution at Niantic is seen merely as a preparation for life in the community center. The average stay in prison is less than five months for a woman involved in the project. When residents of the Niantic model cottage feel she is ready and vote for her to go, the inmate is transfered to the New Haven unit. The hope of the State Corrections Department is that almost all female inmates in the state will be placed in these Community Correctional Alternatives within the next three years.

To sum up, we offer a model of psychological intervention which differs in several respects from past efforts. If offers a program which is rooted in a theory which we believe deals and possibly resolves some of the contradictions inherent in past efforts to use psychology to transform the prison. First, it focuses on changing the broad world view of the inmate, rather than focusing on his achievement of specific insight, or the conditioning of particular behaviors. As well, it offers a moral ideology which we believe is more just than that which is implicit in past psychological efforts. The program, we believe, also addresses the concern of social critics who argue that any efforts to change corrections must be with broad efforts to restructure both the nature of punitive justice institutions and society. While we accept these arguments, we argue that efforts to change inmates and change institutions are not incompatible, but rather each transformation depends upon the other. Only through changing the moral and social awareness of inmates can we change prisons. Only by changing the moral structure of prisons can we hope to raise the moral awareness of inmates. This dialectic of individual and institutional change provides, perhaps, the core concept in our effort. We believe it offers an alternative that the debate on psychological intervention in the prison desperately needs.

REFERENCES

Bandura, A. *Principles of behavior modification.* New York: Holt, Rinehart and Winston, 1969.

Cressy, D. *The prison: Studies in institutional organization and change.* New York: Holt, Rinehart and Winston, 1960.

Dewey, J. *Democracy and education.* New York: Macmillan, 1933.

Empy, R. and Lubeck, S. *Silverlake experiment.* Chicago: Aldine, 1971.

Frazier, T. Transactional analysis and the treatment of staff in a correctional school. Unpublished manuscript, 1972.

Friedlander, K. *The Psycho-analytic approach to juvenile delinquency.* New York: International University Press. 1960.

Hickey, J. Moral change among delinquent youth. Paper presented to the annual meeting of the American Psychological Association, Washington, D.C., 1971.

Jessness, C. *et al.* Search for effective treatment. *California Youth Authority Quarterly,* 1969, Vol. 22.

Jessness, C. *Youth Center Research Paper.* Sacramento: California Youth Authority, 1972.

Jessness, C. Unpublished manuscript, 1974.

Kohlberg, L. Stage and sequence. In D. Goslin (Ed.) *Handbook of socialization theory and research.* Chicago: Rand McNally, 1969.

Langer, J. *Theories of development.* New York: Holt, Rinehart and Winston, 1969.

Mead, G. H. *Mind, self and society.* Chicago: University of Chicago Press, 1934.

Mitford, J. *Kind and usual punishment.* New York: Pantheon, 1973.

National Advisory Commission on Criminal Justice Standards and Goals, *Corrections.* Washington, D.C.: Government Printing Office, 1973.

Piaget, J. and Inhelder, B. *Psychology of the child.* New York: Basic Books, 1969.

Ryan, W. *Blaming the victim.* New York: Patheon, 1971.

Scharf, P. Moral atmosphere of the prison. Paper presented to the annual meeting of the Americal Psychological Association, Washington, D.C., 1971.

Scharf, P. Moral atmosphere and intervention in the prison. Unpublished doctoral dissertation. Harvard University, 1973.

Slavson, S. *Introduction to group therapy.* New York: International Press, 1945.

Studt, E. *et al. C-Unit: Search for community in prison.* New York: Russell Sage, 1969.

Sykes, G. *The society of captives.* Princeton, New Jersey: Princeton University Press, 1958.

Szasz, T. *Law, liberty, and psychiatry.* New York: Macmillan, 1963.

Warren, M. *Center for training in differential treatment: Some history and hopes.* California Youth Authority Quarterly, 1969, Vol. 22.

14
Social Climates in Prison: An Attempt to Conceptualize and Measure Environmental Factors in Total Institutions *[1]

ERNST A. WENK and RUDOLF H. MOOS

Prisons have again become the focus of strong criticism. Critics maintain that not only do prisons fail in their major rehabilitative functions, but also many prisons fail to provide the basic custodial security and safety for the inmates and the needed safety for correctional personnel.

That a prison is a complex social system is often overlooked. People of various psychological make-ups and social and cultural backgrounds interact with each other in fulfilling their respective roles within the boundaries of a highly confined space: the prison environment. Life in these total institutions, including the behavior shown by inmates and staff, is, as elsewhere, a joint function of both the personality factors of the individuals and their interactions with the environment. The quality of this institutional life is determined by both the attributes of the people and the attributes of the environment and the resulting interactions.

Within the institutional environment conflicting attitudes and beliefs about the purposes of a prison system exist, leading to conflicting objectives and philosophies. The attitudes and beliefs of the general public are equally inconsistent, contradictory, and confused. They are communicated to the people in the prison through the courts, politics, and the public media, adding

*Reprinted from *Journal of Research in Crime and Delinquency,* July 1972, 9, 134-148, with permission of the National Council on Crime and Delinquency.

[1] The research reported in this paper was supported by grants MH16461 and MH16026 from the National Institute of Mental Health. Appreciation is due to Robert Shelton and Penny Smail, research assistants in the Social Ecology Laboratory, who aided in the statistical analyses. For a more detailed report on the potential uses of the CIES see Wenk, E.A. and R.H. Moos "Prison Environments: The Social Ecology of Correctional Institutions," *Crime and Delinquency Literature,* 4(4):591-621, December, 1972.

to the contradictions and confusions already existing within the walls. In this complex social and psychological climate the determinants of behavior become difficult to define without relying heavily on scientific methods.

In spite of early recognition of the significance of environmental factors on the behavior of individuals traditionally, social scientists directed most of their attention toward the study of personality factors. The individual became the focus of study, and what was inside the individual was believed to be primarily responsible for his actions. Empirical studies of environmental factors and their contribution to behavior rarely were undertaken.

Recently a shift in emphasis has occurred, and many researchers have conceptualized and measured environmental dimensions. Some studies of institutional environments have attempted to relate environmental factors to behavior occurring in the institution, and others have attempted to relate them longitudinally to treatment outcome through post-release follow-up studies (e.g., Moos and Schwartz [2]).

This paper describes the development of a testing instrument which aims at conceptualizing and measuring some of these environmental factors and attempts to provide the institutional administrator and his staff with a tool to assess an institution's social climate. Specifically, it is hoped that the information resulting from this testing can be used for long-range staff development and ongoing efforts to improve the social climate in the institution. In addition, the instrument should be useful in gauging the social climate periodically as a preventive action, hopefully capable of detecting or bringing to light institutional tensions before a crisis level is reached.

From the beginning of these studies in 1966 the authors intended to relate this research to practical concerns of the institutional administrator, who struggles to fulfill three basic correctional objectives:

1. To reduce infractions of institutional rules, especially individual and collective violence inside the prison.

2. To improve the inmates' personal resources, including education and vocational competence and social problem-solving skills.

3. To reduce recidivism.

The strategy was to develop cooperatively with institutional staff an instrument to empirically measure certain elements or diminsions of significance to social climates and to provide this tool to the institutional administrator to

[2] R. Moos and J. Schwartz, "Treatment Environment and Treatment Outcome," *Journal of Nervous and Mental Disease,* 154(4):264-175, 1972.

help him develop his programs with these significant elements or dimensions in mind. It was believed that the measurement of these environmental elements or dimensions would give staff the opportunity to discuss the concepts represented by these elements and allow staff to formulate improvements. Retesting after a period of improvements would then present evidence of change, if any occurred.

As an example, one dimension assessed by the instrument is the support inmates feel they receive from staff and other inmates. If in a given institution the inmates feel they get little support and staff atempts to improve on this dimension, the kind of improvement achieved after a period of staff efforts can be assessed by readministering the test.

It seems especially important to draw attention to the need for preventive measures in correctional institutions. Acute crisis situations almost always result in physical and psychological damage to the persons involved and in program deterioration because of stricter custodial management which usually follows. Even if a crisis situation arises in an institution with a basically benign social climate, the defusing of the tension will be within reach. In an institution where the precrisis conditions were already comparable to a latent crisis of long standing, the defusing may be a very difficult, if not impossible, task.

For instance, it seems that efforts to introduce honest communications with rioting inmates during an acute crisis may in most cases be doomed if such honest communications traditionally never existed. Such communication efforts have to be established and then maintained day by day as an important concern of the institution. Staff has to be trained to keep communication channels open at all times. Such institutional policy not only may improve the quality of life in an institution but also may provide the most effective crisis control through these preventive steps.

The work reported in this paper should be evaluated with these project objectives in mind. Substantial progress has been made to date, but without doubt we are still at the beginning of the development of some useful aids to the institutional administrator and his staff. While we have reason to be encouraged by the results of our efforts, more work must be carried out if we are to make our correctional institutions more humane, more therapeutic, and safer for all concerned. This is important even in view of the fact that progress has been made in developing alternatives to imprisonment such as community-based correctional services. Prisons still are and will be for some time a very real and substantial part of corrections, and they need our full attention and study.

RELATED STUDIES

Murray[3] developed the concept of environmental press which he saw as the external situational counterpart to the concepts of internalized personal needs. Behavior was seen by Murray as the interactive functions of internal individual needs and the external environmental press. Cooley[4] and Mead[5] have tended to assume that most of the variance in behavior can be explained by situational or environmental differences. Recent research evidence suggests that (a) persons, (b) environments, and (c) person/environment interactions each contribute significantly to variance in behavior.

Raush, Dittman, and Taylor[6] and Raush, Farbman, and Llewellyn[7] studied hyperaggressive children and control children in a psychiatric treatment environment. They found that interactions between the child and the environmental setting were far more important in accounting for behavior that was either the child or the environment alone. These and other studies (Barker,[8] Engel and Moos,[9] Gump, Schoggen, and Redl[10] Moos,[11] Moos and Daniels,[12] Sells;[13] Soskin and John;[14] and Zinner[15] strongly indicate the importance of the environmental setting and of the person's interaction with the environment in accounting for behavioral variance and explain the important differences which may occur in the behavior of the same person in different environments or milieus.

[3] H.A. Murray, *Explorations in Personality*, New York: Oxford University Press, 1938.

[4] C.H. Cooley, *Human Nature and the Social Order*, New York: Scribner's, 1902.

[5] G.H. Mead, *Mind, Self and Society*, Chicago: University of Chicago Press, 1934.

[6] H.L. Raush, A.T. Dittman, and T.T. Taylor, "Person, Setting, and Change in Social Interaction," *Human Relations*, 12:361-378, November, 1959.

[7] H.L. Raush, I. Farbman, and L.G. Llewellyn, "Person, Setting, and Change in Social Interaction: II. A Normal Control Study," *Human Relations*, 13:305-332, November, 1960.

[8] R.G. Barker, (ed.), *The Stream of Behavior*, New York: Appleton-Century-Crofts, 1963; and R.G. Barker, "On the Nature of the Environment," *Journal of Social Issues*, 19:17-38, October, 1963.

[9] T. Engel and R.H. Moos, *"The Generality of Specificity,"* Archives of General Psychiatry, 16:574-581, May, 1967.

[10] P. Gump, P. Schoggen, and F. Redl, "The Camp Milieu and Its Immediate Effects," *Journal of Social Issues*, 13:40-46, 1957.

[11] R.H. Moos, "Situational Analyses of a Therapeutic Community Milieu," *Journal of Abnormal Psychology*, 73(1):49-61, 1968.

[12] R.H. Moos and D.N. Daniels, "Differential Effects of Ward Settings on Psychiatric Staff," *Archives of General Psychiatry*, 17:75-82, July, 1967.

[13] B. Sells, *General Theoretical Problems Related to Organizational Taxonomy: A Model Solution and Its Assumptions*, Fort Worth: Texas Christian University, Institute of Behavioral Research, 1966.

[14] W. Soskin and V. John, "The Study of Spontaneous Talk," in R.G. Barker, (ed.), *The Stream of Behavior*, New York: Appleton-Century-Crofts, 1963, pp. 228-287.

[15] L. Zinner, The Consistency of Human Behavior in Various Situations: A Methodological Application of Functional Ecological Psychology, Houston: University of Houston, unpublished doctoral dissertation, 1963.

Several earlier attempts have been undertaken to measure and compare environmental factors. For example, Stern[16] developed a test which measures college environments in terms of 30 ten-item environmental press scales. Findikyan and Sells[17] studied environmental press chacteristics of various types of campus groups.

Moos and his associates have done extensive work in the development of scales which assess the perceived climates of different social organizations – e.g., psychiatric wards,[18] community-oriented psychaitric programs such as day hospitals and residential treatment centers,[19] university student residences such as dormitories and fraternities,[20] and junior high and high school classrooms.[21] The conceptualization and method used in the present study closely parallel this earlier work.

In the past there has been very little empirical work done toward the development of measures which would differentiate between the social climate of different correctional units. Cressey,[22] in reviewing research about prisons, suggests that many "traits" exhibited by inmates or staff members in correctional organizations may be the result of characteristics of the organization rather than of the person. In an earlier work he points out that it has been customary to assume that "uncooperativeness," "loyalty," "honesty," "aggressiveness," and "paranoia" are characteristics belonging to the person exhibiting the behavior; and he suggests that diagnosis and explanation of various acting out behavior should take into account the environmental context in which the behavior occurs.[23]

The approach closest to the present study is the work by Street,

---

[16]G.G. Stern, *Scoring Instructions and College Norms: Activities Index, College Characteristics Index,* Syracuse, New York: Syracuse University, Psychological Research Center, 1963.

[17]N. Findikyan and S.B. Sells, "Organizational Structure and Similarity of Campus Student Organizations," *Organizational Behavior and Human Performance,* 1:169-190, December, 1966.

[18]R.H. Moos and P.S. Houts, "Assessment of the Social Atmospheres of Psychiatric Wards," *Journal of Abnormal Psychology,* 73(6):595-604, 1968.

[19]R.H. Moos, "Assessment of the Psychological Environments of Community-Oriented Psychiatric Treatment Programs," *Journal of Abnormal Psychology,* 79(1):9-18, 1972.

[20]M. Gerst and R.H. Moos, "The Social Ecology of University Student Residences," *Journal of Educational Psychology,* 1972, in press.

[21]E. Trickett and R.H. Moos, "The Social Environment of Junior High and High School Classrooms," *Journal of Educational Psychology,* 1972, in press.

[22]D.R. Cressey, "Prison Organizations," in J.G. March, (ed.), *Handbook of Organizations,* Chicago: Rand McNally, 1965, pp. 1,023-1,070.

[23]D.R. Cressey, (ed.), *The Prison: Studies in Institutional Organization and Change,* New York: Holt Rinehart and Winston, 1961.

Vintner, and Perrow[24] on the organizational climates of six different juvenile correctional institutions whose goals were oriented toward obedience/ conformity, re-education/development, or treatment. They hypothesized and demonstrated that the differences in institutional goals influenced staff perceptions about: (a) the inmates, (b) the staff/inmate authority relationship, (c) the patterns of social relations, and (d) the leadership that emerged among inmates. The results of this study strengthened the hypothesis that the organizational context of correctional institutions (institutional environment) may shape individual behavior.

METHOD

Instrument Development
Phase One:
Social Climate Scale Form A

The conceptual as well as the methodological basis of other perceived climate scales, particularly the WAS, was used for the new instrument except that items specifically relevant to correctional settings were constructed. The initial 194-item Form A of the Social Climate Scale (SCS) was administered together with the Marlowe-Crowne Social Desirability Scale to inmates and staff in 16 different correctional units in California.[25]

Instrument Development
Phase Two:
Social Climate Scale Form B

Items were then eliminated from the scale (1) if they did not significantly discriminate among units, (2) if they were found to only apply to extreme units, and (3) if the item correlated highly with the Marlowe-Crowne Social Desirability Scale. The result was the Form B which had 120 items which fell into twelve subscales, each characterizing one milieu dimension. Two additional subscales were added, one to assess positive and the other to assess negative halo. The name of the new instrument was changed from Social Climate Scale to Correctional Institutions Environment Scale (CIES), in order to make it clear that it was specifically relevant for correctional settings.

[24] D. Street, R.D. Vintner, and C. Perrow, *Organization for Treatment: A Comparative Study of Institutions for Delinquents,* New York: Free Press, 1966.
[25] R.H. Moos, "The Assessment of the Social Climates of Correctional Institutions," *Journal of Research in Crime and Delinquency,* 5(2):174-188, 1968.

Instrument Development
Phase Three:
Form C (CIES) Final Form

A grant from the National Institute of Mental Health to the NCCD Research Center made it possible to carry out a program of further development and standardization of the instrument. Starting in 1969, project staff from the Research Center of the National Council on Crime and Delinquency tested inmates and staff in various correctional institutions in Arkansas, California, Connecticut, Hawaii, Illinois, Kentucky, Mississippi, New Mexico, New York, Vermont, Washington, and in some institutjions of the Federal Bureau of Prisons. One part of the results of this testing is a shortened instrument: the 86-item Form C of the Correctional Institutions Environment Scale. Utilizing data from six states and the Federal Bureau of Prisons on inmates from 41 correctional units (N = 1,341) and data on staff from 15 correctional units (N = 526), the following steps were taken in obtaining the 86-item CIES Form C from the 140-item CIES Form B:

Step One. Item intercorrelations, item-to-subscale correlations, and subscale correlations, and subscale intercorrelations were calculated for both the inmates and staff sample.

The two subscales, Involvement and Affiliation, were combined into one subscale, Involvement. The items from both the Involvement and the Affiliation subscales with low item-to-subscale correlations and/or with extreme item splits were eliminated from the scale. The best ten items were retained to form the new Involvement subscale.

The Variety subscale was dropped because the items had generally low item-to-subscale correlations. The Aggression subscale, which was originally designed to measure the extent to which inmates are allowed and encouraged to argue with other inmates and staff or to become openly angry and to display other aggressive behavior, was also eliminated because of low item-to-subscale correlations and because some of the items on this scale had relatively extreme item splits. It is interesting to note that aggression, as defined in the Form B version of the instrument, was found not to be a relevant dimension in correctional settings as they function today. The tolerance in correctional milieus for open expression of anger and aggression even in verbal form is rather low. This is quite in contrast to psychiatric treatment units where such expressions are often encouraged and therapeutically utilized.

Both the positive and the negative halo response set subscales were dropped as they appeared to be unnecessary. Stringent criteria for inclusion of an individual's test protocol in a unit sample (less than ten missing items, no obvious patterns of all trues and/or all falses, or specific alternation patterns) was felt to be sufficient to guarantee valid data.

Thus by dropping the two halo response set subscales and the two subscales, Variety and Aggression, and by combining Affiliation and Involvement into one subscale, the step one revision resulted in nine instead of 14 subscales with 96 items instead of the 140 items of Form B. A revised scoring key was obtained, and the data were rescored on these nine subscales.

Step Two. After all the raw data from the inmate and the staff samples were rescored using the new 96-item, nine-subscale scoring key, item-to-subscale and subscale intercorrelations again were calculated. At this point a few items were dropped because of low item-to-subscale correlations or extreme item splits, and a few items which were eliminated in step one were included because they appeared to improve the meaning and/or psychometric consistency of a particular subscale.

The result was a step two scoring key containing 95 items in the nine subscales. The entire inmate and staff sample was rescored using the step two scoring key, and again item-to-subscale and sub-scale-to-subscale intercorrelations were calculated on the basis of this revised step two scoring key.

Step Three. Previous experience had indicated that either nine- or ten-item subscales would be psychometrically adequate. At this point seven items were dropped because each had highly similar content with one other item which was retained. All data were again rescored on the 88-item, nine-subscale step three scoring key; and item-to-subscale and subscale intercorrelations were again calculated.

Step Four. On the basis of the results of these last calculations, an additional shift of two items were made in order to obtain the final 86-item, nine-subscale Form C of the CIES.

During the entire revision procedure attempts were made to keep the meaning of each subscale as broad as possible and to reduce redundancy to a minimum. The reordering and more meaningful organization of the subscales reflect the attempt to develop research tools which not only satisfy scientific requirements but also are useful for the correctional administrator to assist him and his staff in reaching their objectives more effectively.

DESCRIPTION OF THE CIES[26]

CIES Form C has 86 items forming nine subscales which are organized around three principal dimensions relevant to correctional institutions as well as to other social environments: (1) people-to-people relationships, (2) institutional programs, and (3) institutional functioning. Table 1 describes the nine subscales.

---

[26] The CIES and scoring key are available from either author.

Table 1 Correctional Institutions Environment Scale (CIES), Form C
Description of Subscales

1. Involvement	Measures how active and energetic inmates are in the day-to-day functioning of the program—i.e., interacting socially with other inmates, doing things on their own initiative, and developing pride and group spirit in the program.
2. Support	Measures the extent to which inmates are encouraged to be helpful and supportive toward other inmates and how supportive the staff is toward inmates.
3. Expressiveness	Measures the extent to which the program encourages the open expression of feelings (including angry feelings) by inmates and staff.
4. Autonomy	Assesses the extent to which inmates are encouraged to take initiative in planning activities and take leadership in the unit.
5. Practical Orientation	Assesses the extent to which the inmate's environment orients him toward preparing himself for release from the program. Such things as training for new kinds of jobs, looking to the future, and setting and working toward goals are considered.
6. Personal Problem Orientation	Measures the extent to which inmates are encouraged to be concerned with their personal problems and feelings and to seek to understand them.
7. Order and Organization	Measures how important order and organization is in the program, in terms of inmates (how they look), staff (what they do to encourage order), and the facility itself (how well it is kept).
8. Clarity	Measures the extent to which the inmate knows what to expect in the day-to-day routine of his program and how explicit the program rules and procedures are.
9. Staff Control	Assesses the extent to which the staff use measures to keep inmates under necessary controls—i.e., in the formulation of rules, the scheduling of activities, and in the relationships between inmates and staff.

The first three subscales of Involvement, Support, and Expressiveness are conceptualized as measuring **relationship** dimensions.

They assess the extent to which inmates tend to become involved in the unit, the extent to which staff support inmates and inmates tend to support and help each other, and the extent of spontaneity and free and open expression within all these relationships. Thus, these variables essentially emphasize the type and intensity of personal relationships among residents and between residents and staff which exist in the milieu.

The next three subscales, i.e., Autonomy, Practical Orientation, and Personal Problem Orientation, are conceptualized as personal development or **treatment program** dimensions. Each of these subscales assesses a dimension which is particularly relevant to the type of treatment orientation the unit has initiated and developed. Autonomy assesses the extent to which inmates are encouraged to be self-sufficient and independent and to take responsibility for their own decisions. This is clearly an important treatment program variable and reflects a major value orientation by staff. The subscales of Practical Orientation and Personal Problem Orientation reflect two of the major types of treatment orientations which are currently in use in correctional institutions. For example, some units place extremely high emphasis on practical preparation for the inmate's release from the institution, as in training for new kinds of jobs, etc. On the other hand, some units strongly emphasize a personal problem orientation and seek to orient inmates toward increased self-understanding and insight. It is, of course, possible for some correctional units to emphasize both of these dimensions just as some may emphasize neither one.

The last three subscales of Order and Organization, Clarity, and Staff Control are conceptualized as assessing **system maintenance** dimensions. These dimensions are system oriented in that they all are related to keeping the correctional unit or institution functioning in an orderly, clear, organized, and coherent manner.

Each of the 86 items is expressed as a statement to be marked "true" or "false" by the inmates and by the staff. They are worded so that the respondent, by marking "true," indicates that he feels that the expressed behavior or condition is present or encouraged in his unit. A "false" response indicates that he feels it is not present or encouraged. The following items chosen from the nine subscales are presented to give some example:

1. Involvement:
   "Inmantes put a lot of energy into what they do around here."
   "Inmates on this unit care about each other."

2. Support:
   "Staff have very little time to encourage inmates."
   "The staff help new inmates get acquainted on the units."

3. Expressiveness:
   "Inmates are encouraged to show their feelings."
   "People say what they really think around here."

4. Autonomy:
    "Inmates are expected to take leadership on the unit."
    "The staff gives inmates very little responsibility."

5. Practical Orientation:
    "This unit emphasizes training for new kinds of jobs."
    "Inmates here are expected to work toward their goals."

6. Personal Problem Orientation:
    "Staff try to help inmates understand themselves."
    "Discussions on the unit emphasize understanding personal problems."

7. Order and Organization:
    "The staff make sure that the unit is always neat."
    "The staff set an example for neatness and orderliness."

8. Clarity:
    "If an inmate's program is changed, someone on the staff always tells him why."
    "Inmates never know when a counselor will ask to see them."

9. Staff Control:
    "Staff don't order inmates around."
    "All decisions about the unit are made by the staff and not by the inmates."

STANDARDIZATION OF THE CIES

For comparative purposes normative data are needed. This makes it possible to view individual correctional units against a national reference group. Norms were calculated using adult male inmate data from 41 institutional units (N = 1,341) and staff data from 15 institutional units (N = 526) collected with Form B and rescored with the CIES Form C scoring key. Table II shows the national norms of this reference group.

The CIES subscales measure the institutional environment as the individual inmate or staff member perceives it. Persons outside the unit may perceive it quite differently. If the scores of all inmates in one unit are combined and compared to the national norms in profile form, we obtain a picture of the way the group as a whole perceives the unit. Similarly, combining the scores of all unit staff gives us a measure of the consensual

Table 2 National Norms for Adult Males on the CIES Form C

Subscale	Inmates N = 41 Units		Staff N = 15 Units	
	Mean	S.D.	Mean	S.D.
Involvement	4.03	1.36	5.80	1.73
Support	3.38	1.28	6.29	1.43
Expressiveness	2.96	1.28	4.62	1.63
Autonomy	2.74	1.57	5.06	1.94
Practical Orientation	5.38	1.22	7.03	1.29
Personal Problem Orientation	3.76	1.27	5.38	1.60
Order and Organization	3.43	1.50	6.04	0.86
Clarity	3.27	1.11	5.73	0.74
Staff Control	6.44	1.13	4.83	1.69

interpretation by staff of the way they see the social climate of the unit. Four examples will illustrate such comparisons.

Figure 1 shows the profiles of residents and staff of a small open correctional community center. As can be seen, staff and residents perceive their unit very much alike. The agreement between staff and residents is striking and so is the general positive assessment which this unit received. The unit houses selected residents who live at the center until total release into the community. Most of the residents have jobs in the community during the day and a program of group counseling several days each week in the evening. Staff is highly selected and shows a good professional background.

Figure 2 shows the profiles of inmates and staff of an isolated correctional camp facility in a western state. The camp program consists of manual laboring tasks, some machine supported road maintenance work, and a well-developed crafts program. The camp population has recently been declining because of alternative correctional programs supported by the agency's administration. The staff/inmate ratio has been 1:1½ as staff has been maintained in spite of the reduced inmate population. As can be seen, the inmates have a perception of their camp unit that approximates the national norms. In contrast, staff perceives the social climate in the camp quite differently. The greatest discrepancies in Figure 2 occur for the subscales Support, Clarity, and Practical Orientation. Inmates feel that they

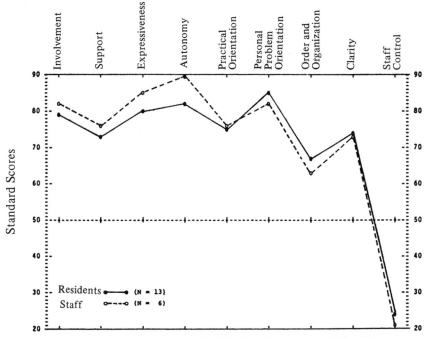

Fig. 1. CIES Standard Score Profiles for Residents and Staff in a Correctional Community Center in a Western State, 1971.

receive little support from each other and from staff, they feel that often they do not know what to expect in the day-to-day routine, and they seem to be somewhat uncertain about the rules and procedures. They also feel that they are not being well prepared for release and that they receive little training of value to them after release from the institution. Staff feels in all these areas that the program which they administer is better than average.

Such discrepancies in perception, if pronounced, may hinder good communication as both groups function in a somewhat differently perceived reality. It should be noted, however, that as a general rule staff scores are somewhat higher than inmate scores (Table 2).

While the first two examples intend to demonstrate how the CIES profiles can be helpful in pointing to staff/inmate congruence or discrepancies in the perception of their environment, the last two examples simply attempt to show how the institutional administrator and his staff could become aware of unit climates not easily obtained through observable unit activities. Such awareness could lead to staff actions aimed at further assessing a particular sector of the institution and finally to corrective measures if conditions seem in need of correction.

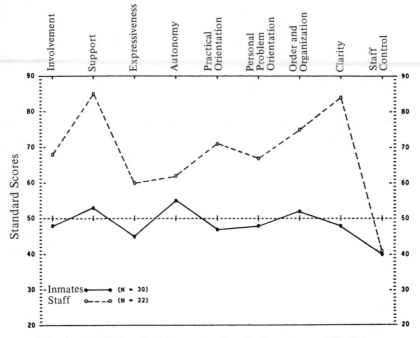

Fig. 2. CIES Standard Score Profiles for Inmates and Staff in a Correctional Camp in a Western State, 1971.

Figures 3 and 4 show the inmate profiles of two units of a southern prison. The most striking feature is the similarity of the two profiles. Compared to the national norms both profiles are quite low on the two relationship dimensions, Involvement and Support, and the two institutional maintenance dimensions, Order and Organization and Clarity. Also low is the institutional program dimension, Practical Orientation.

Perhaps there would be little concern if the two units were similar in their institutional assignments, and the results could be explained by pointing to the similarity of the two groups. The two groups are, however, very different in their composition and in their daily program; and this makes an interpretation more important.

Figure 4 shows the profile of inmates who are assigned to what staff may consider the best program in the institution: a vocational training program in the welding and automotive maintenance trades. Inmates in this program are assigned because of their vocational aptitude and motivation for learning vocational skills. Besides teaching, the program aids the institution by performing work for the agricultural operation of the institution – a major portion of the institution's activities. the program was relatively new when the testing was carried out.

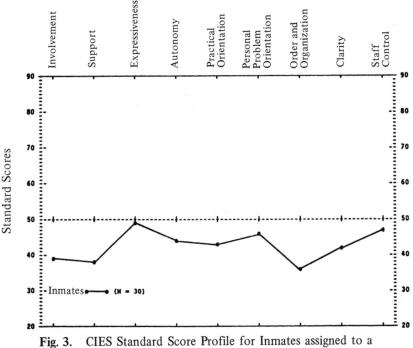

Fig. 3. CIES Standard Score Profile for Inmates assigned to a disciplinary Longline in a Southern Prison, 1971.

Figure 3 shows the profile of inmates who are assigned to a disciplinary Longline, working in the fields under heavy guard by gun-carrying inmate trusties. Inmates in this unit were assigned because of some institutional rules infraction for which they were cited and referred to a disciplinary committee. Their stay in this unit was, therefore, the outcome of a disciplinary action taken by the institutional staff. The testing for this latter group took place in a free-standing school building around which several armed inmate trusties were positioned, and another group of unarmed trusties took up position in the classroom while the testing proceeded. The profile of this group can be expected to show a somewhat depressed picture.

The profile in Figure 4 is unexpectedly low considering the different composition and programs of the two units. The inmates' perception of the social climate in the vocational shop area should lead to study by institutional staff and unit staff as the overall profile seems inappropriately low. Often administrative staff may be unaware of latent difficulties in specific units of their institution. Objective assessment, such as is attempted by the CIES, can provide the first step toward improvement of such situations. Profiles can be discussed and interpreted collaboratively between research staff and institutional staff; and if the profile can be accepted as reflecting accurately environmental factors, steps can be initiated toward correction of certain undesirable conditions.[27]

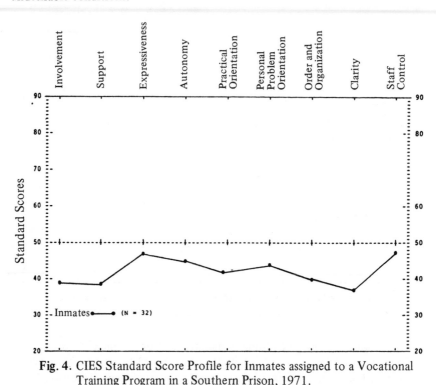

Fig. 4. CIES Standard Score Profile for Inmates assigned to a Vocational Training Program in a Southern Prison, 1971.

COMMENT

If we assume that the way people behave in a given environmental setting is the result of both their personal dispositions and the characteristics of the environment, then the scientific study of environmental characteristics or dimensions is of great significance.

We have reported on the development of a testing instrument which could become a practical working tool for the institutional administrator in helping him to direct the program development and staff training in his institution. Work is in progress on a number of other possible uses of the CIES and other assessment tools. For instance, the CIES Form C, which describes how staff and inmates perceive the unit to be at the time of the

---

[27]It should be noted that these data were obtained in early 1971 and that since then various institutional changes have occurred.

assessment, has a form which describes how staff and inmates think their unit ought to be in order to be an ideal unit. The CIES Ideal Form permits assessment of how staff or inmates envision an ideal unit, and comparison of the real unit climate with the envisioned ideal unit climate provides us with a measurement of how closely the existing conditions approximate the envisioned ideal conditions. Institutional staff could use such data to establish the magnitude of real/ideal social climate discrepancies and through improvement efforts attempt to bring the unit closer to what staff and inmates envision as their ideal unit climate. Thus, the two forms of the CIES can be used to facilitate and evaluate unit change through improvement efforts. Evidence from work in mental health settings indicates that CIES-type profiles, such as the Ward Atmosphere Scale (WAS) profiles, often provide a means to begin staff discussions on some of the environmental dimensions addressed by these instruments. In some of these studies it was observed that staff who, otherwise, seldom take part in staff discussions expressed themselves and actively took part in such training sessions (e.g., Pierce, et al.,[28] and Moos[29])

The CIES provides an opportunity to relate the size of units and their staffing patterns to the social climates prevailing in these various institutional units (e.g., Moos[30]).

In collaboration between project staff and research staff of the United States Bureau of Prisons, the CIES was used as part of the procedure set up to evaluate the efficacy of a demonstration project utilizing an incentive pay program based on actual inmate performance. The data collected during three testings with the CIES over a ten-month period showed that between the first and second testing all groups tested obtained an increase in their scores, pointing to a general improvement in the institution climate. The experimental group was clearly superior in the total number of positive changes in the way they viewed the institution. The third testing revealed a reversal of some of the positive changes noted during the first five months of the project, which was attributed by staff to some incidents in the institution involving intergroup conflicts among inmates around the time of the testing.[31]

Jesness in a California Youth Authority study compared two institutional treatment programs — one applying behavior modification techniques

[28]W.D. Pierce, E.J. Trickett, and R.H. Moos, "Changing Ward Atmosphere Through Staff Discussion of the Perceived Ward Environment," *Archives of General Psychiatry,* 26:35-41, January, 1972.

[29]R.H. Moos, "A Model for the Facilitation and Evaluation of Social Change," *Journal of Applied Behavioral Science,* 1972, in press.

[30]R. Moos, "Size, Staffing, and Psychiatric Ward Treatment Environments," *Archives of General Psychiatry,* 26:414-418, May, 1972.

[31]C. Frank and R. Michel, *Inmate Performance Pay Demonstration Project: Final Report,* El Reno, Oklahoma: Federal Reformatory, January, 1972, mimeo.

and the other transactional analysis methods — and used the CIES to describe the social climates in these units at the beginning of the program and after a two-year period of program application. The results appeared unusually clear in demonstrating that the introduction of new treatment programs had measurable effects on staff's and residents' perceptions of the social climate of each institution.[32]

The above uses of the CIES give some examples of potential application of the instrument. These applications are as relevant for the assessment of adult female correctional units as they are for juvenile correctional units and adult male institutions. As work in correctional settings continues with the CIES and other instruments, additional data will become available of interest not only to the scientific community but also to the correctional practitioner who seeks to utilize some of the research tools available today.

[32] C.F. Jesness, et al. "Program Impact on Social Climate," The Youth Center Research Project. Sacramento, California: American Justice Institute, July, 1972. Chapter IX, pp. 161-175.

15
Community Alternatives to Prison *

NORA KLAPMUTS

Incarceration in closed, security-oriented institutions is rapidly losing popularity as a rehabilitative or control measure for most offenders. The movement toward the expanded use and development of alternatives to the institutionalization of juvenile and adult offenders is spurred by observations that the traditional prison or training school is both excessively costly and ineffective as a rehabilitative tool. Not only has it been shown that imprisonment does not effectively rehabilitate or deter, but the actively destructive potential of most correctional institutions has frequently been emphasized.

It is not that prisons have suddenly become inhumane or destructive to individual lives or even, necessarily, that society has become more sensitive to the plight of those imprisoned. Prisons have never been less than terrible places and the history of prison reform is as long as imprisonment itself. The distinctive characteristic of the current reform effort is its emphasis on abolishing rather than improving the prison: it is no longer popular to hold that imprisonment can be transformed into an effective vehicle of rehabilitation through a massive infusion of manpower or treatment resources. In the light of criminological theory of the past decade, which views crime and delinquency as symptoms of disorganization of the community as much as of individual personalities — or even as a product of an inadequate mesh between the two — imprisonment is coming to be viewed as hopelessly

*Reprinted from *Crime and Delinquency Literature*, June 1973, 5, 305-337, with permission of the National Council on Crime and Delinquency.

anachronistic. It is now widely believed that *reintegration* of the offender with the law-abiding community — the primary goal of the "new" correction — cannot be accomplished by isolating the offender in an artificial, custodial setting.

Reintegration of offender and community was accorded legitimacy as the new direction in correction by the President's Crime Commission, which described the earlier orientation toward treating supposed defects in the individual offender as "a fundamental deficiency in approach." The Commission clearly stated its position that, since institutions tend to isolate offenders from society, "the goal of reintegration is likely to be furthered much more readily by working with offenders in the community than by incarceration."[1]

Since the Commission's report was issued in 1967, the goal of reintegration and the conviction that correction is best undertaken in the community setting have been restated by numerous official planning and policy-making bodies. The Wisconsin Council on Criminal Justice, in its report to the governor, unequivocally established as its study committee's fundamental priority the replacement by 1975 of Wisconsin's existing institutional correction system with a community-based noninstitutional system. The committee stated that all available resources, especially those previously expended for maintaining large correctional institutions, should be devoted to developing offenders' community ties.[2] The President's Task Force on Prisoner Rehabilitation concluded from its study of existing and alternate forms of prisoner rehabilitation that "any offender who can safely be diverted from incarceration ... should be."[3] The single most important recommendation emerging from the California Board of Corrections' study of the correctional system was that the bulk of the correctional effort, its programs and resources, be moved to the community level.[4] The National Council on Crime and Delinquency has issued a policy statement calling for a halt in institutional construction until maximum development and utilization of noninstitutional correction have been achieved.[5] The New Jersey Coalition for Penal Reform has recommended that the state abandon plans for future construction of large-scale custodial prisons while phasing out existing massive institutions.[6] The long-range master plan developed by the John Howard

[1] President's Commission on Law Enforcement and Administration of Justice, *The Challenge of Crime in a Free Society*, Washington, D.C.: U.S. Government Printing Office, 1967, p. 165.

[2] Wisconsin Council on Criminal Justice, *Final Report to the Governor of the Citizens' Study Committee on Offender Rehabilitation*, Madison, 1972.

[3] President's Task Force on Prisoner Rehabilitation, *The Criminal Offender—What Should Be Done?* Washington, D.C.: U.S. Government Printing Office, 1970.

[4] California Board of Corrections. *Correctional System Study—Coordinated California Corrections: The System*. Sacramento, 1971.

[5] Board of Trustees, NCCD, "Institutional Construction: A Policy Statement," Paramus, N.J., 1972.

[6] New Jersey Coalition for Penal Reform, "Position Paper," 1972.

Association for Maryland's Department of Juvenile Services envisions a 50 percent reduction in rates of institutionalization and a tripling of community services.[7] And in Massachusetts a series of bold steps has led to the closing of juvenile institutions and efforts to rapidly develop alternate programs for juvenile offenders.[8]

Disillusionment with the traditional correctional institution as a rehabilitative tool appears justified. Research evaluating institutional treatment has shown that incarceration, and especially lengthy incarceration, does not deter crime or recidivism.[9] The National Advisory Commission on Criminal Justice Standards and Goals notes in its task force report on corrections that treatment program tests have been conducted in a wide variety of incarcerative settings without establishing the rehabilitative value of any. Comments the task force: "The consistency of this record indicates that incarcerative treatment is incompatible with rehabilitative objectives."[10]

An interesting explanation of the counterproductive nature of imprisonment is offered by Robert Martinson in a series of articles on prison reform.[11] In documenting the disintegration of the correctional treatment approach (the offender-oriented medical model of individualized treatment), Martinson observes that efforts over the last 150 years to upgrade the prison environment and to improve and intensify the rehabilitation of inmates have not reduced recidivism rates. He suggests that recidivism rates are not affected by the prison regime itself; that instead they simply reflect the *interruption of normal occupational or life-cycle progress.* In today's highly technological society removal from the community for a period of years, especially at the ages when crime peaks (15 to 25), interferes with the exacting series of moves required to "make it" socio-economically and produces perhaps irreparable "life-cycle damage." While admittedly speculative, Martinson's view has explanatory potential; it suggests why prison reform and the introduction of a range of treatment approaches have not reduced the number of repeaters; it offers an explanation for the observed similarity in recidivism rates among systems with varying correctional practices;[12] it suggests why longer prison

[7] John Howard Association. *Comprehensive Long Range Master Plan: Department of Juvenile Services, State of Maryland.* Chicago, 1972.

[8] Massachusetts Department of Youth Services. *A Stragegy for Youth in Trouble,* Boston, 1972.

[9] California Legislature, Assembly Committee on Criminal Procedures, *Deterrent Effects of Criminal Sanctions.* Sacramento, 1968.

[10] National Advisory Commission on Criminal Justice Standards and Goals, Task Force on Corrections, *Report* (working draft), Austin, Tex., 1972, Ch. 17, "Research and Development, Information and Statistics," p. 8.

[11] Robert Martinson, "The Paradox of Prison Reform" (Parts I-IV), *New Republic,* 166(14):23-25, 1972; 166(15):13-15, 1972; 166(16):17-19, 1972; 166(17);21-23, 1972.

[12] California Legislature, *op cit. supra* note 9.

sentences (for the same offense) are associated with greater recidivism.[13] Prison, Martinson claims, even as it is enriched and improved, produces the paradoxical result of increasing recidivism — not directly by doing or not doing anything to the offender, but simply by removing him from society. He concludes, "Society has outgrown the prison, and deprivation of liberty has come to be a self-defeating measure in a modern industrial economy."[14]

Repeated evidence of the ineffectiveness of imprisonment has led to the radical redistribution of offenders from institutional to community programs in a few jurisdictions. In many others a new interest in community-based correction and a willingness to consider alternatives to incarceration are accompanied by confusion over where and how to reallocate correctional resources. State correction departments and planning groups, conscious of the failure of traditional correctional practices and of the possibilities for greater cost-effectiveness associated with a reorientation toward community-based correction, frequently do not know how to begin. What is meant by community correction? Who should be eligible for community management? What kinds of programs and resources must be developed to absorb the correctional population displaced by the phasing out of prisons and training schools? What programs have been tried and which have been successful? What should be the guiding principles for the use of community resources in lieu of confinement?

The range of programs and resources that should be developed by correctional systems as alternatives to jail, prison, and training school is outlined by the National Advisory Commission on Criminal Justice Standards and Goals in the working papers of its National Conference on Criminal Justice.[15] Its Task Force on Corrections has recommended that each correctional system begin immediately to develop a systematic plan with timetable and scheme for implementing a range of alternatives to institutionalization. Minimum alternatives to be included in the plan are specified: (1) pretrial and presentence diversion programs; (2) nonresidential supervision programs in addition to probation and parole; (3) residential alternatives to incarceration; (4) community resources open to confined populations and institutional resources available to the entire community; (5) prerelease programs; and (6) community facilities for released offenders in the critical

---

[13] Dorothy R. Jaman and Robert M. Dickover. *A Study of Parole Outcome as a Function of Time Served* (Sacrament, Calif: Department of Corrections, 1969); *A Study of the Characteristics and Recidivism Experiences of California Prisoners*. San Jose, Calif.: Public Systems, Inc., 1970.

[14] Robert Martinson, "The Paradox of Prison Reform" (Part I). *New Republic*. 166(14); 23-25, 1972, p. 25.

[15] National Advisory Commission on Criminal Justice Standards and Goals. *Working Papers of the National Conference on Criminal Justice, January 23-26, 1973*. Washington, D.C.: Law Enforcement Assistance Administration, 1973.

re-entry phase, with provision for short-term return as needed.[16] The Commission stresses the need to systematize on a state level the orderly development of community correction, with full consideration of specific local needs. The guiding principles stated by the Commission are supported by others who advocate the most limited possible use of institutionalization: (1) *No individual who does not absolutely require institutionalization for the protection of others should be confined.* (2) *No individual should be subjected to more supervision or control than he requires.*

The trend toward de-institutionalization begins before trial, with alternatives to jailing, or even before arrest, with diversion of noncriminal or marginally criminal cases to social, medical, or other nonjudicial resources. It extends to post-institutional services for parolees and includes a range of partial-imprisonment measures designed to maximize, or at least expand, the community involvement of incarcerated offenders. The principle that no person should be kept in a more secure condition or status than his potential risk dictates or receive more surveillance or "help" than he requires clearly demands the creation of alternatives to institutional handling at every stage of judicial and correctional processing. It implies a special emphasis on the development and use of alternatives at the initial stages of criminal justice and the diversion of more offenders to lower levels of correctional intervention at the earliest feasible opportunity.

Efforts to divert some classes of offenders from the criminal justice system entirely and the use of noninstitutional measures (suspended sentences, fines, probation) for potential jail inmates have been described elsewhere,[17]) as have the programs of partial or graduated release (work release, furlough, halfway houses) for prison inmates and parolees.[18] The present paper deals with community-based alternatives for serious (but not dangerous) offenders who would otherwise be candidates for incarceration in prison or training school. It is an attempt to respond to the questions that arise in connection with recommendations, currently coming from many sources, that the traditional prison or training school be abolished, phased out, or drastically reduced in population and that a large proportion of offenders now sentenced to such institutions be managed in community-based programs.

[16] *Id.,* p. C-140.
[17] Eleanor Harlow. *Diversion from the Criminal Justice System.* Washington, D.C.: National Institute of Mental Health, 1971; William L. Hickey, "Strategies for Decreasing Jail Populations," *Crime and Delinquency Literature.* 3(1):76-94, 1971; William L. Hickey and Sol Rubin, "Suspended Sentences and Fines," *Crime and Delinquency Literature,* 3(3):413-429, 1971.
[18] Eugene Doleschal. "Graduated Release." *Information Review on Crime and Delinquency.* 1(10):1-26, 1969.

Recommendations that prisons and training schools be phased out or abolished generally recognize that a relatively small proportion of offenders — those who are genuinely dangerous to the public and those whose crimes are so repulsive that public opinion demands retribution — will have to be incarcerated even under a reorganized correctional system. But, while the proportion of felony offenders incarcerated varies widely from one jurisdiction to another, probably nowhere are community alternatives being maximally utilized. Estimates of the percentage of offenders who must be imprisoned vary, largely because criteria of "dangerousness" have yet to be stated definitively[19]; but the consensus is that imprisonment is often greatly overused and institutional populations could be significantly reduced without additional risk to the community. Some of the ways in which institutional populations can be or have been reduced include the expanded use of probation, diversion to "intensive" or specialized probation or other non-residential treatment programs, immediate release to special parole services, referral to halfway house, group-home, or other residential programs, and where such centers are a real alternative to prison, placement in a community-based correctional center.

PROBATION PROGRAMS

A considerable proportion of offenders incarcerated in prison or training school probably are no more dangerous than many of those retained in the community on probation.[20] This would imply that the use of probation could be expanded to include many persons now sentenced to an institutional term. There is evidence that this could be accomplished without an increase in probation violation rates. The California Assembly Office of Research examined probation usage and violation data for eighty-eight U.S. district courts, for California superior courts, and for eight California counties. The findings indicated that violation rates are unaffected by the percentage of offenders granted probation. An examination of changes in probation for violation. In the federal district courts, probation usage ranged from 37 percent to 66 percent with no significant variation in violation rates.

[19] The Model Sentencing Act establishes criteria for identifying two groups characterized as dangerous; the assaultive criminal and the racketeer. NCCD Council of Judges, Model Sentencing Act (2nd ed.), Hackensack, N.J., 1972, p. 10.

[20] The California Assembly Office of Research estimates that at least 50 per cent of the men entering prison each year may be no more serious offenders than many of those placed on probation. California Assembly Office of Research. *Preliminary Report on the Costs and Effects of the California Criminal Justice System and Recommendations for Legislation to Increase Support of Local Police and Corrections Programs.* Sacramento, 1969.

There was no support for the assumption that greater reliance on probation as a sentencing disposition is associated with an increase in violations.[21]

These data contradict the belief that offenders now incarcerated could be released to probation in the community only under greatly intensified supervision. Widely divergent rates of probation usage indicate that offenders who are incarcerated in one jurisdiction are retained on probation in another, apparently without adversely affecting crime or other violation rates. And probation appears to do fairly well with those offenders it handles, even under the supposedly adverse conditions of unmanageably large caseloads and little officer time for supervision. Studies of offenders under normal probation supervision have indicated a relatively high success rate. A study of 943 male probationers 16 to 18 years old revealed that about 72 percent were successfully discharged.[22] In a summary analysis of fifteen probation studies in various jurisdictions, Ralph England found reported success rates ranging between 60 and 90 percent; and a survey of probation effectiveness in Massachusetts, California, New York, and a number of foreign countries reports similar results with the modal success rate at about 75 percent.[23]

England explains that many offenders are "self-correcting" and are not likely to recidivate, while others would be dissuaded from further offending merely through exposure to the limited surveillance of the suspended sentence. Empey has suggested that, since the majority of offenders now placed on probation can succeed without much supervision, many of those offenders now incarcerated might succeed under intensified community supervision.[24] Many, apparently, also can succeed under normal or minimal supervision. Certainly no assumption should be made that candidates for institutionalization necessarily require more intensive supervision or "treatment."

Efforts to reduce the use of imprisonment by placing more offenders on probation have often assumed that more officers and smaller caseloads would be prerequisite. The Saginaw Project of the Michigan Council on Crime and Delinquency successfully reduced the percentage of felony offenders imprisoned during the three-year (1957-60) experiment from 36.6 percent to 19.3 percent by increasing the use of probation and other dispositions.[25] The

[21] James Robinson. *The California Prison, Parole and Probation System.* Sacramento: California Assembly Office of Research, 1969, pp. 27-32.

[22] Frank R. Scarpitti and Richard M. Stephenson, "A Study of Probation Effectiveness," *Journal of Criminal Law, Criminology and Police Science,* 59(3):361-369, 1968.

[23] Ralph England, "What Is Responsible for Satisfactory Probation and Post- Probation Outcome?" *Journal of Criminal Law, Criminology and Police Science,* 47(6):667-677, 1957; Max Grunhut, *Penal Reform* New York: Clarendon, 1958.

[24] La Mar T. Empey. *Alternatives to Incarceration.* Washington, D.C.: Office of Juvenile Delinquency and Youth Development, 1967.

[25] Michigan Council, NCCD. *Saving People and Money: A Pioneer Michigan Experiment in Probation.* East Lansing, Mich., 1963.

number of probation officers was increased and caseloads were reduced to the "ideal" maximum of fifty units per officer. This project demonstrated that prison dispositions could be cut in half with no additional risk to the community. However, it is far from clear that small caseloads alone were responsible for the success of this project: research on the impact of reduced caseloads in probation and parole has not supported the assumption that more intensive supervision in small caseloads would reduce violation and offense rates among those supervised.

Caseload Research

Despite the appeal of reducing caseloads to improve supervision, research during the 1960's clearly indicated that merely reducing caseload size does not reduce recidivism. A parole research project in Oakland, Calif., began in 1959 to test whether reducing caseloads of parolees would improve parole performance. Additional agents were employed and ten experimental 36-unit caseloads were established, with five 72-unit caseloads as controls. When the project was terminated in 1961 no overall difference was found in parole performance for reduced and full-size caseloads.[26]

California's Special Intensive Parole Unit (SIPU) studies,[27] conducted in four segments from 1953 through 1963, obtained similar results. Adult parolees were randomly assiged to caseloads of fifteen, thirty, thirty-five, seventy-two and ninety men (the last two serving as controls) and comparisons were made between experimentals and controls and among experimentals. These studies involved several thousand men and follow-ups of at least two years. No significant differences were found in the performances of conventional and any of the three experimental caseloads when offenders were randomly assigned. In the third phase, parolees were classified and assigned according to "risk" categories on base expectancy scores. The results of this experiment were equivocal but there was evidence that, regardless of caseload size, high-risk parolees violated extensively and low-risk parolees seldom violated, while the middle-risk cases performed distinctly better in smaller caseloads. The low-risk cases did as well in very large caseloads as in regular caseloads.

The University of California's San Francisco Project focused on federal probation and parole and the effects of different caseload sizes.[28] Individuals

[26] Bertram M. Johnson. "The 'Failure' of a Parole Research Project," *California Youth Authority Quarterly.* 18(3):35-39, 1965.

[27] California Department of Corrections, Special Intensive Parole Unit, *Research Reports, Phases I-IV,* Sacramento, 1953-64.

[28] University of California School of Criminology. San Francisco Project. *Research Reports.* Berkeley, 1965-67.

placed on probation or parole were randomly assigned to caseloads receiving one of four types of supervision: minimum, intensive, "ideal," and normal. Persons in minimum or "crisis" caseloads were required only to submit a monthly written report to the probation office; no routine contacts occurred unless requested by the offender. Intensive caseloads consisted of twenty units each and contact occurred at least weekly. Ideal caseloads were composed of fifty units, and normal caseloads consisted of one hundred units per month. The results of this experiment indicated that offenders in minimum caseloads performed as well as would be expected had they been receiving normal supervision. The minimum and the ideal caseloads had almost identical violation rates. In intensive caseloads, despite fourteen times the attention provided the minimum cases, the violation rate not only failed to decline but increased with respect to technical violations. Caseload groupings did not differ with respect to nontechnical violations; thus the small caseload was not demonstrated to be more effective in reducing recidivism. The results were interpreted as suggesting (1) that some offenders will succeed under supervision regardless of the type of service while others will violate no matter how much attention they receive; and (2) that with identification of these offender groups, officer time could be allocated to give most attention to those (middle-risk) offenders whose success depends on the presence of certain types of supervision.

These and other studies indicated that reduced caseloads in themselves are of relatively little importance. In both the SIPU studies and the San Francisco Project it was found that good risks could be managed safely in very large, minimally supervised caseloads. Both also found that small caseloads were associated with higher rates of technical violation, a fact which has been attributed to the increased supervision made possible by reduced caseloads.[29] Attention has since shifted away from the study of numbers and toward an emphasis on differential caseload management — that is, toward offender classification and assignment to specialized caseloads identified as appropriate for specific offender (risk-level) types. Experience with differential management in "work-unit" caseloads has suggested that it is feasible to place the more serious offender or the poorer risk on probation without increasing the danger to the community.

[29] James Robison and Gerald Smith. "The Effectiveness of Correctional Programs." *Crime and Delinquency.* 17(1):67-80, 1971.

Differential Caseload Management

In California the work-unit concept has been operative since 1965 when the Work Unit Program was experimentally introduced into parole.[30] This was an experiment in parole programing that provided differential levels of supervision for parolees through a reduction in the size of certain caseloads. The program was designed to provide intensive supervision for selected parolees (such as high violence-potential cases) and less intensive supervision for parolees whose behavior indicated a potential for favorable adjustment. Three levels of supervision were designated with different weights assigned to cases at each level. The sum of weights assigned to the cases supervised by an agent was set at 120 (an average caseload of thirty-five). The Work Unit Program was expected to result in greater use of community resources and in reductions in both parole violation rates and the incidence of new crimes committed by parolees. A follow-up study comparing parole outcomes of work-unit and conventional caseloads (of about seventy cases) indicated a lower return-to-prison rate for the work-unit parole population.[31] A cost savings was also demonstrated for programs based on the workload concept.

A study was initiated in Washington, D.C., to obtain information about the offender population under supervision in the Probation Office of the U.S. District Court for the District of Columbia, and to apply this information in devising a more effective case-management approach based on the needs of the offenders and the resources available to the probation officer.[32] Three major objectives of the study were (1) to classify the entire population under supervision, using a multi-factor instrument designed to predict the outcome of supervision; (2) to attempt to validate the predictive ability of the instrument by comparing all cases that closed successfully with those closed unsuccessfully during all eighteen-month period; and (3) to use the data to set up differential caseload sizes based on high or low success potential.

A total of 1,210 cases were divided into three groups: 43 percent of the entire caseload were rated A for high potential for favorable adjustment; 44 percent were rated B for medium potential; and 13 percent were rated C for

---

[30] The program is briefly described in the *1971 Annual Research Review of the California Department of Corrections,* pp.49-50.

[31] Robison and Takagi take issue with this finding, pointing out that Work Unit caseloads were comprised of better-risk parolees and that when controls for parolee risk level were introduced the difference in parole outcome for work-unit and conventional caseloads was erased. J. Robison and P. Takagi, "Case Decisions in a State Parole System," California Department of Corrections, Research Division, 1968, Administrative Abstract Research Report No. 31.

[32] Robert I. Weiner, "Probation Caseload Classification Study in the United States District Court for the District of Columbia." Washington, D.C.: American University, n.d.

low potential. Each of the seventeen field officers had an unequal distribution of A's, B's and C's in his caseload. Phase II found a closing rate of 63 percent success, with 93 percent of the A group successfully completing their probation while 56 percent of the B group and 17 percent of the C group were successful. Phase III revealed a low number of individuals with a C rating, a result attributed to the screening process employed by the probation staff at the time of the presentence investigation. More than half (52 percent) of those recommended for probation were rated A, while nearly two-thirds (62 percent) of those not recommended for probation were rated C.

On the basis of the findings of this study the following recommendations were made. The Base Expectancy 61-A scoring instrument should be used when preparing the presentence investigation report because of its high accuracy in predicting adjustment. Individuals rated A should be placed in caseloads receiving minimal supervision while C offenders should receive intensive supervision. Officers responsible for supervising those rated A should handle caseloads of at least two hundred cases each. A counseling unit of field officers should supervise offenders rated B and a "crash unit" should be created to work exclusively with low potential offenders in caseloads of a maximum of thirty to thirty-five persons each.

The implications of research on differential or work-unit caseloads for the "deprisonization" effort are clear. If offenders with a high potential for success on probation can be moved out into very large, minimally supervised caseloads (or be given suspended sentences without supervision, fines, restitution orders, or other non-probation dispositions), the probation system will be freed to concentrate its efforts on medium- and poor-risk probationers as well as to absorb that group of offenders now sent to prison or training school because the authorities believe normal probation supervision to be insufficient for them. Not all offenders currently institutionalized are poor risks (in the District of Columbia study, 38 percent of persons not recommended for probation were rated other than C), so not all offenders diverted from incarceration will require placement in the intensive-supervision programs developed for the poor-risk group. Classification must occur before decisions are made as to appropriate disposition.

Probation for the Serious Offender

Many offenders currently are sent to prison or training school because traditional probation supervision is believed insufficient for their control or rehabilitation. Thus, while greater use of suspended sentences, fines, and regular probation will contribute to the reduction of prison populations, any plans to maximize the use of community alternatives will have to deal with the question of what to do with those offenders who appear to need more supervision, services, or assistance in order to remain out of trouble with the law. Although these individuals are not dangerous (the small minority of offenders who are truly dangerous will be incarcerated) they are likely to repeat offenses and to have difficulty adjusting successfully in the community.

A broad range of services and programs has been provided for the treatment of offenders who require more intensive services than regular supervision: group or family counseling may be offered as a service of the court; the offender may be referred to community service agencies for additional assistance; probation officers may meet with selected probationers in frequent group sessions; the juvenile probationer may be required to attend daycare centers or centers providing remedial education or vocational training; and juveniles for whom living with their families is contraindicated because of undesirable home situations may be placed in foster or group homes. Adult offenders also may be required to live in a community residence or halfway house as a condition of probation. Many courts have utilized local volunteers to work with offenders in various capacities, providing tutoring assistance, foster homes, group discussion sessions, counseling, or simply a supportive relationship with a community resident. Most of these programs have not been evaluated. Assessments of effectiveness, where they have been attempted at all, frequently are not very useful: no control group is used, the groups are not comparable, or assignment is not random. Many descriptive studies merely report the subjective judgments of staff or the observed changes over time in arrest patterns of project participants. This means that much of the "community treatment" literature must be interpreted cautiously, although it may still be useful in suggesting the kinds of intervention alternatives that have been tried and that may be duplicated elsewhere.

The variety of services available as an adjunct to probation has permitted some courts greater flexibility in their disposition of offenders for whom neigher institutionalization nor regular probation supervision is considered suitable. However, in many jurisdictions the court simply has no available alternative to incarceration and many offenders are sent to prison or training school who do not need to be there. State subsidy programs have been instituted in an attempt to reduce costs and overcrowding in state institutions by retaining more offenders in the community at the county level. Some of the savings resulting from reduced commitments are diverted to the counties for the purpose of expanding and upgrading probation services for these offenders.

State Subsidy Programs

In 1965 the California State Legislature passed legislation that provided a state subsidy to county probation departments to set up special supervision programs, to increase the degree of supervision of individual cases, and to develop and improve supervisional practices.[33] Reduced commitment of offenders to state correctional institutions was made a mandatory condition for the receipt of subsidy monies. The enabling legislation was the result of the recommendation of a 1964 Board of Corrections probation study undertaken to determine how state costs could be reduced while county probation programs were improved. This study determined that 25 percent of state correctional commitments could be maintained safely and effectively within county systems if probation services were improved. The subsidy plan that was ultimately adopted provided for reimbursement by the state to the counties in proportion to the number of cases retained in the county exceeding the existing rate. A sliding scale was developed to avoid penalizing counties that already had low commitment rates. The following assumptions are among those that influenced the character of the legislation: (1) The most effective correctional services are provided in local communities. (2) Straight probation (without jail) is the least costly service available. (3) Probation is at least as effective as most institutional forms of care. (4) Probation grants can be increased without increasing recidivism. (5) The actual rate of probation grants is determined by the decisions of probation officers and probation decision-making can be altered by rewarding approved behavior. (6) Costs for improved probation supervision can be offset by savings at the state level.

By 1970-71 forty-five counties (over 97 percent of the state population) were operating approved subsidy programs.[34] Commitments to state institutions had decreased markedly: during that year the state received 4,500 to 5,000 fewer commitments than would have been expected had the program not been in operation. Although the more than $18-million in subsidy funds paid to the counties was a new high for the five years of the program, it was still considerably less than what it would have cost to keep these offenders in prisons or training schools. The reduction of commitments also has sharply reduced the need to build new institutions – a potential savings of millions of dollars. Construction of juvenile institutions has come to a halt and several existing training schools have been closed down.

One example of the county programs developed under the California

---

[33]For a description of the origin of state subsidy programs in California and six other states, see Leslie T. Wilkins and Don M. Gottfredson, *Research Demonstration and Social Action*. Davis, Calif.: NCCD Research Center, 1969, pp. 43-70.

[34]Robert L. Smith. *A Quiet Revolution: Probation Subsidy*. Washington, D.C.: Youth Development and Delinquency Prevention Administration, 1971.

state subsidy is the Special Supervision Unit Program of the Santa Barbara County Probation Department.[35] This program provides intensive, individualized supervision as an alternative to institutionalization. Caseloads are limited to forty-two cases per officer. Each officer receives training in classification and diagnosis. All cases are classified by I-Level methods on a scale that determines the individual's level of social integration. Methods of treatment vary with type of offender, but the basic goal of early confrontation and intensive involvement with the probationer is standard. Typically, the offender is seen two to four times per month; in addition, he participates in group counseling, a public agency therapy program, or a special Unit program (such as the Work Project) one-half day per week. Minor violations may be handled in the Unit or by modification of probation, thus serving as a lesson in rehabilitation.

Serious attempts to evaluate the state subsidy program have only just begun. The California Youth Authority (which administers the program for both adults and juveniles) is setting up a basic information system that will provide considerable data on subsidy probationers. Description and some evaluation of the various treatment approaches initiated under the program have also begun. Preliminary reports on some programs have been issued; for example, the Community Oriented Youthful Offender Program (COYOP), one of the Los Angeles County Probation Department's Community Retention Programs.[36] This report notes that the rate of favorable departures from COYOP is at least as good as that of nonsubsidy probation caseloads, even though COYOP caseloads are comprised of more serious offenders. A California Criminal Statistics Bureau study of the statewide subsidy population reports a 55.5 percent success rate for subsidy-caseload probationers, which compares well with the 65 percent success rate for regular caseloads of less serious offenders.[37]

California's probation subsidy program has demonstrated that serious offenders, normally not eligible for probation, can be retained successfully in the community under special supervision programs without jeopardizing public safety and that this can be accomplished at considerable savings of taxpayers' dollars. Other states (e.g., Washington, Pennsylvania, Colorado) have introduced state subsidy programs, not necessarily on the California

[35] Santa Barbara County Probation Department, "Special Supervision Unit Program," Santa Barbara, Calif., 1968.

[36] Lawrence Yonemura and others. *Subsidy Evaluation Project: Community Oriented Youthful Offender Program.* Los Angeles: Los Angeles County Probation Department, 1971.

[37] "Characteristics, Case Movement, Disposition, Experience of Superior Court Probationers in Regular and Subsidy Caseloads." Sacramento, Calif.: Criminal Statistics Bureau, 1971.

model. The Washington program, in operation since January 1970, allows for state subsidy of county probation supervision for juveniles who are eligible for commitment to state institutions. State commitments by participating counties decreased 42.8 percent during the first year, while nonparticipating counties showed increases. Participating counties also implemented new programs and have made better use of existing resources.[38] Not all state subsidy monies have been used to upgrade or modify probation supervision. In Oregon, state funds were used to develop small group-home facilities and in Philadelphia a day center was established.[39] The concept of the state subsidy to county probation departments or, as in Oregon, to the public or private agency operating the program, is a flexible tool that could be used not only to finance improvements in probation service but also to provide the means for developing a wide range of other community programs for offenders.

INTENSIVE INTERVENTION PROGRAMS

When alternatives to incarceration in prison or training school are considered, it is most commonly assumed that some special program of intensive supervision, services, or treatment will be required for the successful handling of offenders who are candidates for institutionalization. Research and experimentation have indicated, however, that there are certain types of offenders (some of those currently on probation and some of those imprisoned) who are likely to fail on probation unless considerable effort is invested in their rehabilitation. Programs developed for this group of serious, habitual, or poor-risk offenders, while they may technically be probation programs in that participation is made a condition of probation, generally entail a much greater involvement with the offender than simple supervision and counseling and may attempt to achieve a considerable modification of attitudes and behaviors that extends beyond the prevention of law violations. More than the probation-plus-services or the small specialized caseload approach, these "intensive intervention" programs are frequently distinguished by their coherent theoretical base or by their very comprehensive approach to changing the lifestyles of offenders assigned to them. Because intensive intervention might easily be construed as interference, and because such programs are certainly more costly than regular probation or other dispositions of lower intervention level, assignment to such programs should

[38] Washington State Institutions Division, "Probation Subsidy in Washington State: Calendar Year 1970." *Research Report.* 3(14):1-24, 1971.

[39] Wilkins and Gottfredson, *op.cit. supra* note 33.

be preceded by a determination that an offender (a) needs the services or treatment and (b) is able to benefit from them.

Intensive intervention programs appear to use either of two approaches to offender rehabilitation or reintegration: one emphasizes *treatment* or attitude and behavior modification; the other focuses on the provision of *services* (vocational training, job-finding, medical care, financial assistance or guidance). There may be an element of both in any given program. The argument for services as opposed to treatment for offenders derives from the observation that treatment programs — at least under the coercive circumstances of the correction system — do not work. A recent survey of 231 treatment program evaluations published from 1945 to 1967 indicated that the outlook for successful *treatment* of offenders is bleak.[40] Others have supported this finding[41] and some have suggested that correction should either reduce its operations to a minimum[42] or concentrate on providing those services that the offender himself identifies as useful to him. One author has even suggested the implementation of a voucher system in which offenders would be given wide discretion in designing their own rehabilitation programs through the voluntary choice and purchase of services.[43] Another has recommended a correctional policy of minimizing harm or interference and maximizing help to the offender (job training, placement services, parole income, free psychiatric help if requested) in a crime-control approach that emphasizes not offender correction but public protection and victim compensation.[44] Intensive intervention programs, whether service- or treatment-oriented or both, must be viewed in the light of current thinking in correction (less — not more — intervention, the inutility of coercive programs, offender participation in selection of services, etc.) and the evidence that no treatment effort has yet been unambiguously successful.

Despite repeated claims that nothing works, intensive community intervention still generates considerable interest, and treatment programs, both residential and nonresidential, have been established and operated with apparent success. The important point that has been made by the operation of such programs is that community-based alternatives to incarceration can handle the institutional candidate at least as effectively as imprisonment,

[40] Douglas S. Lipton, Robert Martinson, and Judith Wilks, *Effectiveness of Correctional Treatment: A Survey of Treatment Evaluations.* New York: State Office of Crime Control Planning, 1970.

[41] Robison and Smith, *supra* note 29.

[42] James Robison. *The California Prison, Parole and Probation System.* Sacramento, 1970. California Assembly Office of Research Technical Supplement No. 2.

[43] David F. Greenberg. "A Voucher System for Correction." *Crime and Delinquency.* 19(2):212-17, 1973.

[44] Martinson, *supra* note 11.

without serious risk to public safety, at less expense, and with less destructive impact on the offender and his family. These community programs may be residential, requiring the offender to live in a group home, halfway house, or community correction center, or they may be nonresidential, enabling the offender to live at home while participating in the program. Because many believe nonresidential programs to be preferred for their less disruptive effect on the normal lives of offenders, the two types of program are treated separately here. Only a few models are highlighted. Representing the nonresidential community program are the California Youth Authority Department's Community Treatment Project, an example of intensive differential treatment of juveniles; the guided group interaction programs, illustrating peer-group efforts to change juvenile behavior and lifestyles; and NCCD's "second-offender" project, which utilizes both treatment and service approaches to deal with second-felony recidivists. Group-home projects and Minnesota's PORT program are residential, as is the Community Integration Project in Easton, Pa.

Many other programs could be mentioned. Massachusetts, in seeking alternatives to the state's now inactivated training schools, has developed a youth advocate system which provides for an alternate residence at the home of a youth advocate, enrollment in school or special education program, assistance in obtaining employment, contact with courts and community agencies, work with families, and participation of youths in developing their own individualized programs. This program and a range of other residential and nonresidential alternatives to training schools were discussed at a conference held in June 1972.[45] An innovative program being developed in Minnesota for offenders rejected for regular probation will provide for the formulation of an explicit restitutjion plan involving the offender, an agent of the criminal justice system, and whenever possible, the victim. Implementation of the plan will include group or individual monitoring of the extent to which the agreement is fulfilled; discharge from custody (and from residence in a community correction center) will immediately follow an offender's completion of the program. Offenders will be offered the option of participating in the program, which is essentially a contractual reconciliation through negotiated settlement by the parties involved, mediated by a representative of the correctional system.[46] The Minneapolis Rehabilitation Center provides a service-oriented program for parolees that could be adapted for probationers who require more extensive assistance to remain out of

[45] Massachusetts Youth Services Department and Fordham University Institute for Social Research. *Conference Proceedings for "The Closing Down of Institutions and New Strategies in Youth Services," June 26-28, 1972.* Boston, Mass., 1972.

[46] David Fogel, Burt Galaway, and Joe Hudson, "Restitution in Criminal Justice: A Minnesota Experiment," *Criminal Law Bulletin,* 8(8):681-691, 1972.

prison. A three-year demonstration project was undertaken to test the impact of comprehensive social, psychological, and vocational services on recidivism rates, vocational stability, and personal adjustment of parolees referred to the Center. The project involved the cooperation of private and public agencies and an interdisiplinary team approach to the coordination of correctional and vocational services. Experimentals were given the services of a social worker, vocational counselor, and clinical psychologist besides referral opportunities to consult with a physician, a psychiatrist, and other professional personnel as needed. Financial assistance was also provided. It was found that experimentals committed significantly fewer and less serious offenses than controls.[47]

NONRESIDENTIAL COMMUNITY INTERVENTION

Community Treatment Project

One of the most widely known experiments in community alternatives to institutionalization, the California Youth Authority Department's Community Treatment Project (CTP), has applied the concepts of offender classification and individualized treatment to a program designed to extend the use of community supervision to offenders who would normally be incarcerated.[48] The original objectives of the project were to test the feasibility of substituting intensive supervision of juveniles in the community for the regular program of institutionalization plus parole and to develop optimum treatment/control plans for each type of offender identified. Since its inception in 1961, the CTP has been investigating many of the questions about differential management raised by its own and other research. While all phases of the project have been based on caseloads of twelve to fifteen clients, the research has suggested that caseload size is only one of many factors responsible for the demonstrated success of the community program. Factors identified as associated with the superior effectiveness of the community-based program include offender classification and differential treatment-relevant decision-making. Intensive or extensive intervention made possible by reduced caseloads and matching of offender types with agent types are also considered important.

Since 1961 the Community Treatment Project has handled seriously delinquent male and female offenders who have been committed from the juvenile courts in California to the state correctional system. Rather than

[47]Richard C. Ericson and Daniel O. Moberg. *The Rehabilitation of Parolees.* Minneapolis, Minn.: Minneapolis Rehabilitation Center, 1969.

[48]California Youth Authority, Community Treatment Project. *Research Reports.* Sacramento, 1961-72.

being institutionalized in state training schools, these youths are placed directly on parole in the community program. After commitment to the reception center, wards are assigned randomly either to a control group, to be given the regular program of institutionalization plus parole, or to the experimental group, to be released immediately to small specialized caseloads in the community. The experimentals, after being classified according to Interpersonal Maturity Level (I-Level) and matched with a parole agent, receive differential or individualized long-term treatment.

The CTP progress reports have been consistently positive in their evaluation of the experimental program. During phase I, the overall success rate of project participants was found to be significantly higher than that of youths in the regular Youth Authority program. Differential success rates were reported: certain types of youth appeared to do especially well under the given treatment conditions while others did about as well as they would have done in an institution or on parole. Additionally, psychological test scores indicated that experimentals achieved greater positive change than control subjects and a higher level of personal and social adjustment. Throughout phase II, follow-up of study subjects from both phases continued to indicate large differences favoring experimentals over controls. Fifteen-month follow-up data showed that 30 percent of male experimentals had violated parole or been unfavorably discharged, as compared with 51 percent of male controls (and 45 percent of regular statewide Youth Authority releasees). At twenty-four months, these outcomes were 43 percent and 63 percent respectively, again favoring the experimental group.

The CTP findings on recidivism, which indicated that the community program is *more* effective than imprisonment, have been challenged by James Robison and others who conclude from analysis of the CTP data that recidivism rates have been managed in such a way as to make the experimentals appear favorable. These authors explain that recidivism rates can be influenced, within certain parameters, by the decision-making authorities and that in the CTP an ideological belief in the effectiveness of community treatment apparently altered the experimental results.[49] In a re-examination of the data, Lerman found that the response to experimentals' offenses was less likely to be revocation unless the offense was of high severity. Experimentals were no less delinquent than controls but they were significantly less likely to have their paroles revoked for offenses of low or moderate severity.[50]

Regardless of the validity of such criticism, the Community Treatment

[49] Robison and Takagi, *supra* note 31. See also Robison and Smith, *supra* note 29.
[50] P. Lerman, "Evaluating the Outcome of Institutions for Delinquents," *Social Work,* 13(3):55-64, 1968.

Project has made some important contributions to both theory and practice in community correction. Providing a composite of diagnostic categories and treatment modalities, the CTP represents an evolving, practical intervention program for delinquency control and a clear alternative to institutionalization for juveniles. The experimental program has been able to handle a large majority of eligible youths (90 percent) *at least as effectively* as the regular institutional program, while 10 percent have been shown to do better in the traditional program.

Phase III (1969-74) of the Community Treatment Project is concentrating on the development of more effective techniques for working with the 25 percent of youths who seem to do poorly in both the traditional and the community-based programs. A CTP residential facility has been utilized to test the impact of an initial residential placement for these youths. Another objective of this phase has been to determine whether the CTP approach can be applied successfully to a wider range of offenders than has been handled to date — such as those committed from adult courts or for seriously assaultive offenses. In this experiment, eligible youths are studied by a clinic team of treatment and research personnel who assign each ward to one of two statuses: Status I youths are predicted to perform better if treatment begins within the CTP residential treatment center; Status II youths are those for whom it is believed treatment should begin within the community. Wards are then randomly assigned to either the community setting or the residential setting. The resulting four separate study groups are later compared on growth, parole adjustment, and other outcome measures. Preliminary analyses have suggested that Status I youths who began their treatment within the CTP residential facility performed considerably better following initial release to parole than Status I youths who began treatment in the community. Status II youths (wards seen as not needing initial residential treatment) who began treatment within the residential facility performed somewhat worse than Status II youths who were released directly to the community.[51] Though tentative, these findings indicate that neither institutionalization nor community treatment is equally effective with all types of juveniles. The CTP thus continues to refine its typologies of offenders and treatment strategies and to expand the application of differential management to include a wider range of both.

Meanwhile, the Community Treatment Project and others such as the Community Delinquency Control Project[52] and the San Francisco Rehabili-

---

[51] Ted Palmer and Eric Werner. *California's Community Treatment Project–The Phase III Experiment: Progress to Date.* Sacramento: California Youth Authority, 1972.

[52] *The Los Angeles Community Delinquency Control Project: An Experiment in the Rehabilitation of Delinquents in an Urban Community.* Sacramento: California Youth Authority, 1970.

tation Project for Adult Offenders[53] have already demonstrated that community programs can effectively handle both juvenile and adult candidates for incarceration. While none of these projects has provided unqualified support for the superior effectiveness of its program, the significant increase in the use of community correction over the last decade in California has been associated with no recorded increase at all in serious crime among those supervised.[54]

Guided Group Interaction Programs

Of the various kinds of nonresidential programs that have been experimented with, one group of programs can be distinguished by a common theoretical orientation. These are the guided group interaction (GGI) programs, which are concerned primarily with peer-group dynamics and the operation of the group in restructuring the offender subculture around socially acceptable norms. These programs also depend to a sometimes considerable extent on the offender's involvement in his own rehabilitation. While other nonresidential programs frequently incorporate the group session into the daily program, less emphasis is placed on the peer group as a major treatment resource.

GGI programs involve the offender in frequent and intensive group discussions of his own and other members' current problems and experiences. Based on the theory that antisocial behavior receives the approval and support of the delinquent peer group and that substituting acceptable norms for delinquent values also requires peer-group support, these programs foster development of a group culture and encourage members to accept responsibility for helping and controlling one another. As the group culture develops and the group begins to show greater responsibility, the staff group leader allows the group a greater degree of decision-making power. Ultimately, the group's responsibility may extend to decisions involving disciplinary measures imposed on members or determination of a member's readiness for release. Peer-group programs have been developed for use primarily with juvenile offenders, although there have been some recent examples of programs for adults that make use of peer-group and behavior-modification principles.

Projects based on the use of peer-group dynamics derive their program content from the Highfields project, established in New Jersey in 1949.[55]

---

[53] Northern California Service League. *Final Report of the San Francisco Project for Adult Offenders.* San Francisco, 1968.

[54] California Assembly, *op. cit. supra* note 20.

[55] Lloyd W. McCorkle, Albert Elias, and F. Lovell Bixby. *The Highfields Story: An Experimental Treatment Project for Youthful Offenders.* New York: Henry Holt, 1958.

Highfields was a short-term residential program for boys involving work during the day and participation in group sessions in the evening. The program was judged to be as successful as training school in controlling recidivism and much less costly. The basic principles of Highfields have been applied in nonresidential settings with apparent success, with Essexfields, Collegefields, and the Provo experiment as the best known examples.

The Provo experiment, initiated in 1959 in Provo, Utah, was divided into two phases. Phase I involved twenty boys at a time in an intensive daily program including work or school and guided group interaction sessions. Each day, following paid employment or school, the boys went to the program center for group sessions, returning at night to their homes. Phase II was designed to aid a boy after release from the intensive phase I program: an effort was made to provide reference group support for the boys and to generate community action to help them find employment. Group development was given high priority since the group, rather than staff alone, was given major responsibility for controlling member behavior and working out solutions to individual or group problems. No length of stay in the program was specified, since release depended not only upon an individual's behavior but on the maturation processes that his group experienced. Release generally occurred between four and seven months. There were no formal rules other than the requirements of appearing each day and working hard on the job. Offenders assigned to the experimental program were compared to two control groups, one under regular probation supervision, the other incarcerated in a training school. Before the experiment, only about 50 to 55 percent of the kinds of persistent offenders who participated in the program were succeeding on probation. Six months after release 73 percent of those initially assigned and 84 percent of those who completed the program had no record of arrest. During the same period the success rate for regular probationers also rose to 73 percent for offenders initially assigned and 77 percent for those who completed probation. Of the offenders sent to training school, however, 58 percent had been rearrested and half of these had been arrested two or more times. Youths released from the reformatory appeared to be nearly twice as likely to commit an offense as were program graduates.[56]

Phase II of the Community Treatment Project was concerned with demonstrating the effectiveness of "Provo-type" treatment and comparing it with differential treatment in the community. Experimentals in San

[56]LaMar T. Empey, Maynard Erickson, and Max Scott, "The Provo Experiment: Evaluation of a Community Program." *Correction in the Community: Alternatives to Incarceration.* Sacramento: California Department of Corrections, 1964, pp. 29-38.

Francisco were assigned randomly to either a Differential Treatment Unit (DTU) or a GGI Unit. The GGI Unit did not use differential diagnosis as a basis for treatment, although I-Level classification was made for research purposes. Wards in GGI Units participated in full-time school or work and attended guided group interaction meetings. Average caseload size was fifteen. Detailed analyses of the rap-sheets (presenting a rundown of all police contacts, etc.) of all DTU and GGI males who were part of the San Francisco Community Treatment Project (1965-69) study sample revealed that DTU discharges performed better than their GGI counterparts on twelve-month follow-up, although most of the differences had washed out by the eighteen-month follow-up. Combining the results of the two follow-up cohorts, DTU subjects performed slightly but not significantly better than GGI subjects, but a large difference was found with respect to severe offenses. By twelve months the percentage of discharges who had committed at least one severe offense was more than six times greater within the GGI sample and by eighteen months 55 percent of the GGI group and only 10 percent of the DTU group had been involved in at least one severe offense. A 24-month follow-up is being made to test the reliability of this finding.[57]

The Essexfields Rehabilitation Project was established in 1959 in Essex County (Newark), N.J., on assumptions similar to those of the Provo experiment. The program was limited to twenty boys at a time who had been referred to the program as a condition of probation. Five days a week the boys participated in the program from seven in the morning to ten at night, working during the day and attending group sessions in the evening. Length of stay in the program was indeterminate, but was usually from four to five months. The program was evaluated by comparing recidivism rates of Essexfields boys with the rates of groups on probation, in residential group centers, and in the state reformatory. Despite the potential hazards of the high-delinquency area in which it was located, Essexfields demonstrated a rate of inprogram failure that was slightly lower than that of the residential group centers. Recidivism rates indicated that reformatory boys would do not worse and might do better at Essexfields or in the group centers.[58]

Collegefields, established in Newark, N.J., in 1965, developed out of the same theoretical base as Essexfields and Provo, but in addition, a major goal of this project was to alter the educational experience of delinquent boys. Each weekday twenty-five boys attended academic classes in the

[57]Ted Palmer and Alice Herrera, *CTP's San Francisco Experiment (1965-69); Post-Discharge Behavior of Differential Treatment and Guided Group Interaction Subjects.* Sacramento: California Youth Authority, 1972.

[58]Richard M. Stephenson and Frank R. Scarpitti, "Essexfields: A Non-Residential Experiment in Group Centered Rehabilitation of Delinquents," *American Journal of Correction,* 31(1):12-18, 1969.

morning and group sessions in the afternoon. The basic curriculum of the public school system was modified to meet individual student needs and remedial instruction was provided. During stays of from four to seven months in the program, boys advanced in achievement by as many as three academic years. Comparison of outcome of experimental subjects with two control groups on probation demonstrated greater gains for the Collegefields boys on IQ, attitudes toward school, realistic self-assessment, and achievement motivation, but no difference in recidivism rates was found.[59]

Despite the somewhat uncertain nature of the findings on effectiveness of guided group interaction, none of the research results contradicts the overall conclusions that intensive intervention in the community is at least as effective as incarceration or that offenders normally sent to an institution can be retained in the community as safely when special services are provided.

The Kentfields program of the Kent County (Mich.) Juvenile Court, initiated in 1970, is demonstrating the cost-effectiveness of behavior modification techniques with "hard-core" delinquents. The cost of treating a boy at Kentfields for one year is about $400 – several thousand dollars less than the cost of training school placement. In addition, the program provides labor for local units of county government at the $1.60 minimum or $3 average wage rates. Follow-up information collected from probation officers and validated by parents showed that, of the fifty-four boys who graduated from the program during the first year, only two had committed offenses serious enough to warrant commitment to training school. A majority were at home and working or attending school.[60] The data suggest that behavior modification techniques can be used successfully with serious delinquents and that it is not always necessary to spend large amounts of money to deal effectively with chronic juvenile offenders.

Community Treatment for Recidivists

The National Council on Crime and Delinquency, in conjunction with the Oakland County (Mich.) Circuit Court, established the Community Treatment for Recidivist Offenders Project in 1971 to demonstrate that second-felony adult offenders can be retained and treated in the community at no greater risk to public safety and with considerable savings in resources.

---

[59] Saul Pilnick and others, *Collegefields: From Delinquency to Freedom.* Newark, N.J.: Newark State College, 1967.

[60] William S. Davidson. *Kentfields Rehabilitation Program: An Alternative to Institutionalization.* Grand Rapids, Mich.: Kent County Juvenile Court, 1971.

It was believed that concentrating on offenders who have already demonstrated a tendency toward repeated offending, rather than on the first-offender group (many of whom will not commit another offense), would have a greater impact on the system of correctional services. The target group consists of adult offenders who have been convicted of at least one prior felony, or whose prior conviction was for a misdemeanor reduced from a felony charge. For purposes of evaluative research, 50 percent of second-felony offenders are sent to prison and 50 percent are referred to the project. A special service unit was created within the probation department to implement the project. Intensive casework and group services are provided as needed for offenders in caseloads not exceeding thirty-five cases per officer. Peer-group influence toward positive change is accomplished by means of peer task groups which meet to assist members in identifying problems, planning remedial treatment, and monitoring progress toward stated goals. Project staff function as service brokers, obtaining individual and group services to meet identified offender needs. Community resources are inventoried to assist in the matching of offenders with appropriate resources. Citizen volunteers are utilized whenever their special services will contribute to offender reintegration. Services are purchased when they cannot be obtained from volunteers or social service agencies.

Referrals to the project as of December 1972 totaled 290, of which 144 had been selected randomly for project supervision and 146 for either regular probation or prison. The 144 cases assigned for project supervision include eighty-one offenders who would have received regular probation and sixty-three who would have been incarcerated. Initial trends indicate that the project is achieving positive results. It has had only nine failures as of December 1972, with failure defined as a prison sentence for a new offense or a probation violation during project supervision. Of particular significance is the fact that only one of the nine failures was from the group of offenders diverted from prison.[61]

The Community Treatment for Recidivist Offenders Project will merit careful attention. Community intervention programs have not been utilized frequently for adult prison candidates, especially for second-felony recidivists. Evaluation of the project will run from termination in June 1973 to December 1973. Comparisons will be made with control groups derived from the selection process, and a retrospective sample or all offenders released from probation from 1968 through 1970 will be taken. The data will be examined to ascertain criminal patterns, characteristics of successes and failures, and the effectiveness of conventional probation.

[61] Community Treatment for Recidivist Offenders Project. *Annual Report: 1972.* Pontiac, Mich.: NCCD and Oakland County Circuit Court, 1973.

RESIDENTIAL COMMUNITY PROGRAMS

Group Homes for Delinquents

Jurisdictions in which the courts do not have access to sufficient resources frequently institutionalize juveniles whose homes are not considered conducive to their rehabilitation, simply because the judge sees no alternative. Group-home programs for delinquents have been devised to provide such alternatives. These programs are developed and adminstered under various arrangements. The contract group home is operated by an organization such as a church or civic group or by private individuals and financed through a contract with the state agency. Agency-operated homes are staffed by employees of the agency responsible for placing the offenders in the program.[62] Most of the latter are halfway houses for parolees from institutions, but there is an increasing use of such facilities as the initial placement in lieu of incarceration. Many states are currently considering opening group homes and halfway houses as alternatives to the increasingly unpopular correctional institution. Many Model Cities utilized funds made available under that program to develop such facilities.[63]

The Silverlake Experiment in Los Angeles was a group-home project providing a program similar to that of Provo, Highfields, and Essexfields in that an effort was made to create a nondelinquent culture through peer-group interaction and to involve offenders in decision-making. Seriously delinquent boys, ages 16 to 18, were diverted from training school and placed in a large family residence in a middle-class neighborhood. Up to twenty boys at a time lived in the residence during the week and attended school daily; weekends were spent at home. The daily group meeting was the major formal mechanism for implementing program goals. The objective was to structure a social system in which emerging norms, and their observance, were a function of collaborative client-staff decision-making. A study of the extent of actual collaboration between staff and boys found that information about problem behavior was shared freely and that the effectiveness of the program culture as a social control measure increased over time.[64]

---

[62] Experience in Illinois with both state-operated and contract group homes suggests the superiority of the latter with respect to both operational and financial considerations. Illinois Department of Corrections, Juvenile Division. *Project Group Homes: A Report.* Springfield, Ill., 1972.

[63] Eugene Doleschal, "Criminal Justice Programs in Model Cities." *Crime and Delinquency Literature.* 4(2):292-328, 1972.

[64] LaMar T. Empey and George E. Newland, "Staff-Inmate Collaboration: A Study of Critical Incidents and Consequences in the Silverlake Experiment." *Journal of Research in Crime and Delinquency.* 5(1):1-17, 1968.

The Attention Home program of Boulder, Colo., which opened its first group home in 1966, is a distinctly different kind of group-home program in concept, organization, and operation. The major difference is that the program is completely locally supported. The homes are operated by a nonprofit, nongovernmental corporation and managed by a board of directors composed of interested county residents. The basic idea is broad community involvement in and support of programs to curtail delinquency without resorting to institutionalization. Because of extensive volunteer support in services and materials, the Attention Homes cost considerably less than comparably sized government-supported group-home programs.[65]

The Group Home Project of the California Youth Authority was undertaken to develop and test temporary confinement facilities with varying and controllable atmospheres. This prject was an integral part of the Community Treatment Project, which has made wide use of out-of-home placements to facilitate the emergence of nondelinquent patterns in CTP wards; The objectives of the project were to classify home environments according to structure, nature of rewards and penalties, and type of houseparents and to evaluate the effectiveness of each type of home and of group homes generally. The study sample consisted of adolescents committed to the state correctional system after an average of five police arrests and placed in the CTP. Eight boys' homes (six for long-term placement and two for temporary care) and one girls' home were established. The homes were operated by nonprofessionally trained husband/wife teams who worked in conjuction with one or more CTP parole agents. During the three years (1966-69) of the project, ninety-three separate placements were made (fifty-one for long-term and forty-two for temporary care).

The temporary-care home appeared to have definite advantages over most other placement alternatives (e.g., independent placement, relatives, foster homes). From an operational standpoint there appeared to be two quite successful boys' group homes, while others were moderately successful and at least two were unsuccessful. The final report of the Group Home Project outlines the differential effectiveness of the various group-home models, provides descriptions of home atmospheres and personnel types and identifies problems encountered in establishing and operating these homes.[66]

[65] John E. Hagardine. *The Attention Homes of Boulder, Colorado.* Washington, D.C., Juvenile Delinquency and Youth Development Office, 1968.

[66] Ted Palmer. *The Group Home Project: Differential Placement of Delinquents in Group Homes.* Sacramento: California Youth Authority, 1972.

Probationed Offenders Rehabilitation Training

Probationed Offenders Rehabilitation Training (PORT), established in 1969 in Rochester, Minn., is a live-in, community-based, community supported and directed program for both juvenile and adult offenders.[67] The program provides an alternative for those offenders who require greater control and attention than probation can offer and who, without PORT, would have been sent to training school or prison. Through December 1971 PORT has accepted sixty male residents ranging in age from 13 to 47 and in offenses from truancy to armed robbery. All but three would have been incarcerated. Entrance into the program is voluntary: the candidate spends a three-week evaluation period in residence at PORT while he and the screening committee determine whether the program is the choice of both. The committee performs more of a catalytic than a screening function and so far it has not rejected any applicant.

The core of the program is a combination of group treatment and behavior modification. Behavior modification was added after a year of operation when it was found that the group alone was insufficient. A point system is used to mete out levels of freedom systematically, based on measured performance in tangible areas. The newcomer starts out at the lowest level of a group-evolved classification system, with categories ranging from I (minimum freedom) to V (freedom equal to that of an individual of the same age in the community). Through a process of demonstrating performance to the group and earnings on the point system, the resident gradually gains the freedoms and responsibilities accorded a normal person of his age. The "peer group" of PORT residents assists its members in identifying problems and setting goals and evaluates each individual's readiness for increased freedom and eventual release. Twelve to fifteen resident counselors, mostly college students, live in the building and room with the offenders, in effect replacing the guard/counselor staff of the institution.

A key to the success of the program is the involvement of the community and the heavy use of existing local resources. Educational, vocational, employment, and mental health services and other resources are not duplicated in PORT as they are in an institution. The community actually runs PORT through a corporate board of directors which hires staff and sets policy. Public support and voluntary service contributions to PORT programs are obtained through the PORT Advisory Committee, a group of about sixty-five Rochester citizens.

[67] Kenneth F. Schoen, "PORT: A New Concept of Community Based Correction." *Federal Probation.* 36(3):35-40, 1973.

While it is too early to state with complete assurance that the concepts employed at PORT are effective, the program appears promising. Of the sixty residents served by the program as of December 1971, thirty-four have been discharged, six as failures (sent to institutions) and twenty-eight who are now living in the community. The following conclusions have been drawn from experience to date: (1) The mixing of juveniles and adults is not only practical but preferred. (2) Community involvement and support from the start is essential. (3) Most existing community resources can be utilized and need not be duplicated. (4) The program can be operated at a cost of less than $3,000 per year per bed. (5) The dual treatment method of group therapy and behavior modification seems to be the most successful both in affording control and in achieving individual goals.

It is the intention of PORT not only to provide an effective correctional service in Rochester but to develop a model program that can be transferred to other communities throughout the state and nation.[68] Three other Minnesota communities have already set up programs modeled after PORT.

Community Integration Project

The Community Integration Project in Easton, Pa., is an experimental research project with the goal of proving that convicted young adult offenders who meet stringent selection criteria can be controlled and treated more effectively and less expensively in a community residence than in prison. Offenders classed as eligible for the project are randomly assigned to the residence group or the control group (sent to prison). Each participant lives in the residence for about six months, after which he becomes an out-resident and lives at home. All participants are employed in the metropolitan area in jobs that pay the federal minimum wage. Program staff members help residents to find and maintain career-oriented positions. From wages earned, residents pay room and board, make at least partial restitution to victims, contribute to the support of their dependents, and pay taxes. Therapeutic, vocational, and academic counseling are provided as needed. The research/evaluation component of the three-year project, which was designed and is being operated by the National Council on Crime and Delinquency, will examine cost-effectiveness and the impact on family stability and community safety.

The Community Integration Project is intended to serve as one among

---

[68] See *PORT Handbook: A Manual for Effective Community Action with the Criminal Offender* (St. Paul: Minnesota Corrections Department, 1972.

several alternatives to incarceration. There are probably many offenders who do not need and cannot benefit from the degree of control and supervision provided by the program. On the other hand, functioning as a kind of work-release center or halfway house, it can play a useful role in demonstrating that viable alternatives to the traditional prison do exist.

The Community Correction Center

As federal and state governments begin to turn away from the traditional prison and training school and toward community alternatives to institutionalization, one of the alternatives most frequently put forward as a model for future development is the community correction center. One of the strongest pushes in this direction has come from the Federal Bureau of Prisons, whose ten-year building program is aimed at replacing existing prisons with smaller ones. In addition, the Bureau operates more than a dozen Community Treatment Centers which function primarily as halfway houses for offenders on prerelease status but also accept selected short-sentence prisoners and female offenders.[69] The states have also begun to incorporate "community-based" treatment facilities (small, minimum-security institutions) into their overall correctional systems. Illinois has selected locations for four new community correction centers for adult male felons. It is expected that the creation of these new centers will reduce overcrowding in the state's three maximum-security prisons and provide opportunities for offenders to move from maximum- to medium- to minimum-security facilities as they are prepared to do so. Location of these new facilities in the more densely populated areas of the state is designed to facilitate community involvement and citizen participation as volunteers.[70]

Washington State, which has expressed its intention of not financing large institutions any longer than necessary, views the small institution, located in the community it serves, as the model for future correction facilities. The Washington Corrections Center at Shelton is an ultra-modern facility surrounded by a fence instead of a wall. Inmates live in individual rooms instead of cells, and there are many activities to combat idleness. Younger first offenders are sent there and the center serves a reception and diagnostic function for all sentenced inmates. At the Treatment Center for Women, residents occupy private rooms in residence cottages with all the

[69] *The Residential Center: Corrections in the Community.* Washington, D.C.: U.S. Bureau of Prisons, 1968.

[70] Illinois Department of Corrections, Planning Task Force on Community-based Treatment Facilities. *Planning for Community-Based Corrections.* Chicago, 1972.

modern conveniences. Each woman has a key to her room and many of them leave the institution during the day to work or attend classes in nearby communities.[71] These facilities are products of a new trend toward attractive, home-like, nonsecure correctional institutions that are placed in the community in order to overcome the disadvantages of isolation from community resources and opportunities. An institution situated in the locale which supplies the offender population is better able to draw upon the social, educational, employment, and health services and resources of that community and to involve community residents and the offender's family in the reintegration process.

Despite the vast improvement over the maximum-security prison represented by these new facilities, the rapid development of these "non-prisons" could present a real threat to the movement to deinstitutionalize correction. With modern, well-equipped facilities readily available, will the development of noninstitutional community programs be viewed as essential? How many potential prison inmates will be diverted to probation when the pressures of unbearable prison conditions are lifted? Will some of those persons now placed on probation be referred instead to "community residences" for that extra degree of supervision and control? Will these new institutions be plagued by many of the same problems now facing prisons? Are they any more effective than (less expensive) nonresidential programs? *Are they necessary?*

The community correction center or community-located institution may have a place in a fully diversified correction system. As a minimum-security institution it may provide the degree of supervision and control that some offenders require. But care should be taken that, in reallocating correctional resources, investment in these small institutions is not made at the expense of the development of community resources at a lower level of intervention.

CONCLUSION

In the California study of the effects of criminal penalities it was concluded that since severe penalties do not deter more effectively, since prisons do not rehabilitate, and since the criminal justice system is inconsistent and has little quantitative impact on crime, the best rehabilitative possibilities would appear to be in the community.[72]

[71] Robert Schuman. "Washington's Institutions: Rehabilitation Stressed in Programs, New Units." *American Journal of Correction.* 34(6):29, 37, 1972.

[72] California Legislature, *op. cit. supra* note 9.

This reasoning typifies much current thinking in correction and illustrates the kind of cognitive leap on which enthusiasm for "community treatment" is based. If prisons do not rehabilitate, and if the goal of correction is to reduce recidivism through integration of offender and community, it seems axiomatic that treating the offender without removing him from society will be more effective. Unfortunately, while one may express the opinion that, since prisons are not effective (a validated observation) then one *might as well* retain offenders in the community, one cannot assume without the support of adequate research that the best rehabilitative possibilities are to be found in the community. The most rigorous research designs generally have found that offenders eligible for supervision in the community in lieu of incarceration do *as well* in the community as they do in prison or training school. When intervening variables are controlled, recidivism rates usually appear to be about the same.

This is not to derogate community alternatives to institutionalization, since it is a most important finding: a large number of offenders who are candidates for incarceration may be retained in the community as safely, as effectively, and at much less expense. Additionally, the observed effects of the overcrowded and isolated institution on the personal and social adjustment of the individual are avoided. It is unnecessary to demonstrate, as most experimental projects appear to feel pressured to do, that recidivism rates are *lower* when offenders are retained in the community. Given the fact that expensive and overcrowded institutions are not doing the job they are supposed to be doing, it is appropriate to expect that less costly, less personally damaging alternatives will be utilized whenever they are at least as effective as imprisonment.

The historical trend in correction is toward the expansion of community-based alternatives to imprisonment. This has come to mean limiting the use of incarceration to dangerous offenders and diverting all others to the least drastic alternative at the earliest feasible opportunity in criminal justice processing. The goal of reducing institutional populations is furthered by legislation decriminalizing victimless crimes, by the informal handling of minor deviance without resort to the courts (e.g., the youth service bureau), by the expanded use of alternatives to jail and detention (release on recognizance, bail), and by increased reliance on deferred prosecution, suspended sentences, fines, restitution orders, and probation. For many offenders who make it as far as an institutional sentence, alternatives such as those described above have been shown to be at least workable alternatives.

A fully diversified correctional system, in which resources are optimally allocated, would provide a range of alternatives sufficient to insure that no individual is subjected to greater control or treatment than he requires or can benefit from, not merely because such a system would concur with modern conceptions of justice but because it would be maximally cost-effective. Because the vast majority of offenders apparently do not require and cannot benefit from imprisonment, this would entail a reallocation of correctional resources to reverse the present 90 percent investment in institutional programs. It will not be sufficient simply to build smaller prisons or community-located institutions, although such institutions might be one component of an overall plan. Because the proportion of offenders who must be incarcerated is as yet unknown, it would appear reasonable to begin by diverting as many offenders as possible to community programs and resources of greater cost-effectiveness, leaving the construction of correctional institutions until it is known how many and what kinds of offenders must be served by institutional programs.

Isolation and banishment have not worked. It is coming to be recognized that unless society is willing to keep a large and growing number of offenders in permanent custody, it must begin to accept greater responsibility in the areas of social control and correction. The evidence obtained from experimental work in community correction — and supported by the results of experience with partial imprisonment and graduated release the treatment of mental illness, and alternatives to criminal justice processing — makes it clear that a vast proportion of offenders can be managed in the community or diverted from the justice system entirely, thus returning to the community its responsibility for dealing with behaivor it defines as antisocial or deviant.

Until alternatives to institutionalization are demonstrated to be *more* effective than imprisonment in preventing further crime, an important rationale for the use of community programs will be that correctional costs can be reduced considerably by handling in the community setting a large number of those offenders normally institutionalized. Experimental projects have shown that, for a large proportion of institutional candidates, incarceration is apparently unnecessary. If, in light of this evidence, society is still determined to keep these offenders in prisons and training schools, it must be willing to pay the price. The central question thus becomes: Are the goals of punishment and temporary incapacitation worth the high costs of constructing and maintaining correctional institutions, as well as the personal and social costs incurred through exposing individuals to the institutional experience?

16
Short-Term Behavioral Intervention with Delinquent Families: Impact on Family Process and Recidivism [*][1]

JAMES F. ALEXANDER and BRUCE V. PARSONS

Throughout the history of psychotherapy, evaluation of the effects of intervention have been notoriously absent. When evaluation has been attempted, most studies have failed to utilize control groups that really controlled for such major alternative hypotheses as attention placebo, maturation, and other intervening experiences. Other studies have used dependent measures of questionable relationship to overt behavior, such as projective devices, self and therapist reports, personality inventories, and Q sorts (Bergin, 1971). The field of family therapy also suffers from these deficiencies, with most reports characterized by enthusiastic program description and little or no data (Parsons and Alexander, 1972).

In response to this problem, the present investigation adopted the philosophy that family therapy research should involve four main goals. These goals, pursued in this project, are: (a) to provide a clear description of the intervention techniques; (b) to describe and evaluate the behavioral changes in family process expected from intervention (process measures); (c) to use clearly defined and essentially nonreactive behavioral criteria to evaluate the effects of intervention (outcome measures); (d) and, of course, incorporate adequate controls for maturation and professional attention.

The intervention program (designated short-term behavioral family

[*]Reprinted from *Journal of Abnormal Psychology*, 1973, 81, 219-225, with permission. Copyright 1973 by the American Psychological Association.

[1]Portions of this paper were presented to the meeting of the Rocky Mountain Psychological Association, Albuquerque, New Mexico, May 1972. This study was supported by a grant from the United States Department of Health, Education, and Welfare (No. 72-P-40061/8-01) entitled Intake Services for Detained Children.

intervention) involved a set of clearly defined therapist interventions with delinquent families designed to: (a) assess the family behaviors that maintain delinquent behavior; (b) modify the family communication patterns in the direction of greater clarity and precision, increased reciprocity, and presentation of alternative solutions; (c) all in order to institute a pattern of contingency contracting in the family designed to modify the maladaptive patterns and institute more adaptive behaviors.

To evaluate the impact of these interventions and control for the effects of maturation and professional attention, families receiving the program (described below) were compared to families receiving alternative forms of family intervention and families receiving no formal intervention. It was hypothesized that families in the short-term behavioral family program, in contrast to these comparison groups, would demonstrate changes in family interaction (process measures) in the direction of less silence, more equality of speech, and greater frequency of positive interruptions. Further, reflecting these adaptive changes in family process, it was hypothesized that families receiving the program would demonstrate significantly lower recidivism rates than comparison groups on follow-up.

METHOD

Selection of Subjects

During the project, a total of 99 families were referred by the Salt Lake County Juvenile Court to the Family Clinic at the University of Utah from October 1970 to January 1972. Subsequent to the program, follow-up records were available only on 86 families of 38 male and 48 female delinquents, ranging in age from 13 to 16 years, who had been arrested or detained at the Juvenile Court for a behavioral offense. Such offenses included adolescents who had: (a) run away; (b) been declared ungovernable; (c) been habitually truant; (d) been arrested for shoplifting; (e) been arrested for possession of alcohol, soft drugs, or tobacco. With minor exceptions caused by program availability, families were randomly assigned upon detention to either the treatment program, comparison groups, or a no-treatment control condition.

Treatment Condition

Forty-six families were randomly assigned to the short-term behavioral family intervention program. Systems theory (Coles and Alexander, 1971;

Watzlawick, Beavin and Jackson, 1967) provided the theoretical underpinning for the program, with the general proposition that families of delinquent teenagers represent maladaptive, disintegrating systems (Alexander, 1973). In this model, deviant behavior is seen as a function of the entire system in which the individual is embedded. The fact is, however, the systems theory represents more of a model, or point of view, than a specific theory, and does not include a set of clearly derived specific techniques for changing maladaptive patterns of family interaction. Thus, the specific treatment techniques, as well as the goals of intervention, were based on prior family interaction studies which have found that deviant families, as compared to normals, are more silent, talk less equally, have fewer positive interruptions, and in general are less active (Alexander, 1970; Duncan, 1968; Mischler and Waxler, 1968; Stuart, 1968; Winter and Ferreira, 1969). These manifestations of maladaptive interactions may be subsumed under the general concept identified by Patterson and Reid (1970) as lack of reciprocity in family interaction. Specifically, Patterson and Reid have demonstrated that when the amount and balance of mutual positive reinforcement has been altered (i.e., made more equitable by therapeutic intervention), families have moved from "bedlam" to relatively low rates of disruptive behavior.

Utilizing this concept, the present investigation was aimed at systematically extinguishing maladaptive interaction patterns and instituting reciprocity instead. Based on a matching to sample philosophy (Parsons and Alexander, 1972), the goal was to modify the interactions of deviant families so that they would approximate those patterns (described above) characteristic of "normal," or "adjusted" families. To meet this goal, therapists emphasized the removal of the circumstances (interactions) that elicited the behavioral offense, and replacing them instead with a process of contingency contracting (Stuart, 1968). In this process, therapists actively modeled, prompted, and reinforced in all family members: (a) clear communication of substance as well as feelings, and (b) clear presentation of "demands" and alternative solutions; all leading to (c) negotiation, with each family member receiving some privilege for each responsibility assumed, to the point of compromise.

In most cases, one or more family members were initially unwilling to negotiate about the major issue(s) that led to the delinquent offense (e.g., curfew times, choice of friends, etc.). Thus in general therapists chose a less crucial issue to use in training family members in contingency contracting (e.g., staying away after school until dinner in return for washing dishes). Generally, success in resolving such "minor" issues led to a willingness to deal with the major issues. To assist therapists in identifying the major issues, a training manual describing major "themes" in delinquent families was developed, together with a series of specific "do's" and "don'ts."[2]

To facilitate training in reciprocity of communication and behavior management skills, several specific manipulations were applied to all treatment families. First, therapists differentiated rules from requests. Rules were defined as limits designed to regulate the control the action and conduct of the family. Requests, on the other hand, were defined as "asking behavior" designed to prevent response constriction, that is, the person being requested to perform an act could reply in the affirmative or the negative without fear of negative sanction. By differentiating rules from requests, an unambiguous structure was placed upon the family system. Research in the area of delinquency development indicates that parents often set too many rules and are inconsistent with their use of punishment when these rules are broken. In doing this, a general lack of structure is built into the home and an environment for adolescent acting out is fostered. The aim of this treatment manipulation, then, was to make rules explicit, thus aiding in the development of an understandable environment in which the family could deal with one another.

A second major manipulation involved the systematic application of social reinforcement. In order to increase the family's ability to be variable in their communication patterns (negotiate for change constructively), it was necessary to train the family members in labile, solution-oriented communication patterns while they negotiated the specific content of the rule-request/ token economy features of the program. Specifically, these communication patterns were categorized as: (a) interruption for clarification; (b) interruptions designed to increase information about the topic or about one's self in relationship to the topic; and (c) interruptions designed to offer informative feedback to other family members. This training consisted of having the therapist explicitly state the meaning and purposes of interruptions and the manner in which he would reinforce those behaviors. This was done because prior research (e.g., Mischel, 1958; Mischel and Grusec, 1967; Rotter, 1964) indicates that informational feedback about the situation and contingencies that will confront the subject in the future critically affect his behavior. Additionally, most experiments fail to obtain performance gains in the absence of accurate or at least partially correct hypotheses regarding the reinforcement contingencies (Adams, 1957; Dulany, 1962; Spielberger and DeNike, 1966). This explanation was followed with the subsequent dispensing of social reinforcement (e.g., verbal and nonverbal praise) by the therapist for the elicitation of the above types of communication variability.

Two additional manipulations were applied to some but not all families. A family training manual was designed for the project, basically consisting of

---

[2] Reprints and copies of training manual may be obtained from the senior author.

a behavior modification primer aimed at the acceleration and extinction of behaviors on a systems level. This manual was a modification of a manual developed by Patterson and Gullion (1968) entitled *Living With Children*. It was felt that by alerting the family to the treatment rationale, they would be better able to incorporate and utilize the basic tenets of the treatment program. Unfortunately, few families read the entire manual, and experience demonstrated that the therapist time taken to insure reading could be more efficiently spent directly modifying the family's interaction patterns.

Token economy programs were also occasionally used, particularly with younger teenagers displaying home-specific behaviors in a context of high family contact. In designing the token system, each family member was asked to specify exactly what responses he would like to see accelerated in the other members. In addition to specifying three such responses, each family member identified the way in which he would like to be rewarded by the other. When a means was developed for the exchange of these responses, the family members were assisted in achieving reciprocity in their interactions.

Selection and Training of Therapists

Therapists consisted of 18 first- and second-year graduate students in clinical psychology participating in a clinical practicum series emphasizing family treatment, each of whom (with a few exceptions) saw two families. These students had little previous training and thus were more or less unbiased as to theoretical treatment regarding family therapy. Later, two selected undergraduate paraprofessionals were also assigned families after serving an "internship" as cotherapists with more experienced therapists.

Training included: (a) an initial four weeks of group training including role playing, discussions of therapist training manuals, and live observation (one-way mirrors) and group observation of therapists as they saw families; (c) biweekly group supervision of therapists to discuss and role-play interventions with families. In general, therapists received 6 hours of training and supervision each week. In addition, a session by session description of a "model" treatment program was developed (Parsons and Alexander, 1972), though therapists were allowed to spend more or less time on each phase of training as needed (e.g., some families were initially reasonably clear and precise concerning demands, while other families required several sessions of training in this preliminary skill).

Comparison Conditions

To provide comparison groups to control for the effects of maturation and professional attention, an additional 30 families were randomly assigned (with minor exceptions due to program availability) to one of three comparison groups:

Client-centered family group program. Nineteen of the families were assigned to a program representative of treatment in many juvenile centers; a basically didactic group discussion context focusing on attitudes and feelings about family relationships and adolescent problems based on the client-centered model. These families met for the same total time as families in the short-term behavioral treatment program. The two therapists, hired by the court to see families, were of course unaware that they represented a "comparison" condition. These therapists, one a fifth-year graduate student, one a recent PhD, did differ from therapists in the treatment condition in terms of having more clinical experience. However, it was assumed that any resulting bias would operated in favor of the comparison group.

Psychodynamic family program. An additional 11 families were referred to a (Mormon) church sponsored family counseling program, which represents exactly the form of treatment a significant proportion of teenagers in Salt Lake County receive upon referral to the court. Because these referrals were made through local clergy to a separate agency, specific information on treatment parameters in this condition was impossible to obtain. However, one master's of social work (MSW) staff member (personal communication, April 1971) described the program as placing emphasis on insight as a vehicle for therapeutic change based on an eclectic psychodynamic model. Average treatment duration was estimated at 12-15 sessions, with considerable variation from family to family. The therapy staff, consisting of MSWs and PhDs, generally represented a more experienced group than in the experimental treatment condition.

No-treatment control. An additional 10 randomly selected families were released from the court with no formal treatment but were contacted for testing on process measures (described below) 5-6 weeks after intake (comparable to posttesting interval for treatment families).

Procedure: Process Measures

As described in greater detail elsewhere (Parsons and Alexander, 1973), the first 20 treatment families completing the program, 10 client-centered family program families completing their program, and the 10 no-treatment controls were tested on family interaction tasks upon completion of their programs. Families were met in the waiting room of the Counseling Center by an experimenter naive as to their group designation and escorted into the interviewing room. After being seated in a prearranged order (father, child, mother), the family was given a series of three tasks: (a) behavior specificity phase; (b) vignette phase; and (c) interaction phase.

Accuracy of perception (behavior specificity phase). Each family member was given a pencil and clipboard with two mimeographed sheets attached. The family was then instructed by the experimenter to list, in an independent fashion, the three behaviors each would like to see changed in each of the other members. Each family member was also asked to list the three behaviors each other member might want him to change.

Accuracy of perception (vignette phase). Each family member was then asked by the experimenter to record independently, in writing, his responses to each of three situations calling for parental action in relation to the child's behavior (e.g., the child's coming home long after curfew time). Both parents and child defined the type of action he would expect each of the other members to take.

Interaction phase. Upon completion of these tasks the family was instructed to discuss, for a period of 20 minutes, their responses made during the behavior specificity phase and vignette phase. Families were told that they need not reach an agreement on the task. The experimenter then left the room after informing the family that during this time their interactions would be observed and recorded on an audiotape.

Dependent measures: Changes in family process. The three interaction measures were based on the 20-minute audiotape sample of families discussing the accuracy of perception tasks. To obviate problems of reliability, all data were automatically recorded on event recorders by means of voice actuated microphones worn by each family member.

As described above, the treatment manipulations, designed to increase reciprocity and clarity of communication, were hypothesized to produce changes in three dependent measures found in prior research to differentiate adaptive from nonadaptive family systems. Specifically, it was hypothesized that families receiving the program, as opposed to the comparison groups, would demonstrate: (a) more equality of interaction as measured by lower average within family variance of talk time across groups; (b) less silence, reflecting greater family activity; and (c) a greater frequency of interruptions, measured by overlapping event recorder deflections. This measure was derived from recent work by Duncan (1968) and Mischler and Waxler (1968), who found (contrary to early findings in family research) that high rates of interruptions were characteristic of normal families, while deviant families demonstrated low interruption rates. An increase in such interruptions, as a function of therapy was expected as a reflection of increases in both general activity level and attempts at clarity of communication.

Outcome Measures

As discussed above, even if changes in family process could be demonstrated as a function of intervention, such changes by themselves may not relate to the ultimate goal of intervention, reducing problematic (i.e., delinquent) behavior. Thus for the present report, juvenile court records were examined following termination of treatment for recidivism, that is, rereferral for behavioral offense. It was hypothesized that congruent with the positive changes in family interaction, treated families would demonstrate a significant reduction in recidivism, while controls who were not expected to show changes in family interaction patterns would also demonstrate no reduction in recidivism.

RESULTS

To insure that random assignment of families resulted in comparability of groups, subjects were compared on demographic variables (i.e., age, socioeconomic status, and distribution of sex), prior recidivism rates, and pretest scores on the three interaction measures. As described elsewhere (Alexander and Parsons, 1972; Parsons and Alexander, 1973), no differences of any of these variables were found.

Process Measures

Table 1 contains the group means for each of the three process variables. As can be seen, statistically significant differences were found on each dimension, with families receiving short-term behavioral family intervention, as hypothesized, demonstrating significantly lower variance (i.e., more equality) in talk time, less silence, and more interruptions.

Note that one-way analyses of variance were run and found to be significant. However, severe heterogeneity of variance, skew, and sample sizes raised serious doubts about the appropriateness of F tests. Thus significance values are presented for the rank-sum test for several samples (Dixon and Massey, 1957).

Table 1 Process Measures: Posttest Means on Three Interaction Variables

	Variance of talk time[b] (in seconds)	Silence (seconds)	Frequency of interruptions
Short-term family behavioral treatment ($N = 20$)	1194.8	154.4	65.9
Client-centered family groups ($N = 10$)	1494.6	220.1	18.5
No-treatment controls ($N = 6$)[a]	2099.5	237.0	20.2
H value[c] ($df = 2$) of differences	11.19*	11.70*	13.75*

[a] Four families were unavailable for testing.
[b] Lower score indicates more equality of speech.
[c] Rank sum test for several samples.
* $p < .05$.

Outcome Measures: Recidivism

At a 6- to 18-month interval following termination of the various treatment programs and control condition, juvenile court records of 86 families were examined for recidivism. (Note that the follow-up period for individual families varied widely, but across groups the period was comparable). Table 2 presents recidivism rates for the four groups, plus data on two additional comparison groups.

Specifically, 46 cases were randomly selected from several hundred court cases referred during the project period but not assigned treatment due to program availability. These families were randomly selected during the same periods as the referrals on the treated families, in a yoked control fashion. Demographic and prior recidivism variables were comparable to treated families. The second additional "comparison group" represents recidivism rates for 2,800 cases seen county wide during 1971, some of whom received various treatments (i.e., community mental health, church-sponsored counseling, private therapy, etc.) while many did not. Because these two latter groups were examined only on a post hoc basis, they were not included in the statistical analysis.

As can be seen in Table 2, the randomly assigned no-treatment controls

Table 2 Outcome Measures: Recidivism Rates for Treatment and
Comparison Groups

Condition	N	No. of cases of recidivism	No. of non-recidivism cases	% recidivism
Groups compared statistically				
Short-term family behavioral treatment	46[a]	12[c]	34[c]	26
Client-centered family groups treatment	19[b]	9[c]	10[c]	47
Eclectic psycho-dynamic family treatment	11	8[c]	3[c]	73
No treatment controls	10	5[c]	5[c]	50
Groups not included in statistical comparison				
Post-hoc selected no-treatment controls	46	22	24	48
County-wide recidivism rates, 1971	2800			51

[a] Includes 12 cases who dropped the program before completion
[b] Includes 9 cases who dropped the program
[c] Differences between samples: $X^2 = 10.25, df = 3, p < .025$.

demonstrated a 50 percent recidivism rate and the (comparison) family groups program a 47 percent rate comparable to the county wide 51 percent rate and the 48 percent demonstrated by the post hoc selected no-treatment controls. Further, the electic psychodynamic family program demonstrated a 73 percent rate, while the short-term behavioral family program demonstrated a significant (tested by chi-square) reduction in recidivism to 26 percent.

In addition to recidivism in behavioral offense, subsequent criminal offenses (i.e., felony, hit and run, etc.) were also evaluated. In a comparable direction to the behavioral data, though not significant, the treatment group demonstrated the lowest rate (17 percent) of subsequent criminal referral. The other groups ranged from 21 percent to 27 percent.

Two additional comparisons are of interest. First, although the treatment group had the lowest recidivism rates and the "best" scores on process measures, the hypothesized relationship between the two had still not been directly and statistically demonstrated. To do this, cases were divided into recidivism versus nonrecidivism groups, independent of treatment category. As expected, the nonrecidivism cases compared to recidivism cases, domonstrated significantly lower variance ($\overline{X}$s = 801.9 and 2143.8, respectively, t = 3.97, df = 34, p < .01), significantly less silence ($\overline{X}$s = 171.5 and 203.3, respectively, t = 2.94, df = 34, p < .01) and significantly more interruptions ($\overline{X}$s = 58.7 and 28.5; respectively, t = 4.17, df = 34, p < .01).

Finally, time to recidivism was evaluated for the treatment group, the two comparison treatment groups, and the no-treatment controls. For families in which recidivism did occur, these average times were equivalent (2.4, 2.4, 2.8, and 2.7 months, respectively). Thus the program seemed to be effective in reducing the rate of recidivism but not in delaying its onset given its occurrence.

DISCUSSION

The results clearly demonstrate the efficacy of a short-term, specific, behavioral family treatment program for delinquent teenagers. Although the program was not completely successful in eliminating recidivism, a significant (both statistically and economically) reduction was demonstrated. Further, the inclusion of the control and comparison groups suggests that the beneficial effects of this form of treatment cannot be attributed to the effects of attention placebo or maturation. Finally, the fact that the comparison groups received forms of therapy representative of existing treatment procedures suggests that the threatment program utilized in the present project provides an efficient and economical alternative to existing practices.

The results also support the philosophy of therapy evaluation adopted in the project. Specific therapist interventions were found to significantly modify family interaction patterns, while nonspecific interventions did not. More importantly, however, these changes in interaction were related to decreased recidivism rates, while families that demonstrated no changes in interaction also demonstrated no reduction in recidivism. These results, of course, have important implications not only for implementing family treatment programs, but they also suggest directions for prevention.

Concerning the issue of outcome evaluation, it should be noted that the recidivism rates reported above included families who had dropped out of the program. All too often, psychotherapy outcome research involves only clients who have completed the program or have met some criterion such as attending four or five sessions. The inclusion of all referrals in outcome data, in contrast, provides a more meaningful, and honest, evaluation of the particular therapy program in question. For example, dropout information was available for the treatment group, the client-centered family groups program, and the no-treatment controls. With dropouts excluded, the recidivism rates for these groups were 22 percent, 50 percent, and 50 percent, respectively suggesting (somewhat unfairly) an even greater positive impact of the treatment program.

One final point must be emphasized. The fact that treatment and two comparison conditions involved some form of "family therapy" emphasizes that a focus on families per se is not sufficient to modify family interaction patterns or reduce rates of delinquency. Instead, it appears that family intervention programs may profitably be focused on changing family interaction patterns in the direction of increased clarity and precision of communication, increased reciprocity of communication and social reinforcement, and contingency contracting emphasizing equivalence of rights and responsibilities for all family members. This, of course, does not mean that other forms of therapy, not evaluated here, might not be as effective. Nor do the results imply the forms of family therapy used for comparison might not be considerably more effective in different contexts (i.e., different client populations, problem natures, therapists, etc.) However, at this stage of development in family therapy techniques, the burden of proof rests with the adherents of these alternative models.

REFERENCES

Adams, J.K. Laboratory studies of behavior without awareness. *Psychological Bulletin,* 1957, **54**, 393-405.

Alexander, J.F. and Parsons, B.V. Short term behavioral intervention with the meeting of the Rocky Mountain Psychological Association, Salt Lake City, May 1970.

Alexander, J.F. Defensive and supportive communications in normal and deviant families. *Journal of Consulting and Clinical Psychology,* 1973, in press.

Alexander, J.F., and Parsons, B.V. Short term behavioral intervention with delinquent families: Impact on family process and recidivism. Paper presented at the meeting of the Rocky Mountain Psychological Association, Albuquerque, May 1972.

Bergin, A.E. The evaluation of therapeutic outcomes. In A.E. Bergin and S.L. Garfield (Eds.), *Handbook of psychotherapy and behavior change.* New York: Wiley, 1971.

Coles, J.L. and Alexander, J.F. Systems theory and family behavior: Principles and implications. Paper presented at the meeting of the Rocky Mountain Psychological Association, Denver, May 1971.

Dixon, W.J. and Massey, F.J. *Introduction to statistical analysis.* New York: McGraw-Hill, 1957.

Dulany, D.E. The place of hypotheses and intentions: An analysis of verbal control in verbal conditioning. In C.W. Eriksen (Ed.), *Behavior and awareness—A Symposium of Research and Interpretation.* Durham, North Carolina: Duke University Press, 1962.

Duncan, P. Family interaction in parents of neurotic and social delinquent girls. Unpublished doctoral dissertation, University of Wisconsin, 1968.

Haley, J. *Changing families: A family therapy reader.* New York: Grune & Stratton, 1971.

Mischel, W. The effect of the commitment situation on the generalization of expectancies. *Journal of Personality,* 1958, **26**, 508-516.

Mischel, W. and Grusec, J. Waiting for rewards and punishments: Effects of time and probability on choice. *Journal of Personality and Social Psychology,* 1967, **5**, 24-31.

Mischler, E. and Waxler, N. *Interaction in families.* New York: Wiley, 1968.

Parsons, B.V. and Alexander, J.F. Short-term family intervention: A therapy outcome study. *Journal of Consulting and Clinical Psychology,* 1973, in press.

Patterson, G.R. and Gullion, M.E. *Living with children. New methods for parents and teachers.* Champaign, Ill.: Research Press, 1968.

Patterson, G.R. and Reid, J.B. Reciprocity and coercion: Two facets of social systems. In C. Neuringer and J. Michael (Eds.), *Behavior modification in clinical psychology.* New York: Appleton-Century-Crofts, 1970.

Patterson, G.R., Reid, J.B. and Shaw, D.A. Direct intervention in families of deviant children. *Oregon Research Institute Research Bulletin,* 1968, Whole No. 8.

Rotter, J.B. *Clinical psychology.* Englewood Cliffs, N.J.: Prentice-Hall, 1964.

Spielberger, C.D. and DeNike, L.D. Descriptive behaviorism versus cognitive theory in verbal operant conditioning. *Psychological Review,* 1966, **73**, 306-326.

Stuart, R.B. Taken reinforcement in marital treatment. In R. Rubin and C. Franks (Eds.), *Advances in behavior therapy.* New York: Academic Press, 1968.

Watziawick, P., Beavin, J.H. and Jackson, D.D. *Pragmatics of human communication.* New York: Norton, 1967.

Winter, W.D. and Ferreira, A.J. Talking time as an index of intrafamilial similarity in normal and abnormal families. *Journal of Abnormal Psychology,* 1969, **74**, 574-575.

Part IV
Legal and Ethical Issues

The final part of this book concerns the legal and ethical issues which are inevitably raised when mental health and criminal justice agencies interact. McGarry and Kaplan begin this section by providing a broad overview of recent developments in the rapidly developing field coming to be known as "mental health law". A solid grounding in this area is an essential prerequisite to mounting meaningful programs on the interface of mental health and criminal justice (see also Schwitzgebel, 1971, 1973; Mental Health Law Project, 1974; and Brooks, 1974).

Shah considers both legal and ethical issues when he relates community mental health to the problems of the criminal justice system. He argues that many traditional mental health concepts are inadequate in community settings, and more emphasis needs to be placed on environmental manipulation. In the same vein, Judge David Bazelon (1973) has recently asked whether mental health professionals in the correctional system have adequately confronted the moral issues inherent in their work. In addressing a conference of correctional psychologists, he stated:

> Instead of facing up to the true dimensions of the problem and society's social and economic structure, we prefer to blame the problem on a criminal class — a group of sick persons who must be treated by doctors and cured. Why should we even consider fundamental social changes or massive income redistribution if the entire problem can be solved by having scientists teach the criminal class — like a group of laboratory rats — to march successfully through the maze of our society? In short, before you respond with

enthusiasm to our plea for help, you must ask yourselves whether your help is really needed, or whether you are merely engaged as magicians to perform an intriguing side-show so that the spectators will not notice the crisis in the center ring. In considering our motives for offering you a role, I think you would do well to consider how much less expensive it is to hire a thousand psychologists than to make even a miniscule change in the social and economic structure. (p. 152).

Silber cogently analyzes the "paradigm clash" currently taking place at the border of mental health and criminal justice, with one camp seeing psychological treatment as the most humane and effective way to treat offenders, and the other fearing a "Therapeutic State" and the demise of civil liberties. Critiquing each of these positions, Silber sets his own course by suggesting new roles for mental health professionals in criminal justice settings.

Finally, ethical issues come squarely to the fore when Abramson and Monahan debate whether California's recent community mental health law, which restricted involuntary civil commitments, is "criminalizing" mentally disordered behavior or "psychiatrizing" criminal behavior. It is only by such frank and open airing of issues that the intricate legal and ethical dilemmas which characterize community mental health interaction with the criminal justice system will ever be resolved. Further reading in this area would include Szasz (1963, 1970), Halleck (1967), Mitford (1973), Zusman and Shaffer (1973), Peszke and Wintrob (1974), and Opton (in press).

REFERENCES

American Friends Service Committee. *Struggle for justice: A report on crime and punishment in America.* New York: Hill and Wang, 1971.

Bazelon, D. Psychologists in corrections — Are they doing good for the offender or well for themselves? In S. Brodsky, *Psychologists in the criminal justice system.* Urbana, Illinois: University of Illinois Press, 1973.

Brooks, A. *Cases and materials on law, psychiatry and the rights of the mentally disabled.* Boston: Little, Brown, 1974.

Ennis, B. and Siegel, L. *The rights of mental patients: The basic ACLU guide to a mental patient's rights.* New York: Avon, 1973.

Halleck, S. *Psychiatry and the dilemmas of crime.* New York: Harper and Hoeber, 1967.

Mental Health Law Project, *Legal rights of the mentally handicapped.* Mimeo, 1974 (3 volumes).

Mitford, J. *Kind and usual punishment: The prison business. New York:* Alfred Knopf, 1973.

Opton, E. Psychiatric violence against prisoners: When therapy is punishment. *Mississippi Law Journal,* in press.

Peszke, M. and Wintrob, R. Emergency commitment – A transcultural study. *American Journal of Psychiatry,* 1974, **131**, 36-40.

Schwitzgebel, R. *Development and legal regulation of coercive behavior modification techniques with offenders.* Washington, D.C.: U.S. Public Health Service, 1971.

Schwitzgebel, R. Right to treatment for the mentally disabled: The need for realistic standards and objective criteria. *Harvard Civil Rights – Civil Liberties Law Review,* 1973, 8, 513-535.

Szasz, T. *Law, liberty, and psychiatry.* New York: Macmillan, 1963.

Szasz, T. *The manufacture of madness.* New York: Harper and Row, 1970.

Zusman, J. and Shaffer, S. Emergency psychiatric hospitalization via court order: A critique. *American Journal of Psychiatry,* 1973, **130**, 1323-1326.

17

Overview: Current Trends in Mental Health Law *[1]

A. LOUIS McGARRY and HONORA A. KAPLAN

In recent years there has been extraordinary activity in the courts and legislatures of America relating to mental health law. A major new legal thesis is that adequate treatment for the institutionalized mentally ill and mentally retarded is a constitutional right. In particular, the class action suit, which we will discuss in greater detail later, has emerged as a mechanism with the potential for unprecedented and accelerated change in mental health systems.

Implicit and, in some cases, explicit in this activity is the requirement that the states reorder their priorities in order to provide adequate resources for the care and treatment of the mentall ill and retarded. It is ironic that such a charge should come at a time of financial austerity in the states, indeed at a time when a number of the states have been forced to cut their mental health budgets. It remains to be seen what the impact of all of this activity will be. The recent landmark case on the right to treatment in Alabama (1) has been appealed to the 5th Federal Circuit Court of Appeals. At stake here, among other important issues, are the degree of authority and the breadth of the remedies a federal court can impose on a state government.

This paper will not exhaustively examine all of the recent legal activity relating to mental health. Rather, we will be describing and analyzing what we regard as the major trends in representative states and courts and the implications of these trends. In doing so we may only succeed in grasping a

*Reprinted from *American Journal of Psychiatry,* 1973, **130,** 621-630, with permission. Copyright 1973, the American Psychiatric Association.
[1]This work was supported by Public Health Service grant 6813-2 from the Center for Studies of Crime and Delinquency, National Institute of Mental Health.

tiger by the tail, since what will be described is a rapidly evolving, dynamic process subject to significant change tomorrow or, indeed, today.

HISTORICAL BACKGROUND

In earlier times the primary concern of legislation relating to mental illness was the protection and security of society. In colonial America there were laws relating only to the violent and indigent insane. The violent insane were generally treated as common criminals and incarcerated in jails so "that they do not damify others" (2, p. 80). The indigent or dependent insane were dealt with no differently than paupers. Going as far back as 1639, communities enacted repressive settlement laws that penalized paupers and vagabonds, and the dependent insane often roamed the countryside, literally without a home.

During the second half of the 18th century and during the early 19th century, when local communities began to deal with mental illness in a more organized fashion, jails and poorhouses were again used as solutions for the violent and indigent insane. There were, however, no statutes during this period that related to commitment of the mentally ill. Since only the violent or indigent were involved, commitment was easily accomplished. "A few words hastily scribbled on a chance scrap of paper . . . and the deed was done" (3, p. 62).

The early 19th century and the Age of Reason brought significant reform, albeit short-lived, to the treatment of the mentally ill. Due in large part to the ideas of Rush, Pinel, and Tuke, treatment and cure (rather than incarceration and punishment) seemed possible. The philosophy of "moral treatment" advocated the resocialization of the mentally ill individual within an institutional setting where his social and physical environment could be completely and therapeutically structured.

To carry out the precepts of moral treatment a few asylums or special institutions exclusively for the insane were developed in a number of states.[2] In response to the warm and open therapeutic milieu of these facilities, as well as to selective admission policies, the asylums providing moral treatment achieved impressive success. This "cult of curability," coupled with the effective humanitarian crusades for better care and treatment for the insane led by Dorothea Dix, resulted in the establishment of a network of public

---

[2]The first private facilities were Friends Hospital, Philadelphia (1817); Bloomingdale Asylum, N.Y. (1817); and McLean Asylum, Mass. (1818). Among the early public institutions were the hospital at Williamsburg, Va. (1773), Eastern Kentucky State Hospital and South Carolina State Hospital (1824), and Worcester State Hospital, Mass. (1833).

facilities for the insane in addition to those under private auspices. However, procedures for commitment remained undefined by statute.

The assumption by the government of broad responsibility for the mentally ill, who were viewed as a distinctly separate group, represented a significant change in public policy. However, public institutions for the mentally disabled could no longer be selective in their admission policies. Within a short period of time public hospitals exceeded their bed capacities, while patient turnover was almost nonexistent. State facilities thus evolved into custodial, rather than therapeutic, entities, differing a little from other kinds of custodial institutions, such as jails and poorhouses.

During this period of rapid growth of public asylums, a concern for the rights of the individual who had been committed to such a facility began to develop. This interest resulted more from public anxiety over the wrongful commitment of the sane than from a desire to protect the rights and liberty of the mentally ill. A vigorous campaign for strict commitment laws to prevent wrongful detention was led by Mrs. E.P.W. Packard, who herself had been confined in a mental hospital in Illinois for three years. Consequently, during the 1870s a number of states enacted fairly rigorous commitment laws, some of which included a jury determination of insanity. (Ironically, the jury trial resulted in more commitments of sane individuals than had ever been the case under any other procedure [4].) Legally, this period has been characterized as the "romance with the criminal law" (5). The overly legalistic approach to mental illness and civil commitment "contributed in no small degree to the stigma attached to mental disease" (3, p. 438). Because these statutes utilized the criminal-judicial model, they promoted the public's identification of civilly committed persons with criminals and thus created anxiety and isolation in the management of these patients.

Despite the advances in psychiatric knowledge and treatment that ensued in the 20th century, there was no major impetus for changing commitment laws until the middle of the century. After World War II, there was a growing conviction in the psychiatric community that the criminal law features of commitment statutes, including such concepts as notice and judicial hearings, were detrimental to the treatment of mental illness. During this period of "the romance with psychiatry" (5), model legislation was drafted that dispensed with criminalistic terminology, jury trials, and judicial procedures to decide the issue of commitment (6, pp. 454-475). New statutory provisions permitting commitment for varying periods of time based wholly on psychiatric certifications (rather than on judicial determinations) reflected this approach.

More recently there has been another shift, involving a "significant disenchantment ... with both restrictive and punitive legal barriers and excessive reliance on psychiatric judgment" (5). There has been a growing attack on what is regarded as paternalism, particularly on the part of institutional administrators and clinicians. In contrast to the law of the past hundred years, which focused primarily on commitment procedures, increasing attention is now being paid to the rights, treatment, and living conditions of the mentally ill and retarded *after* they have been admitted to mental health facilities.

With the widespread growth of the open-door policy in mental health facilities and with the increase in voluntary admissions during the past two decades, we have entered an era in mental health law that might be called a "romance with the community." Increasingly, the relationship between the mental patient and the mental health facility is taking on a contractual character with options on both sides of the contract. Thus at least eight states (6, p. 19) now provide "informal" or unconditional voluntary admissions in which either the patient or the facility can terminate treatment at any time. All states but one provide for conditional voluntary admission, in which the patient agrees to give notice of his intention to terminate treatment (6, p. 19). The facility may then initiate judicial proceedings to commit the patient involuntarily if the commitment standards are met. Thus the courts are being used less frequently, the dignity and autonomy of the patient are enhanced, and mental hospitalization is further decriminalized.

JUDICIAL DECISIONS

Law is interpreted, modified, changed, and expanded both through statute and through judicial decision. As a general rule, broad, prospective legal change is effected through legislation; decisional or case law is traditionally more limited and remedial, determining the rights and obligations of particular persons or parties. Only in recent years have the courts been used to any significant degree as a forum for the mentally ill and mentally retarded. While historically there have been decisions relating to wrongful detention in mental hospitals (7, 8), the status, rights, and treatment of the mentally disabled have only recently become a matter of judicial concern.

The last two decades have been characterized by the establishment and expansion of civil (9), criminal (10), and consumer (11) rights through judicial decision. This general model of heretofore powerless and neglected groups in society, utilizing the judicial system as both a forum for the expression of legitimate grievances and as an effective and responsive vehicle for social change, is now being adopted by and for the mentally disabled.

Class Actions

Legal efforts on behalf of the mentally ill and retarded have been procedurally facilitated by use of the "class action" mechanism in particular. In essence, class actions are representative law suits brought by a group of individuals who stand in the shoes or represent the interests of an indeterminate number of persons sharing the same legal claim against an alleged common wrongdoer or defendant. In 1966, as part of a general revision of the Federal Rules of Civil Procedure, Rule 23 was rewritten to permit broader application of the class suit. Subsequently, 44 states patterned their state procedural rules, on the federal model, creating greater uniformity in and accessibility of class actions at both the state and federal levels. (Mississippi, New Hampshire, Rhode Island, Tennessee, Vermont, and Virginia do not currently have statutory provisions governing class actions.) Generally speaking, these revisions in the procedural requirements for class actions give the courts greater discretion to permit such suits when it is in the interests of justice to do so. Recent examples of permissible classes of plaintiffs include shareholders in a company, consumer groups, and mental patients.

Class suits were originally utilized to provide legal recourse to persons who had relatively small but legitimate claims and who lacked the financial resources to pursue such an action unless they were able to amalgamate claims with similarly injured persons. However, "the modern approach to class actions is encouraging litigation where a remedy is theoretically, but not practically available—as in consumer class actions where each class member has been injured in a small way, but where the aggregate injury is great indeed" (12). The current emphasis is thus placed on the potential impact of the remedy, rather than on the financial ability to bring suit (although this continues to be of concern).

There is no uniform standard or rule of thumb for how many individuals are necessary to bring a class suit. "Of far greater importance is the adequacy of representation by those who would be representative plaintiffs" (12). This requires an "ascertainable class" or a clearly defined group of persons with common interests (13). The facts and law that would permit recovery to one member of the class bringing the suit must permit recovery to all members of the class. This is essential because of the operation of the legal principle of res judicata, which makes the court's decision binding on the entire class, whether it is favorable or not.

The type of issue involved in the case may be determinative of the appropriateness of the class action mechanism: "A civil rights case is much more likely to gather judicial support in borderline cases than is an ordinary suit for fraud" (12). Moreover, underlying the concept of the class action is a notion of equalizing the positions of the parties: "To permit the defendants to contest liability with each claimant in a single, separate suit would, in many cases, give the defendants an advantage which would be almost equivalent to closing the door of justice to all small claimants. This is what we think the class suit practice was [designed] to prevent" (14, p. 90).

In terms of recovery, the class action is more effective in obtaining injunctive relief (i.e., a court order that the defendant either cease or take particular actions) than in awarding compensation or monetary damages. This is determined in large part by the nature of the action: those persons whose interests are represented and in fact litigated in a class suit may, in reality, be unknown and therefore unable to share in their legitimate portion of a monetary award. The difficulty of determining a single sum as damages in cases where the divider is unknown is obvious. In the area of mental health and retardation the legal relief sought by mental patients has most often been injunctive in nature (e.g., that the physical facilities and treatment services of institutions be improved): therefore the class action can be a particularly appropriate and effective vehicle for such purposes.

While a comprehensive compilation of judicial decisions relating to the mentally disabled is beyond the scope of this paper, we will attempt to categorize and evaluate the impact of some of these decisions. It should be pointed out that case law is wholly binding only within the jurisdiction of the court rendering the decision; consequently, a decision of one state need not be followed in another. On the other hand, the common law is based on precedent: the influence and impact of a particular decision, especially in a substantive area where there is little case law, can be impressive.

Right-to-Treatment Decisions

Of major significance is the recent line of cases recognizing the right to treatment of institutionalized mentally ill and mentally retarded persons. Beginning with the landmark decision in *Rouse v. Cameron* (15) in 1966, the District of Columbia Circuit Court of Appeals held that mental patients committed by criminal courts had the right to adequate treatment. The mental condition of such persons had resulted in their being found not guilty by reason of insanity: in the absence of criminal responsibility, punishment and incarceration were precluded. Although criminal commitment to a high-security mental hospital for therapeutic care and treatment would be both appropriate and constitutional, such confinement *without adequate treatment* was held tantamount to incarceration, thus transforming the hospital into a penitiary. The *Rouse* decision stated that "the purpose of involuntary hospitalization is treatment, not punishment": adequate treatment was in effect held to be the sine qua non of such criminal commitments. Two years later, again in the context of criminal commitments to mental hospitals, Massachusetts extended the right to treatment to persons found incompetent to stand trial (16).

In 1971, in response to a class action, an Alabama Federal District Court further extended the right to adequate treatment to *all* mentally ill and mentally retarded persons who were in institutions involuntarily, whether their commitments were under civil or criminal procedures (1). Moreover, the court based its decision on a constitutional guarantee of the right to treatment: "To deprive any citizen of his or her liberty upon the altruistic theory that the confinement is for humane therapeutic reasons and fail to provide adequate treatment violates the very fundamentals of due process" (1, p. 1785).

Dissatisfied with the state plan for improvement of facilities required by the court in its first order (1, p. 785) and utilizing contributions and suggestions of a panel of national mental health experts, the court issued an order in April 1972 (17) that detailed the criteria for adequate treatment in three areas: 1) a humane psychological and physical environment, 2) a qualified staff with a sufficient number of members to administer adequate treatment, and 3) individualized treatment plans. However, the focus in the 1972 *Wyatt v. Stickney* order is exclusively on the allocation and expenditure of state funds for mental health institutions. Given limited resources for mental health services, the widespread application of the explicit and comprehensive *Wyatt* standards and requirements could be antithetical to the general movement toward community alternatives to institutional care. In October 1972, Judge Johnson, who wrote the *Wyatt* opinion, further applied its holding to require adequate medical treatment, including psychiatric services for prison inmates (18). In sharp contrast to these holdings a federal district court in the same Circuit (Georgia) held that determinations regarding the quality of mental health services and the adequacy of treatment rest with the "elected representatives of the people" and not with the courts (19).

These cases involved patients involuntarily committed under civil or criminal law. The increasing utilization of voluntary admissions to mental hospitals substantially mitigates the "incarceration" component of involuntary hospitalization. However, while the issue of adequacy of treatment for voluntarily admitted patients has not yet been addressed by the courts, there is no medical, legal, or ethical justification for compromising the quality of care and treatment at a mental health facility because of the legal status of the recipient. Minimum standards for adequate treatment should be no different, and certainly no lower, for voluntary patients than for involuntary patients. The constitutional guarantee of equal protection under the laws, particularly when one is dealing with state facilities, should mandate such a result.

Mental Retardation Law Suits

While *Wyatt v. Stickney* encompassed the rights of both the mentally ill and mentally retarded, there have been a number of recent cases that have specifically focused on the legal interests of the mentally retarded. Class actions on behalf of mentally retarded residents in state facilities have been brought in New York (20, 21), in Massachusetts (22), in Illinois (23, 24), and unsuccesfully (pending appeal) in Georgia (19). As in the *Wyatt* model, the plaintiffs seek the establishment and implementation of standards for adequate treatment and the improvement of the physical plant and treatment services. In the area of patient labor, class suits are under way in Tennessee (25) and in Florida (26) alleging the unconstitutional servitude of mentally retarded residents required to perform services in state facilities.

In an important decision in Pennsylvania in 1971, a federal court ordered that all mentally retarded children there be accorded access to a free public education program appropriate to their learning capacities (27). The potential impact of this decision on the custodial mental retardation facility could be enormous. In the District of Columbia plaintiffs in a class action had been suspended from school because of mental, behavioral, physical, or emotional handicaps or deficiencies. The court initially ordered the reenrollment of the named plaintiffs and the identification and readmission of other members of the class. In March 1972, judgment was made in favor of the plaintiffs, although the detailed order has not yet been handed down (28). In California a suit is currently being brought on the grounds of denial of educational to a mentally retarded child in response to the state's attempt to terminate her placement in a state facility because of her "noneducability" (29). To date, the court has enjoined the state from interfering with the child's education until a final judicial determination is made.

Inaccurate and arbitrary classification and placement of mentally retarded children and the denial of their right to education is the basis for pending law suits in California (30). Louisiana (31), and New York (32). Other pending right-to-education suits are being brought in Michigan (33) and in North Carolina (34); others deal with autistic children (California)(35), special education in general (Delaware) (36), and emotionally disturbed children (Massachusetts) (37).

In addition to the broad categories of the right-to-treatment and mental retardation cases discussed here there have been several decisions delineating other rights of the mentally disabled. In *Commonwealth v. Wiseman* (38) the Massachusetts Supreme Judicial Court established the right to privacy of institutionalized mental patients and prohibited their commercial exploitation. This was particularly significant since there had been no legal recognition of the right to privacy for anyone in Massachusetts until this decision (39, 40). In New York a federal court held that an involuntarily committed mental patient whom the court had not found incompetent was constitutionally guaranteed the right to refuse certain kinds of treatment because of religious beliefs (41). Still another court held that it would not permit the sterilization of a mental retardate who had given birth to two illegitimate children because the patient was unable to give consent (42).

While there are decisions and statues in other jurisdictions that conflict with and contradict these cases, the examples cited here do represent some of the current judicial thinking in the area of mental health and retardation. Moreover, it is suggested that these decisions will have an impact beyond their jurisdictions. While the *Rouse* decision was narrowly grounded in a statutory right to treatment, subsequent decisions have not been legislatively derived.[3] Partially in response to the right-to-treatment decisions, legislative proposals have begun to reflect this legal concept (43) [Fla Stats ss 394.459 (1), (2), (3)].

The initial *Wyatt v. Stickney* order (1) required the State of Alabama to devise and submit a plan to the court for upgrading state institutions for the mentally disabled. This mechanism of administrative response and solution under judicial supervision has been emulated elsewhere (22, 44). In New York State the public furor resulting from the Willowbrook expose and lawsuit (20) apparently resulted in the restoration of $5 million to the state budget. While such measures cannot be exclusively attributed to recent decisions protecting the legal rights of the mentally disabled, the impact of these landmark cases has most likely been significant.

As noted before, case law is essentially a response to past injustices and wrongs: appropriate redress is traditionally made to particular persons in particular situations. Thus judicial solutions, while occasionally broadly and innovatively applicable, are ordinarily limited in scope and tied to the past.

STATUTORY CHANGE[4]

Comprehensive and prospective legal change in protecting the rights of and providing services to the mentally disabled can be found primarily in legislative measures. In the past few years a number of states have enacted new legislation or have recodified and amended their existing statutes relating to mental health and mental retardation. An examination of some of these

---

[3] *Wyatt v. Stickney* (1) was based on constitutional grounds.

[4] Mental health legislation in the following states was reviewed and regarded as representative for purposes of the statutory section of this paper: California, Florida, Georgia, Illinois, Massachusetts, Minnesota, Missouri, New York, and Pennsylvania.

new laws has suggested several trends, or at least common problem areas for which legislative solutions have been undertaken. There is clearly no single or uniform method of dealing with these areas: what these new statutes have in common is a comprehensive attempt to correct the deficiencies of the past. "It is one of the happy incidents of the federal system that a single . . . State may, if its citizens choose, serve as a laboratory . . ." (45, p. 311). Here we see a number of legislative "experiments" going on simulataneously, with the potential of providing us with a number of innovative ways to improve the mental health system.

While the new mental health laws discussed in this paper deal with many of the same problem areas, they vary greatly in their length and degree of detail. Massachusetts, following the suggestion that "less law rather than than more law may be the answer for the future" (46), recently enacted a relatively short mental health statute. This statute, in many instances, assigns regulatory authority to administrators to establish detailed standards, criteria, and requirements. For example, the definition of mental illness for the purposes of admission and involuntary commitment to mental health facilities is left to articulation in administrative regulations [Mass Gen Laws, ch 123 s 2:Mass Dept of Mental Health Regulation 1]. After promulgation, such administrative regulations have the force of law (47, p. 309). In addition, they are a more flexible mechanism and more easily amended than statutory law.

On the other hand, states such as New York and California have relatively lengthy and specific statutes, in addition to which regulations are also promulgated. While public hearings are required for the adoption of rules and regulations, it is probably fair to assume that legislation is subject to greater accessibility and public scrutiny and to more rigorous accountability than are regulations.

No value judgment should be made regarding the length and specificity of a statute. There are advantages and disadvantages to each approach. What is of primary importance is careful drafting, consistency, and comprehensiveness.

Areas of Change

The trends and changes in the new mental health statutes are generally in response to two broad problem areas: 1) the debilitative and dysfunctional effects of long-term custodial institutionalization, and 2) the neglect and, indeed, the abrogation of the rights and personal dignity of individuals committed to hospitals for indeterminate periods of time. The thrust of new mental health legislation has thus been toward shorter hospital stays, community alternatives to institutionalization, legal protection of the patient's rights, and substantial guarantees of the quality of treatment while under the care of the facility. We shall consider these changes in greater detail later in the paper.

New Statutory Trends Related to Institutionalization

Variety of admission statuses. Less than 25 years ago "the World Health Organization reported that only 13,848 of 138,353 admissions to state mental hospitals in the United States, slightly more than 10 percent, were voluntary" (6, p. 17). Stated conversely, almost 90 percent of these patients had been involuntarily committed to mental institutions. In contrast to this almost monolithic system of hospitalization, more recent statutes provide a number of alternative routes to hospitalization and a variety of admission statuses. In addition to involuntary admissions there are the informal voluntary admissions based on the general hospital model [e.g., Pa Stats Title 50 s 4402; Ill Stats ch 91½ s 4-1; NY Mental Hyg Law s 31.15]. Another (and more common) voluntary admission status is a limited or conditional one in which release requires written notice and a lapse of generally three to ten days [e.g., Pa Stats Title 50 s 4403; Fla Stats s 394.465; Ga Code s 80-503; NY Mental Hyg Law s 31.13]. There are also pretreatment statuses such as emergency [e.g., Fla Stats s 394.463 (1); Ga Code s 88-504; Ill Stats ch 91½ s 7-1; Minn Stats s 253A.04], diagnostic [Pa Stats Title 50 s 4406], and evaluative [Fla Stats s 394.463 (2); Ga Code s 88-505.2; Calif Welf & Instits Code ss 5200, et seq] admissions that are usually of short duration and often precede admission for planned care and treatment.

Several legislative provisions explicitly state a presumption or a preference for voluntary admissions. "It shall be the duty of all state and local officers . . . to encourage any person suitable therefor and in need of care and treatment for mental illness to apply for admission as a voluntary or informal patient" [NY Mental Hyg Law ss 31.21(a), 31.23; see also Fla Stats s 394.465; Ga Code s 88-503]. In Massachusetts the right to conditional voluntary status and notice of that right on admission are absolute [Mass Gen Laws ch 123 s 12(c)].

The diversity in admission statuses, as well as the documented increase in the numbers of voluntary admissions to mental hospitals (6, pp. 17, 48), indicates substantial legislative effort to put an end to hospital stays of unlimited duration in which the patient could not initiate his discharge or his release. It also represents an increasing sophistication and an accommodation of the hospitalization episode to the particular needs of the particular patient. Finally, it represents enhanced emphasis on the rights of mentally disabled persons to freedom of movement and to self-determination.

Classification of mentally ill and mentally retarded persons. One of the disparate elements of the new mental health statutes is their inconsistent manner of classifying or categorizing mentally ill and mentally retarded persons. Nowhere is the terminology uniform from one state to another. This is partly the product of the differential variety of admission statuses available under the new laws. There are other distinctions as well. For example, eligibility for consenting admission to facilities often depends on age, ranging from 14 years to Georgia [Ga Code s 88-503] and Florida [Fla Stats s 394.465] to 18 years in most states [e.g., Pa Stats Title 50 s 4402, et seq; Ill Stats ch 91½ s 5-2; Minn Stats s 253A.03]. This disparity reflects the ambiguity in classifying adolescents as either children or adults.

In the past the law has generally not differentiated among disabilities; mental illness, epilepsy, mental retardation, and senility have often been jumbled together into a single statutory provision. Of special significance in recent legislative reform has been the degree of awareness and sophistication in particularizing these disabilities. For example, mental retardation has been clearly differentiated from mental illness: "A mentally retarded person may be considered mentally ill provided that no mentally retarded person shall be considered mentally ill solely by virtue of his mental retardation" [Mass Gen Law ch 123 s 1]. Moreover, the new laws specifically require the development of services that are adapted and appropriate to the needs of the mentally retarded (rather than acquiescing to watered-down mental health programs). Finally, there is awareness of variations within mental retardation: levels or degrees of retardation have now been recognized in statute and regulation [Mass Gen Laws ch 123 s 2; Mass Dept of Mental Health Regulation MR 116].

Few of the recent mental health statutes have reformed procedures relating to the category of the psychiatric offender, i.e., the mentally ill person who is within the criminal law system. Generally, provisions relating to this area will be found in the criminal statutes. With few exceptions [e.g., Pa Stats Title 50 ss 4407, et seq; Mass Gen Laws ch 123 ss 13-19] procedures governing the mentally ill criminal offender have tended to be neglected even in those states which have undergone substantial revision of their mental health statutes. There is a risk here that when civil statutes governing the mentally ill become procedurally complex or when standards for civil commitment become more restrictive, recourse to simpler criminal procedures may increase. Thus in California, with its new, restrictive civil procedures, an increase in the use of criminal procedures has been reported (49). It is a relatively simple matter to allege "disorderly conduct" or "disturbing the peace" against a mentally ill person and bring about commitment in a mental hospital based on the question of his competency to stand trial.

However, attention is being focused on this area in case law (50, 51). Indeed, a recent decision by the United States Supreme Court stated: "Considering the number of persons affected, it is perhaps remarkable that the substantive constitutional limitations on this power [to commit mentally ill persons] have not been more frequently litigated" (51, p. 747). It is likely that statutory reform will eventuate in the area of the mentally ill offender.

Limitations on involuntary commitment. Closely linked to the greater variety of admission statuses and to the increasing use of voluntary admission have been significant limitations on the wholesale use of involuntary commitment. Indeed, a primary purpose of the new California mental health law is "to end the inappropriate, indefinite and involuntary commitment of mentally disordered persons . . ." [Calif Welf & Instits Code s 5001(1)]. The statutory standard for involuntary commitment has become somewhat more stringent in a number of states, contributing to a decreasing number of involuntary commitments. In 1959, only five states restricted involuntary hospitalization to those who were "dangerous." Ten years later nine states utilized dangerousness as the sole criterion for involuntary commitment, while 18 others permitted the need for care and treatment (or the welfare or best interests of the patient or society) to serve as alternative bases to dangerousness for involuntary hospitalization (6, p. 36). In 1971, Massachusetts adopted the concept of "likelihood of serious harm" (i.e., dangerousness) as its standard for commitment [Mass Gen Laws ch 123 ss 7, 8, 12]. It should be noted that in 1971, Massachusetts specifically rejected the concept of "social harm" (other than physical harm) as a basis for commitment; prior to this time, Massachusetts had been alone in its use of this standard (6, p. 36). New York, in a statute that became effective January 1, 1973, utilizes the standard of "likelihood of serious harm" for some commitments [NY Mental Hyg Law s 31.37], while Missouri in a 1969 law introduced "dangerousness" as one of its standards for commitment [Mo Stats s 202.800].

New statutory restrictions on involuntary commitment have had an effect on the institutionalization of the mentally retarded. In Massachusetts, for example, there can be no involuntary commitment of mentally retarded persons who are not also mentally ill [Mass Gen Laws ch 123 ss 1, 7(1)]. In some of the newer statutes providing for the involuntary commitment of the mentally retarded, the standard for commitment is distinct from that for commitment of the mentally ill; in New York it is limited to a person ". . . in need of inpatient care and treatment as a resident in a school, [where] such care and treatment is essential to his welfare, and [where] his judgment is so impaired that he is unable to understand the need for such care and treatment" [NY Mental Hyg Law s 33.01].

Procedurally, involuntary commitment may be accomplished through the courts or through the medical certification of mental disability by a psychiatrist. In some of the new statutes a variety of commitment mechanisms have evolved, each appropriate to the particular involuntary status involved. For example, medical certification is often utilized for brief periods of involuntary hospitalization, such as emergency care [e.g., Pa Stats Title 50 s 4405 (ten days); Mo Stats s 202.795 (five days); Minn Stats s 253.04 (three days)]. (One court has held that involuntary commitment by medical certification for an indeterminate period of time is unconstitutional [52].) Judicial commitment usually relates to longer commitments and is accompanied by the full panoply of legal protections such as notice, hearing, representation by counsel, and so forth [Mass Gen Laws ch 123 s 5; Minn Stats s 253A.07; Ill Stats ch 91½ ss 8.9; Ga Code s 88-507, et seq; Fla Stats s 394.67]. Falling somewhere between these procedures is a quasi-judicial or administrative commitment carried out by hearing officers [Fla Stats s 394.457 (6); Ga. Code s 88-506]. It should be noted that administrative commitment is subject to judicial review [Fla Stats s 394.547 (6) (e)] (6, p. 57).

These statutory measures serve to restrict the availability and unnecessary utilization of involuntary commitment for long periods of time. In so doing they force closer scrutiny of the clinical status and particular needs of the mentally disabled individual and militate against the neglect of institutionalized patients.

Orientation of facilities toward the community. A number of the new mental health laws reflect the general shift in mental hospital treatment toward "open-door" policies and the effort to abolish locked and neglected back wards. New statutory provisions set forth explicit internal procedures for patient management and for administration of the institutions. For example, some provisions were designed to result in shorter patient stays, as we discussed previously. Others mandate periodic clinical review [Ill Stats ch 91½ s 10-2; Minn Stats s 253A.17-(7); NY Mental Hyg Law s 15.03; Mass Gen Laws ch 123 s 4]. This involves a close, individualized evaluation of a patient's progress, with a view toward discharge and continued treatment in the community rather than in the institution. The Massachusetts statute specifically requires the consideration of alternatives to hospitalization in is periodic review provision [Mass Gen Laws ch 123 s 4], while the Illinois law sets forth a similar requirement in its commitment hearings [Ill Stats ch 91½ s 9-6]. It is likely that these provisions will contribute to an increasing patient turnover and a decreasing hospital census. This should make possible a reallocation of resources, perhaps directed toward community alternatives.

As a result of the impetus of the federal Community Mental Health Centers Act of 1963 (53, 54), more than 300 community mental health centers have been established throughout the country. Some recent statutes have recognized the halfway house and community residence as viable and homelike alternatives to the traditional hospital as well [Minn Stats s 245.691; Calif Welf & Instits Code ss 5115, 5705.5; NY Mental Hyg Law s 11.29; Mass Gen Laws ch 19 s 29; Mass Dept of Mental Health Regulation 5.2; Mo Stats s 202.645; Fla Stats s 393.015; Minn Stats s 252.021]. Advocates of the community residence model argue that rigorous state regulation and licensure of these programs risk their conversion into "mini-institutions." On the other hand, legislative recognition and approbation of their intermediary function further encourage a change in the role of the state hospital and state school. Rather than providing custodial care for chronic patients, the large mental institutions may well be transformed into crisis-oriented facilities for more acutely ill patients.

The orientation of mental health programs toward the community, as well as the increasing use of voluntary hospitalization, represents acceptance into and by society of its mentally ill citizens and narrows the differences in legal and social status between the mentally healthy and the mentally ill.

Trends Related to Patients' Rights

Explicit statutory recognition in recent legislation of the civil and personal rights of the mentally ill and mentally retarded not only constitutes significant and needed reform, but also indicates the kinds of discrimination and illegal restrictions that had been placed on the mentally disabled in the past. Enumerated in recent legislation are such rights as that to communicate with persons outside the facility (via correspondence, telephone, and visits) [e.g., Pa Stats Title 50 s 4423; Mo Stats s 202.847; Fla Stats s 394.459 (4); Ga Code s 88-502.5; Ill Stats ch 91½ s 12-2; Minn Stats ss 253A.05, 253A.17; Calif Welf & Instits Code s 5325; NY Mental Hyg Law 15.05; Mass Gen Laws ch 123 s 23]; to keep clothing and personal effects [e.g., Fla Stats s 394.459 (5); Ga Code s 88-502.6; Calif Welf & Instits Code 5325; NY Mental Hyg Law s 15.07]; to religious freedom [e.g., Pa Stats Title 50 s 4423; Minn Stats s 253A.17]; to vote [Fla Stats s 394.459 (6); Mo Stats s 202.847; Ga Code s 88-502.7; Ill Stats ch 91½ s 9-11; NY Mental Hyg Law s 15.01; Mass Gen Laws ch 123 s 25]; to be employed if possible [e.g., Pa Stats Title 50 s 4423; Ga Code s 88-502.8; NY Mental Hyg Law s 15.09]; to manage or dispose of property [Mo Stats s 202.847; Ill Stats ch 91½ s 9-11; Minn Stats s 253A.18]; to execute instruments such as wills [Mo Stats s 202.847; Minn Stats s 253A.18; Mass Gen Laws ch 123 s 25]; to enter contractual relationships [Mo Stats s 202.847; Ill Stats ch 91½ s 9-11; Minn Stats s 253A.18; Mass Gen Laws ch 123 s 25]; to make purchases [Mo Stats s

202.847; Minn Stats s 253A.18] ; to education [Fla Stats s 394.459 (7); Ga Code s 88-502.9; NY Mental Hyg Law s 15.11]; to habeas corpus [e.g., Pa Stats Title 50 s 4426; Ill Stats ch 91½ s 10-6; Calif Welf & Instits Code s 7250]; to independent psychiatric examination [Pa Stats Title 50 s 4423; Fla Stats s 394.459 (3)(b)] ; to civil service status [Ill Stats ch 91½ s 9-11; NY Mental Hyg Law s 15.01] : to retain licenses, privileges, or permits established by law such as a driver's or professional license [Minn Stats s 253A.18; Ill Stats ch 91½ s 9-11; NY Mental Hyg Law s 15.01] : to sue and be sued [Minn Stats s 253A.18]; to marry [Minn Op AG 1008 Sept 22, 1968; Mass Dept of Mental Health Regulation MH 16]; and not to be subject to unnecessary mechanical restraints [Mo Stats s 202.843; Ga Code s 88-502.4; Minn Stats s 253.17].

Mental illness does not necessarily impute incompetency in exercising one or more of these rights, and incompetency requires specific judicial determination. A number of statutes clearly differentiate between mental illness and mental incompetency [e.g., Mo Stats s 202.847; Mass Gen Laws ch 123 s 25; Fla Stats s 394.459 (1)] and make reference to this distinction in their catalog of patients; rights [e.g., Ill Stats ch 91½ s 9-11; NY Mental Hyg Laws s 29.03].

The right to legal representation. The constitutional guarantee of the right to counsel or legal representation, which originated in the area of criminal law (55), has been incorporated into a number of new mental health statutes to protect the rights of patients in commitment hearings, including the appointment of counsel for indigent persons [e.g., Fla Stats ss 394.467 (2) (d), 394.467 (3), 394.473; Ga Stats ss 88-502.12, 88.503.3, 88.506.6; Ill Stats ch 91½ s 9-4]. The participation of an attorney representing the interests of the patient precludes the reality or the appearance of railroading commitment and establishes a true "adversary" setting, ensuring close adherence to statutory commitment standards.

Mechanisms for review, appraisal, and explanation of patients' rights are being introduced in several states. New York, for example, has established the Mental Health Information System, a court-affiliated service to review the admission and retention of all patients and to inform and advise patients of their rights [NY Mental Hyg Law s 29.09]. A California court has instituted the use of a nonprofit legal services group to apprise involuntarily certified patients of their legal rights (56). In Minnesota, review boards examine the admission and detention of patients [Minn Stats s 253A.16], while Massachusetts requires the designation of a "civil rights officer" in each mental health facility to assist the patient in exercising his rights [Mass Dept of Mental Health Regulation MH 16]. In addition, apart from traditional guardianship and conservatorship provisions, new and more flexible forms of patient representation or patient advocacy have been statutorily established

[Calif Welf & Instits Code s 5350; Fla Stats s 394.459; Ga Code s 88-502.19; Ill Stats ch 91½ ss 9-6, 9-7].

Legal representation of patients' rights and interests indicates a fundamental change in attitudes toward the mentally disabled: no longer is the mental patient passively subject to the legal, economic, and personal consequences of his illness, but may, with legal assistance if necessary, affirmatively and actively continue to control his own life.

Privacy and confidentiality. Protecting the privacy of mental patients, as well as the confidentiality of their communications and medical records, has become a significant legal concern. The "right of privacy" implies the right of the individual to keep some information about himself or access to his personality (as by a photograph or personality test) completely secret from others. "Confidentiality," on the other hand, presupposes disclosure of certain information to another person; however, the communication of such information is limited to specifically authorized parties. "Privileged testimonial communication" is an evidentiary concept, permitting the patient or client to prevent his physician, psychologist, etc., from disclosing confidential communications in court or in other legal proceedings.

All but three states (Rhode Island, Texas, and Wisconsin) recognize the right of privacy in some form (57, footnote 3), while approximately two-thirds of the states have enacted physician-patient testimonial privilege statutes (58). Interestingly enough, physician-patient testimonial privilege statutes in Connecticut [Gen Stats of Conn Title 52-146 (d), (e), (f)] (59, footnote 8) and in Massachusetts [Mass Gen Laws ch 322 s 203] protect only communications between psychotherapists and patients—one of the few areas where the legal interests of the mentally disabled have been given priority. In addition, mos of the new mental health statutes specifically protect the confidentiality of patient records [Pa Stats Title 50 s 4602; Fla Stats s 394.459 (8); Ga Code s 88-502.10; Ill Stats ch 91½ s 12-3; Minn Stats s 246.13; Mass Gen Laws ch 123 s 36; Calif Welf & Instits Code s 5328 (cf. s 5328.2); NY Mental Hyg Law s 15.13]. The Massachusetts statute goes on to protect patients "from commercial exploitation of any kind. No patient shall be photographed, interviewed or exposed to public view without either his express written consent or that of his legal guardian" [Mass Gen Laws ch 19 s 29 (f)].

Informed consent. Another issue relating to patient rights is the ability or capacity of the mentally disabled individual to give informed consent to his "voluntary" admission, to particular kinds of treatment or therapy, to surgical procedures, or to scientific research (including interviews, behavioral observation and testing, administration of drugs, and so forth). The case law regarding a mental patient's capacity to consent is ambiguous, and decisions support almost any position.[5] There are a few statutory provisions requiring patient consent to surgery and to specific modalities of treatment such as electroconvulsive therapy [Minn Stats s 253A.17; Calif Welf & Instits Code ss 5325, 5325.5; NY Mental Hyg Law s 15.03; Mass Gen Laws ch 123 s 23].

With regard to capacity to give informed consent to voluntary admission, some states have avoided the issue and created admission statuses such as "nonobjecting" [Ga Code s 88-506; NY Mental Hyg Law s 33.25] or "voluntary commitment" [Pa Stats Title 50 s 4403]. Finally, there is almost no statutory or case law relating to consent to scientific research (62). Federal (63) and state (64) guidelines requiring patient consent to participation in research are essentially hortatory but may indicate the direction of future statutory or regulatory amendment.

Statutory right to treatment. Corresponding to the growing body of case law relating to the right to treatment, recent legislation has begun to articulate substantive guarantees of adequate and humane treatment:

> Each patient in a facility shall receive treatment suited to his needs which shall be administered skillfully, safely, and humanely with full respect for his dignity and personal integrity. Each patient shall receive such medical, vocational, social, educational, and rehabilitative services as his condition requires to bring about an early return to his community [Fla Stats s 394.459 (3); also see Mo Stats s 202.840; Ga Code ss 88-502.2, 88-502.3; Ill Stats ch 91½ s 12-1; NY Mental Hyg Law s 15.03].

Such guarantees would appear to be enforceable in court, if necessary. However, criteria for judicial assessment of the adequacy of treatment received remains a problematic area (65).

CONCLUSIONS

In one sense we have now come full circle in mental health law since the days of the "moral treatment" of the mentally ill. In those days admission to mental hospitals was selective and the unresponsive patient was turned away. Treatment was adequate, but only for the few. Now we are required to provide adequate treatment, but for the many. Fortunately, with the significant advances in the treatment of the mentally ill in the past 20 years, we should be able to make accelerated progress toward such a desideratum. This will require increased allotment of public resources for the

---

[5] Compare *Wilson v. Lehman* (60) and *Lester v. Aetna Casualty & Surety Co.* (61).

mentally ill and thymentally retarded. However, much can be accomplished by the reallocation and more productive utilization of the resources we now have.

The role of the law that has emerged in recent years may be regarded as catalytic toward improving care and treatment for the mentally disabled. If some of the new statutes and case law appear to be excessively rigid or burdensome in their implementation, or if these reforms appear at times to be advanced by overly aggressive and overzealous lawyers, it is well to remember that there is no conflict regarding the ultimate ends to which all this energy is directed. Change is painful, but we know that it is both necessary and inevitable if we are to have progress.

It matters greatly, however, what the impact of change really is. It is of fundamental importance that the effects of these changes on the quality of people's lives and health be monitored carefully. Empirical follow-up of changes in mental health law is badly needed, and little has appeared in either the psychiatric or the legal literature. It is of great significance that the United States Supreme Court itself, beginning with the landmark school desegregation decision of 1954 (9) and most recently in *Jackson v. Indiana* (51) found such empirical studies to be persuasive in its decision making.

In closing we again underscore the dynamic, evolving nature of mental health law and the complex series of "experiments" that are now going on in this area. What we have written in this paper will therefore become dated rapidly. One can only wonder what new legal "romance" awaits us.

REFERENCES

1. Wyatt v Stickney, 325 F Supp 781 (MD Ala 1971)
2. Records of the Governor and Company of the Massachusetts Bay in New England, vol. 5, 1854
3. Deutsch, A. *The mentally ill in America: A history of their care and treatment from colonial times,* 2nd revised ed. New York, Columbia University Press, 1949
4. Dewey, R. The jury law for commitment of the insane in Illinois (1867-1893), and Mrs. E.P. W. Packard, its author, also later developments in lunacy legislation in Illinois. *Am J Insanity* 69:571-584, 1913
5. Curran, W.J. Community mental health and the commitment laws: a radical new approach is needed. *Am J Public Health* 57:1565-1570. 1967
6. Brakel, S.L. and Rock, R.S. *The mentally disabled and the law,* revised ed. Chicago, University of Chicago Press, 1971
7. Matter of Josiah Oakes, *8 Law Reporter* (Mass Sup Ct 1845)

8. Whitree v State of New York, 290 NYS 2d 486 (1966)
9. Brown v Board of Education of Topeka, 349 US 294 (1954)
10. Miranda v State of Arizona, 384 US 4861 (1966)
11. Vasquez v Supreme Court, 94 Cal Rptr 796 (1971)
12. Ashe, L. The class action: Solution for the seventies. *New England Law Review* 7:1-23, 1973
13. Darr v Yellow Cab Co. 65 Cal 2d 695 (1967)
14. Weeks v Bareco Oil Co. 125 F 2d 84 (7th Cir 1941)
15. Rouse v Cameron, 373 F 2d 451 (DC Cir 1966)
16. Nason v Superintendent of Bridgewater State Hospital, 233 NE 2d 908 (Mass 1968)
17. Wyatt v Stickney, 344 F Supp 373 (MD Ala 1972)
18. Newman v State of Alabama, Civil Action No. 3501-N (MD Ala 1972)
19. Burnham v Department of Public Health of the State of Georgia. Civil Action No. 16385 (ND Ga 1972)
20. New York State Association for Retarded Children et al v Rockefeller, 72 Civil Action No. 356 (ED NY 1972)
21. Paresi et al v Rockefeller, 72 Civil Action No. 357 (Ed NY 1972)
22. Ricci et al v Greenblatt et al, Civil Action No. 72–469F (D Mass 1972)
23. Wheeler et al v Glass et al, Civil Action No. 71-1677 (7th Cir 1971)
24. Rivera et al v Weaver et al. Civil Action No. 72C 133 (Ill 1972)
25. Townsend v Treadway, Civil Action No. 6500 (Tenn 1972)
26. Roebuck et al v Florida Department of Health and Rehabilitative Services, et al, Civil Action No TCA 1041 (ND Fla. Tallahassee Division 1972)
27. Pennsylvania Association for Retarded Children v Commonwealth of Pennsylvania, 3341 Supp 1257 (ED Pa 1971)
28. Mills v District of Columbia Board of Education, Civil Action No. 1939-71 (DDC 1972)
29. Lori Case et al v State of California Department of Education et al. Civil Action No. 101679 (Cal Superior Ct. Riverside Cy 1972)
30. Larry P, MS, MJ et al v Riles et al. Civil Action No. c-71-2270 (ND Calif 1972)
31. LeBanks et al v Spears et al, Civil Action No. 71-2897 (ED La. New Orleans Division 1972)
32. Reid v. New York Board of Education, Civil Action No. 71-1380 (SD NY 1971)
33. Harrison et al v Michigan, Civil Action No. 38557 (ED Mich 1972)
34. North Carolina Association for Retarded Children, Inc. et al v State of North Carolina et al (ED NC 1972)
35. Michael Burnstein, Fred Polk et al and Alan Miller, Jonathan Booth et al v Board of Education and Superintendent of Contra Costa County School District (Cal Superior Ct. Contra Costa Cy 1972)
36. Catholic Social Services, Inc. et al v Delaware Board of Education et al (Del 1972)

37. Association for Mentally Ill Children, Lori Barnett et al v Greenblat, Lee et al, Civil Action No. 71-3047-J (D Mass 1971)
38. Commonwealth v Wiseman, 249 NE 2d 610 (Mass 1969)
39. Themo v NE Newspaper Publishing Co. 27 NE 2d 753 (Mass 1940)
40. Kelly v Post Publishing Co. 98 NE 2d 286 (Mass 1951)
41. Winters v Miller, 446 F 2d 65 (2d Cir 1971)
42. Frazier v Levi, 440 SW 2d 393 (Texas 1969)
43. Senate Bill 1274, House Bill 2118, General Assembly of Pennsylvania, 1968
44. Williams v Lesiak, Civil Action No. 72-571 W (D Mass 1972)
45. New State Ice Co v Liebmann, 285 US 262 (1932)
46. Curran, W.J. Community mental health: New legal concepts. *N. Engl J Med* 271:512-513, 1964
47. Yiatchos v Yiatchos, 376 US 306 (1964)
48. McGarry, A.L., Greenblat M. Conditional voluntary mental hospital admission. *N Engl J Med* 287:279-280, 1972
49. Abramson, M.F. The criminalization of mentally disordered behavior: possible side-effect of a new mental health law. *Hosp Community Psychiatry* 23:101-105, 1972
50. Baxstrom v Herold, 383 US 107 (1966)
51. Jackson v Indiana, 406 US 715 (1972)
52. Dixon v Commonwealth of Pennsylvania, 325 F Supp 966 (MD Pa 1971)
53. United States Code Annotated, Title 42 ss 2681-2687 (1964)
54. United States Code Annotated Supp (1969)
55. Gideon v Wainright, 372 US 335 (1963)
56. Thorn v Superior Court of San Diego County, 464 P 2d 56 (1970)
57. Medical practice and the right to privacy. *Minnesota Law Review* 43:943 963, 1959
58. Curran, W.J., Sterns,B., Kaplan, H. Legal considerations in the establishment of a health information system in greater Boston and the State of Massachusetts (unpublished). Available upon request from Prof. William J. Curran, Harvard School of Public Health, 55 Shattuck St., Boston, Mass. 02115
59. Felber v Foote, 321 F Supp 85 (DC Conn 1970)
60. Wilson v Lehman, 379 SW 2d 478 (Ky 1964)
61. Lester v Aetna Casualty & Surety Co. 240 F 2d 676 (5th Cir 1957)
62. State ex rel Carroll v Junker, 482 P 2d 775 (Wash 1971)
63. Department of Health, Education, and Welfare. The Institutional Guide to DHEW Policy on Protection of Human Subjects. DHEW Publication No. (NIH) 72-102. Washington, D.C., US Government Printing Office, Dec. 1, 1971
64. Massachusetts Department of Mental Health: Policies and Procedures Concerning Access to Subjects and Data Within the Massachusetts Department of Mental Health. Boston, MDMH, Sept. 1, 1972
65. Robitscher, J. Courts, state hospitals and the right to treatment. *Am J Psychiatry,* 129-298-304, 1972

18
Community Mental Health and the Criminal
Justice System: Some Issues and Problems *[1]

SALEEM A. SHAH

This presentation will focus on a few of the important issues, problems, and challenges pertaining to the handling of social deviance by the community mental health and criminal justice systems. Since both systems are very much concerned with the definition, labeling, and handling of a wide range of social deviance, numerous points of interaction and collaboration are inevitable. Some outstanding problems with traditional mental health concepts and practices will be noted, a few community mental health principles and approaches will briefly be outlined, and some specific points of interaction will be discussed.

Historically the basic objectives of mental health and the criminal justice system have become intertwined. While previously the mentally ill were regarded and treated much like criminals, at the present time an increasingly wide range of deviants defined as criminals are being regarded by many as suffering from mental disease or illness. (34) The evaluation of criminal behavior as reflecting mental illness appears often to be predicated, at least in part, on a desire to provide more humane and therapeutic handling for such persons. Many commentators have noted, however, that the benign aims and remedial intentions have not often been followed by consequences which could be judged as therapeutic and humane. (3, 7, 9, 11, 15, 17, 27, and 32)

*Reprinted from *Mental Hygiene*, 1970, **43**, 1-12, with permission of the National Association for Mental Health.

[1]This article is a condensed version of a paper delivered at the Seminar on Law and Community Mental Health held in Zion, Ill. June 11-13, 1969. It was sponsored by the NIMH, the Illinois Department of Mental Health and the University of Illinois.

More humane treatment in the handling of deviants has generated certain problems involving a gradual confusing and confounding of the "social control" or deterrent functions and objectives of the criminal law with the "therapeutic" and remedial objectives of mental health.

This mixture of social control with mental health and social welfare objectives and ideologies appears to have been a significant factor in the development of the philosophy and procedures of the juvenile court, especially within the United States.

The legal proceedings were defined as "civil" rather than "criminal," and instead of criminal convictions the judicial findings led to status adjudications.

Within the past three decades certain other categories of adult offenders have also been viewed as requiring "remedial" and "therapeutic" handling instead of regular criminal sanctions. Thus, varieties of offenders, mainly sex offenders, have been covered by special statues aimed at persons designated as "sexual psychopaths," "sexually dangerous persons," and the like. Here again, legal proceedings have been designated as "civil" rather than "criminal," and status adjudications have replaced criminal convictions. The particular concepts and labels that are applied tend to determine the manner in which the person will be handled. Thus, if we were to consider the rules defining the intended meaning of certain labels, juvenile delinquents are not supposed to be "punished" but "treated." Their involuntary confinement does not constitute "incarceration," but is believed to "residential care and treatment." Likewise, "sexual psychopaths" are so designated in order that they may receive "remedial," "curative," and other "therapeutic" services. Hence, even though they may end up with long and indeterminate confinement in marked contrast to the more limited penal sanctions allowed by criminal statutes, such handling is not supposed to be construed as "punitive" since the stated aims are therapeutic and the red brick buildings in which such persons are confined are often referred to as "hospitals." As we all are supposed to know, "hospitals" provide "treatment" while prisons provide "punishment." Finally, since such proceedings have been clearly labeled as "civil", in those instances where the individual is later subjected to "criminal" prosecution for the same deviant behavior even after his apparent recovery in the "remedial" institution, such actions cannot be construed to violate the constitutional prohibitions against double jeopardy.

These are some of the "word games" which result from the confusion of social control and therapeutic objectives in the handling of certain types of social deviants.

Despite the professed good intentions and idealistic rhetoric which typify "civil" procedures of the kind described, in view of the actual consequences that individuals subjected to such procedures experience, there is reason to believe that the societal motives involved have been and continue to be less than wholly benign and therapeutic. The stated "therapeutic and remedial" intentions may, in fact be designed in large measure to avoid the Constitutional prohibitions against preventive detention.

SOME TRADITIONAL MENTAL HEALTH CONCEPTS AND THEIR LIMITATIONS

Mental health professionals typically come from a background of clinical training and experience. When these professionals work in community mental health settings a number of weaknesses become apparent in the clinical concepts and intervention strategies commonly utilized.

Three major weaknesses which have been noted in traditional mental health concepts (23) will be discussed briefly.

1. Behavior has traditionally been viewed largely as a function of the individual's inner or "intrapsychic" life. The treatment approaches derived from this conceptualization have typically involved the one-to-one therapeutic interaction. And, since such treatment is largely mediated through verbal communications, the ability to talk about oneself and one's feelings, to form verbal abstractions, and to introspect, were necessary for such therapy suitably to be conducted. Thus, not only have social class variables been involved in the practice of psychotherapy as demonstrated by Hollingshead and Redlich (13) but it has been suggested that many of the basic concepts and principles of traditional psychotherapy tend to be class-linked. (25 and 34) These therapeutic techniques are not very applicable with lower class persons, a category which encompasses the bulk of convicted offenders. Given the available evidence for the effectiveness of psychotherapy and the manpower situation in regard to mental health professionals, such one-to-one therapeutic interventions are extremely costly in addition to being very inefficient.

2. A second conceptual weakness of traditional mental health approaches is the tendency to psychologize a variety of social problems, i.e., the tendency to assign psychological causes to such phenomena. We hear talk, for example, about "sick communities," "castrated people," "pathological families," and sick societies" — all of which adds little or nothing to our understanding of the complexities of a community, a social system, or the socio-political struggles involved in social movements.

Moreover, by applying psychodynamic and mental health terms and concepts, the impression may be given that we really understand the phenomena, that psychodynamic concepts are relevant and applicable, and that we can also somehow pinpoint the necessary "therapy" for such societal ills.

3. Perhaps the most important conceptual weakness relates to the illness model borrowed from clinical medicine. There has been much discussion of the problems associated with the concept of "mental illness." (23, 28 and 34)

It is the psychiatric or mental health model of illness which has inherent in it many conceptual weaknesses. The major problem results from the tendency to view deviant behavior as abnormal, and then to consider such deviations from the norm as indicative of psychopathology or illness.

Medicine approaches the notion of abnormality in line with the dictionary meaning of the term, viz., "not average, typical, or usual, deviating from a standard, extremely or excessively large." In medicine, abnormality is not necessarily associated with illness. A seven foot basketball player may reflect abnormal growth, but he is not thereby considered ill. It could be, however, that certain abnormalities may be the result of pathology, while other abnormalities may increase the likelihood of one's becoming ill even though they are not pathological in themselves.

In mental health, however, the notion of illness has been used to describe (label) and also "explain" a veritable host of deviant and disturbing behaviors, e.g., crime, delinquency, promiscuity, marital infidelity, racial prejudices, political fanaticism, general unhappiness and discontent, sometimes even the behavior of those whom we happen not to like, and also those who do not fit into the prevailing togetherness that we may like to think characterizes middle-class American life.

Essentially, the difficulty with the psychiatric or mental health concept of illness has to do with the confusion resulting from the rough formula: behavioral deviancy=abnormality=mental illness. It could be that clinicians tend to have an occupationally trained incapacity to look at problems of the individual in terms of the broader and non-pathological social context.

SOME CONCEPTS RELATED TO COMMUNITY
MENTAL HEALTH

Reiff (23) has suggested three ideas as basic to the concept of community psychology which are closely related to the concept of community mental health. The three ideas are the following: major emphasis is placed upon social system intervention to bring about changes in individual behavior; the social interventions should go beyond the clinical case or the individual toward influencing in some degree the behavior of all people in the sub-system or system; as opposed to the notion of the therapist working with particular disturbed individuals, the community mental health worker is expected to assume the role of a participant-conceptualizer. The "participant-conceptualizer" stresses the activist component in professional life and indicates the active and close involvement of the mental health professional with various social systems influencing the behavior of troubled or troublesome individuals.

Obviously, the state of our present knowledge about complex social systems and available intervention strategies finds us at some distance from the above community mental health objectives. Quite obviously, too, community mental health professionals need greatly to broaden their knowledge through studies in the fields of sociology, anthropology, ecology, political science, politics, law, community planning, and all forms of social action.

THE CONCEPT OF SOCIAL COMPETENCE

Related to the aforementioned developments in community mental health, the notion of social competence has also been gaining attention as a more viable and less problematic concept than that of mental illness. (10 and 22) Social competence has been viewed as developing along three major dimensions, all closely interrelated.

First is the ability to learn or to use a variety of alternative pathways or behavioral responses in order to reach a given goal. Second, the socially competent individual comprehends and is able to use a variety of social systems within the society, moving within these systems and utilizing the resources they offer. Third, social competence depends upon effective reality testing. Reality testing involves not merely the lack of psychopathological impairment in perception of the world, but also a positive, broad and sophisticated understanding of this world.

Intervention approaches based upon a social competence model follow the premises that: 1. The psychologically or socially inadequate person needs to learn success-oriented ways of behaving in society, in addition to alleviation of his anxieties and correction of maladaptive behaviors; 2. With growing competence and social achievement an individual also grows in general psychological strength—which can enable him to then cope with formerly serious emotional problems; 3. Social competence will most effectively be achieved when intervention is directed at the level of the ecological unit — consisting of the individual and his immediate and relevant social environment; and 4. The ecological unit can have a range of definition from the very narrow immediate context of treatment to the breadth of an entire community. However, throughout the intervention process one must be concerned both with the individual's competence and also with the design of social pathways through which he will travel and in which he will learn additional personal and social skills. (10)

A BEHAVIORAL CONCEPTUALIZATION
AND MODEL

In contrast to the "intrapsychic" conceptualization discussed earlier, in which behavior is viewed as largely a function of the individual's inner or mental life, a behavioral conceptualization has a different emphasis. Behavior is viewed and defined as involving an interaction between an individual and a particular environment. For example, one does not behave on the job as he does in church, the New Year's party, the poker game, or in the privacy of the home. Biochemical factors relating to the consumption of alcohol or other drugs can also markedly alter and influence behavior. To varying degrees the environment influences and controls the kind of behavior displayed. It is not surprising, therefore, that offenders described as highly impulsive, explosive, and dangerous while in the community, may later be described as "model inmates" within correctional institutions.

Since behavior is viewed as representing an interaction between the individual and a particular environment, emphasis is placed upon understanding the factors which currently maintain and influence the relevant behavior. Much attention is given toward influencing the physical and social environment in order to facilitate and bring about changes in the behavior of the individual.

The above conceptualization is most relevant in the assessment of behavior. A person's functioning is inadequate or deficient in reference to some specific task or situation. Inadequacy of behavior relates both to the available skills (repertoires) possessed by the person, and also to the complexity of the situation (environment) in which he has to function. For example, a young man who may be described as lazy, shiftless, lacking in interest, and with a low tolerance for frustration, may in some other situations display remarkable patience, interest, persistence, and ingenuity; e.g., when working on his hot rod, training as an athlete, courting a girl, or planning a heist.

In regard to predictions, clinicians tend mainly to consider the characteristics of the individual in assessing future behavior. Sufficient attention is generally not given to the particular settings, situations, and environments which will interact in different ways with the individual variables. Thus, certain social settings and environments may tend to inhibit, suppress, and control deviant behavior, while others might encourage, elicit, and even provoke such behavior. (25, 26)

SOME SPECIFIC ISSUES AND COMMUNITY
MENTAL HEALTH CONTRIBUTIONS

Societal Definition and Handling of Deviance

Our society defines a very wide range of problems as the concern of the juvenile and criminal justice systems. Yet, in terms of volume, most of the cases in the criminal courts involve essentially violations of moral norms or instances of annoying behavior, rather than dangerous crime. Almost half of all arrests are on the charges of drunkenness, disorderly conduct, vagrancy, gambling, and minor sexual violations. (33) Moreover, the President's Crime Commission has pointed out that a major factor in the predicament faced by the criminal system involves the too ready acceptance of the notion that the way to deal with almost any kind of reprehensible conduct is to make it a crime. (33) As Morris and Hawkins, (20) among many others, (1, 33) have pointed out, this "overreach" of the criminal law is extremely costly – in terms of the harm that is done and the secondary deviance that is generated; also in terms of the neglect of the proper tasks of law enforcement and more effective utilization of the criminal law.

To decrease the number of deviants funneled into the juvenile and criminal justice systems, efforts need to be directed at influencing societal tolerance and labeling so that non-dysfunctional deviant behavior might better be tolerated, the range of deviances defined as delinquency and crime be reduced, and other alternate community programs and facilities developed to address these social problems.

Another critical need in this regard pertains to the development of appropriate consultative and training services to law enforcement officers and prosecutors, i.e., persons who are key "gatekeepers" to the criminal justice system. A rather critical function of community mental health agencies should be to provide these "gatekeepers" with reliable and accurate information to assist them in their decision-making functions. A variety of research needs is glaringly apparent. A number of other programs can also be developed with law enforcement agencies to assist them in various aspects of their activities.

Diversion From the Criminal Justice System

Another way of decreasing the load on the criminal justice system is to screen out and divert to other social institutions and agencies deviants who might more appropriately be handled in other systems. For example, it has been suggested that persons accused of crime and found to be suffering from emotional and related problems, could be screened and diverted, at the pre-trial or even pre-charge stage, to appropriate treatment and rehabilitative agencies. (27, 33)

Based on some detailed recommendations to the President's Crime Commission on this subject, (27) a pilot project supported by NIMH is currently undertaking a program to develop and carefully evaluate the pre-trial diversion of mentally disturbed persons from the criminal process.

Mental Health Diagnostic and Predictive Procedures

In various community programs as well as in correctional institutions, a good deal of the time and effort of mental health professionals is taken up with diagnostic evaluations. Often little time is left for providing other and more useful mental health services. One might question whether the traditional test battery, or mental status evaluations, or detailed social histories which may go as far back as to describe the erotic interests of the patient's grandparents, are very relevant to the intervention strategies needed within a community mental health framework. In view of the recurring commonalities in the life histories and clinical pictures obtained from many chronic offenders, one might as easily diagnose them as suffering from "low incomism, superimposed on cultural deprivation, chronic undifferentiated type".

The above comments reflect serious concerns about the use of scarce mental health professionals to provide traditional diagnostic studies, especially when the reliability, validity and general efficiency of such efforts remains relatively undetermined. However, the impression among many persons in the criminal justice field seems to be that assessments provided by psychiatric and mental health professionals are in some way akin to pronouncements by the proverbial Greek oracles. An increasing number of difficult decisional problems, e.g., determinations pertaining to release on bail or on recognizance, are seen by some persons to require psychiatric and mental health assessments, even though the relevance and demonstrated reliability and predictive validity of such evaluations remains to be determined.

Community-based Treatment and Rehabilitative Programs

It has frequently been stated that large numbers of confined offenders and delinquents could quite satisfactorily be treated and supervised in the community. It is noteworthy that along with having one of the most moralistic criminal laws in the Western world, the United States also stands very high in reference to the frequency and severity of penal confinement.

While there has been much movement toward diversified programs of community corrections, the need for carefully developed and systematically evaluated programs is still great. A program which shows much promise in this regard is California's Community treatment Project (CTP), partially supported by NIMH. (21) Based at least in part on the results of the CTP, in 1966 California launched a rather unique Probation Subsidy Program designed to markedly increase community supervision and handling of convicted youth offenders. (30 and 31) Simply stated, the plan encourages counties to reduce their rates of commitment to state correctional institutions in return for a subsidy (up to $4000 for each uncommitted case) which is commensurate with the over-all degree of reduction achieved. Consistent with a state-approved plan, the subsidy (derived from savings by the state for cases previously cared for by the state) has to be used by the counties to improve and expand probation supervision and other community facilities for delinquents and offenders.

Among other promising innovations in community corrections is the increasing use of support-professionals and non-professionals (including ex-offenders) to provide a variety of services. For example, the Probation Case-Aides Project in Chicago, being supported in part by NIMH, is utilizing carefully selected indigenous non-professionals (including some ex-offenders) in the supervision of probationers. Many other programs are utilizing citizen volunteers to assist in probation supervision and also to get more directly and meaningfully involved in addressing the delinquency and crime problems of their community. A good example of such a program is the one being conducted by Judge Keith Leenhouts in Royal Oaks, Michigan. (16)

To date, mental health agencies have not exactly distinguished themselves by their eagerness to provide treatment and related services for offenders. It would appear that the poor motivation of offenders for treatment is further compounded by the equally poor motivation of many mental health professionals to get involved with these difficult cases.

Some Issues Pertaining To Law and Mental Health.

Previous remarks have already pointed to some of the undesirable consequences resulting from confusion of social control and therapeutic objectives in the handling of law violators who are also believed to be suffering from mental disorders. There are a number of other situations and legal procedures in which similar problems arise. It has been only during the past two or three years that a number of landmark Supreme Court and appellate decisions have required greater attention to "due process" and other safeguards in civil commitment procedures; these decisions have also addressed the issue of "right to treatment" when persons are involuntarily confined supposedly for purposes of treatment.[2]

A study of psychiatric examinations in connection with civil commitment proceedings found that the psychiatric interviews ranged in length from 5 to 17 minutes, with a mean time of 10.2 minutes. Despite the perfunctory nature of the examinations, the examiners appeared to make the presumption that mental illness was present and usually recommended commitment. These recommendations were very speedily rubber-stamped by judges—the mean time observed in one court was 1.6 minutes. (24) A number of studies have also suggested that mental health examiners often confuse legal issues with mental health issues, confuse different legal issues such as fitness to plead and criminal responsibility, and tend to use irrelevant and unnecessarily strict criteria in recommending release from the hospital.

One also finds that with striking regularity questions and issues that are basically and clearly legal come to be re-defined or are interpreted within mental health terms and concepts. For example, the legal determination of incompetency to stand trial somehow becomes synonymous with medical and psychiatric criteria justifying automatic commitment to a mental hospital. Similarly, an adjudication of not guilty by reason of insanity—basically and essentially a moral and social value judgment—often leads automatically to involuntary and indeterminate commitment to a hospital; this without a specific finding as to the current need for such confinement.

In both of the above situations it is difficult to understand why outpatient examinations and community based treatment could not be used in a number of situations. In a noteworthy decision in the District of Columbia,[3] the court upheld the defendant's argument that the inpatient commitment for mental examination violated his right to pre-trial bail under the Bail Reform Act. The court also held that if a defendant so requests, his commitment shall be limited to examination on an outpatient basis, unless hospital authorities set forth reasonable grounds for believing that inpatient commitment is necessary for an effective examination.

Studies such as the NIMH supported research currently being conducted by McGarry and Lipsitt on the issue of pre-trial incompetency, offer much hope that the criteria for such determinations can be made more precise and objective. It appears on the basis of initial findings that, given

---

[2] For example: *Baxstrom v. Herold* 383 U.S. 107 (Feb. 23, 1966), *Rouse v. Cameron,* 125 U.S. App. D.C.366, 373 F 2d 657 (1966), *Lake v. Cameron,* 124 U.S. App. D.C. 264, 364 F 2d 657 (1966). *Millard v. Cameron,* 125 U.S. App. D.C. 383, 373 F 2d 486 (1966), *Nason v. Supt. of Bridgewater State Hosp.,* 233 N.E. 2d 908 (Mass. 1968).

[3] *Marcy v. Harris,* 400 F 2d 722, U.S. Ct. App. D.C., 1968.

careful and relevant examinations and with the close involvement of legal consultants, a much smaller number of persons would properly be found incompetent to stand trial. Lacking adequate examinations by mental health professionals who have a clear and accurate understanding of the legal questions and criteria involved, thousands of persons found incompetent to stand trial spend many years on the back wards of state hospitals across the country. It should be remembered, of course, that these accused persons are presumed to be innocent and that they have not had their day in court. Furthermore, often the offenses involve misdemeanors which upon conviction would bring sentences of less than a year.

There is a great need to develop training programs for lawyers and mental health professionals in order that they might be more alert to some of the problems and dangers in the above situations, be better informed about legal and mental health issues, and thus function more effectively. It is also most essential to provide community based programs for mental examinations and also treatment for the categories of persons discussed above.

Another serious problem is that of trying to assess and predict "dangerousness". It it quite common to find mental health professionals making predictions as to the future dangerousness of an individual. What is very hard to find, however, are systematic evaluative studies to determine the accuracy of predictions which lead to preventive incarceration. The follow-up study by Hunt and Wily (14) of cases released following the Baxstrom decision,[4] revealed that clinicians typically tend to over-predict the likelihood of dangerous behavior. Other writers on this subject (7, 17, 28) have also noted the limited accuracy of the aforementioned predictions, as well as the great technical difficulties in predicting low frequency events.

Finally, it is most important to note the critical value of key legal decisions which can bring about vast and nation-wide changes in institutional practices. As compared to the relatively limited range of efforts directed at particular individuals or facilities, landmark decisions can influence the handling of thousands of persons across the country. For example, in New York State alone the Baxstrom decision led to 969 persons being removed from security hospitals to civil hospitals and released to the community.

Mental health professionals need to work closely with lawyers to develop test cases which could lead to important and far reaching improvements in the handling of mentally disturbed persons and those accused or convicted of crimes. Likewise, legislative means also need to be used to bring about changes and improvements in larger social systems.

---

[4] *Baxstrom v. Herold* , 383 U.S. 107 (Feb. 23, 1966).

CONCLUSIONS

This presentation has indicated some of the problems with traditional clinical concepts in mental health practice, especially in relation to various interactions with the criminal justice system. A variety of alternate concepts and approaches have been mentioned which relate to community mental health programs. It should be emphasized that, while the concepts and principles are fairly clear, mental health professionals have a long way to go in order to acquire the necessary knowledge and expertise about the community, various social systems, the socio-political power structures, and other skills relevant to the effective utilization of community mental health intervention strategies.

Those of us in the mental health field need to be alert that we do not become prematurely enamored of new concepts and slogans, while ignoring or under-emphasizing the careful development of sound programs. There is also the danger that new programs may tend to become institutionalized before an adequate knowledge base has been developed and the value of such programs has systematically been demonstrated.

Following their very detailed and monumental study of the crime problem in the United States the President's Commission on Law Enforcement and Administration of Justice (33) provided a rather grim picture regarding our handling of the problems of delinquency and crime. In commenting upon the general state of our criminal justice system the Commission set forth a very clear challenge to mental health and other social systems to make their full contribution toward addressing a major societal problem. The Commission remarked:

> In sum, America's system of criminal justice is over-crowded and overworked, undermanned, underfinanced, and very often misunderstood. It needs more information and more knowledge. It needs more technical resources. It needs more coordination among its many parts. It needs more public support. It needs the help of commumity programs and institutions in dealing with offenders and potential offenders. It needs, above all, the willingness to re-examine old ways of doing things, to reform itself, to experiment, to run risks, to dare. It needs vision.

REFERENCES

1. Allen, F. *The borderland of criminal justice.* Chicago, Illinois: University of Chicago Press, 1964.
2. Bard, M. and Berkowitz, B. Training police as specialists in family crisis intervention: a community psychology action program, *Community Mental Health Journal,* 3:315–317, 1967.
3. Bazelon, D.L. The promise of treatment, address delivered at the Judge Baker Guidance Center, Boston, Mass., April 14, 1967. (mimeo.)
4. Becker, H.S *Outsiders: Studies in the sociology of deviance,* New York: The Free Press, 1963.
5. Cohen, H.L., Educational therapy: The design of learning environments. In J. Shlien (Ed.) *Research in psychotherapy.* Vol. III, Washington, D.C., American Psychological Association, 1968.
6. Cohen, H.L. et al. Training professionals in procedures for the establishment of educational environments. Silver Spring, Maryland: Educational Facility Press, 1968.
7. Dershowitz, A.M. Psychiatry in the legal process: A knife that cuts both ways, *Trial Magazine,* February–March 1968.
8. Dunham, H.W. Community psychiatry: The newest therapeutic bandwagon, *Archives of General Psychiatry,* 12:303–313, 1965.
9. Goldstein, J. and Katz J. Dangerousness and mental illness; Some observations on the decision to release persons acquitted by reason of insanity, *Yale Law Journal,* 70:225–235, 1960.
10. Gladwin, T. Social competence and clinical practice, unpublished report, NIMH, March 1966.
11. Hess, J.A. and Thomas, T.E. Incompetence to stand trial: Procedures, results and problems, *American Journal of Psychiatry,* 119:715–720, 1963.
12. Hobbs, N. Helping disturbed children: Psychological and ecological strategies, *American Psychologist,* 21:1105-1115, 1966.
13. Hollingshead, A.B. and Redlich, F.C. *Social class and mental illness.* New York: Wiley & Sons, 1958.
14. Hunt, R.C. and Wiley, E.D. Operation Baxstrom after one year, *American Journal of Psychiatry,* 124:134-138, 1968.
15. Kutner, L. The illusion of due process in commitment proceedings, *Northwestern Law Review,* 57:383-399, 1962.
16. Leenhouts, K. Concerned citizens and a city criminal court, seventh annual report, April 1960-April 1967, General Board of Christian Social Concerns of the Methodist Church, Washington, D.C., 1967.
17. Livermore, J.M., Malmquist, C.P., and Meehl, P.E. On the justifications for civil commitment, *University of Pennsylvania Law Review,* 117:75-96, 1968.
18. McGarry, A.L. Competency for trial and due process via the mental hospital, *American Journal of Psychiatry,* 122:623-630, 1965.

19. Morris, N. Psychiatry and the dangerous criminal, *Southern California Law Review*, 41:514–547, 1968.
20. Morris, N. and Hawkins, G. The overreach of the criminal law, *Midway*, 9:71–90. 1969.
21. Palmer, T. California's Community Treatment Project in 1969: An assessment of its relevance and utility to the field of corrections, paper prepared for the Joint Commission on Correctional Manpower and Training, March 1969. (mimeo.)
22. Rae-Grant, Q.A., Gladwin, T. and Bower, E.M. Mental Health, social competence, and the war on poverty, *American Journal of Orthopsychiatry*, 36:652-664, 1966.
23. Reiff, R. Social intervention and the problem of psychological analysis, *American Psychologist*, 23:524–531, 1968.
24. Scheff, T.J. The societal reaction to deviance: Ascriptive elements in the psychiatric screening of mental patients in a midwestern state, *Social Problems*, 11:401–413, 1964.
25. Shah, S.A. Treatment of offenders: Some behavioral concepts, principles, and approaches, *Federal Probation*, 30:29–38, 1966.
26. Shah, S.A. Preparation for release and community follow-up: Conceptualization of basic issues, specific approaches, and intervention strategies, in, Cohen, H.L. et al.(Eds.) *Training professionals in procedures for the establishment of educational environments*, Silver Spring, Md., Educational Facility Press, 1968.
27. Shah, S.A. The mentally disordered offender, in, Allen, R.C., Ferster, E.Z. and Rubin, J., (Eds.) *Readings in law and psychiatry*, Baltimore: The Johns Hopkins Press, 1968.
28. Shah, S.A. Crime and mental illness: Some problems in defining and labeling deviant behavior, *Mental Hygiene*, 53:21–33, 1969.
29. Smith, M.B. and Hobbs, N. The community and the community mental health center, *American Psychologist*, 21:499–509, 1966.
30. Smith, R.L. Probation supervision: A plan of action, *California Youth Authority Quarterly*, Vol. 18, Summer 1965.
31. Smith, R.L. Probation subsidy: Success story, *California Youth Authority Quarterly*, Vol. 20, Winter 1967.
32. Szasz, T.S. *Law, liberty, and psychiatry*, New York: Macmillan, 1963.
33. The challenge of crime in a free society, a report by the President's Commission on Law Enforcement and Administration of Justice, U.S. Government Printing Office, Washington, D.C., February 1967.
34. Wootton, B. *Social science and social pathology*. London: George Allen & Unwin, Ltd., 1959.

19
Controversy Concerning the Criminal Justice System and its Implications for the Role of Mental Health Workers *

DAVID E. SILBER

The old debate over how to view criminal offenders, always lively and occasionally acrimonious, has taken a new turn in the past decade or so. They argument used to be over whether criminals were sick (and thus ought to be treated instead of punished) or bad. The new dimension is concerned with the consequences of a psychiatric conception: (a) Is it an encroachment of civil liberties? and (b) Is the treatment conception psychologically sound? The issues are complicated and interlocked, emotionally charged, and important to society. Before going to the question of treatment and roles for treatment workers, it would be worthwhile to review the arguments; what follows is an attempt to separate the main hypotheses of both camps.

CRIMINAL BEHAVIOR IS SYMPTOMATIC OF PSYCHOLOGICAL DISTURBANCE

This *was* the enlightened liberal position. Many psychiatric writers (Abrahamsen, 1967; Alexander and Healty, 1935; Alexander and Staub, 1956; Halleck, 1967; and Lindner, 1946; among others) have characterized criminals as having the same traumatic developmental difficulties, leading to similar deficient personalities, as neurotic individuals. Often the explanations hypothesize the same psychosexual connections between adult criminal behavior and infantile fixations as are assumed to operate in the formation of

*Reprinted from the *American Psychologist,* 1974, **29**, 239-244, with permission. Copyright 1974 by the American Psychological Association.

neurotic behaviors: "We direct our regard back to the fog-enshrouded days of infancy and early childhood, when were laid down the irrevocable patterns of our lives" [Lindner, 1946, p. 58]. The most passionate advocate of the psychoanalytic-psychodynamic interpretation of criminals as "mentally ill" is probably Menninger (1968). Menninger argued that society's response to criminals (as evil and immoral persons) is as misguided as earlier notions that mental illness is a sign of satanic possession.

Most interpretations of criminal behavior as disturbed are made in a reformist spirit, usually coupled with appeals to radically change the criminal justice system. Proposals usually include changing the court system, changing the role of mental health worker, and transforming the prison system: "We [the public] commit the crime of damning some of our fellow citizens with the label 'criminal' and having done this, we force them through an experience that is soul searching and dehumanizing" [Menninger, 1968, p.9]. Their alternative proposals may be summarized as follows:

1. *Precriminal detection.* Delinquency-prone youths should be detected prior to contact with the police, to allow preventative measures (unspecified) to be instituted. Presumably this might entail enforced treatment for uncooperative juveniles and/or their families.

2. *The substitution, in most cases, of informal nonadversary proceedings (either civil or criminal) for the formal adversary proceedings now characteristic of criminal trials.* Others (e.g., Glueck, 1962) have argued for some informal method of determining guilt or innocence that would not take *mens rea* ("evil intent") into account, in much the same way that juvenile court is supposed to work.

3. *The substitution of indefinite sentences*[1] *for fixed or indeterminate sentences.* Along with an indefinite sentence, the person would be remanded to a treatment center rather than to prison for incarceration. Institutionalization would be mandatory, but the aim would be correction of psychological disturbance and social rehabilitation.

4. *Treatment.* Psychotherapy in one form or another would be widely used, along with environmental manipulation, guidance, and education. It is recognized that some persons might have to remain in such confinement programs on a more or less permanent basis. Interestingly, most commentators do not mention using the newer behavior modification techniques in their proposals for such treatment centers, although psychologists in prison settings often do (Brodsky, 1972).

In short, the general purpose of these proposals would be to provide settings where the man, rather than the deed, is adjudicated and treated.

---

[1]The indefinite sentence lasts until the person is pronounced "cured," as in the case of civil commitments to a mental hospital. The indeterminate sentence is a penalty sentence, usually with a maximum and minimum time specified.

THE NEW OPPOSITION

To a growing body of civil libertarians, these proposals are appalling and pose a challenge to personal freedom occasioned by the growth of what they call the "Therapeutic State." Kittrie (1971) has admirably clarified the threats to traditional legal safeguards posed by nonadversary civil commitment proceedings. Szasz (1963) has attacked the intrusion of psychiatric thought into the legal arena as a curtailment of liberty. Treatment in specialized corrective facilities and mental hospitals has been attacked by Spece (1972) on the same grounds. In the process, the concept of the mental health worker as a helper of persons takes a dreadful beating. We come off, instead, as wanting a piece of the legal action (Christie, 1971), ill-informed and judgmental (Szasz, 1963), sloppy in thought and hasty in action (Kittrie, 1971), or unreflective and mildly sadistic (Spece, 1972). It would be wise to take close heed of the main points raised by these writers.

1. Informal, civil proceedings jeopardize a person's basic rights ordinarily guaranteed under criminal law. Such rights include the right to counsel, specified indictment, time to prepare a defense, trial by jury, be present during the proceedings, confront adversary witnesses directly, and be judged solely on the basis of innocence or guilt.

2. Civil commitment for indefinite periods is a judgment against the person, not the deed, and as such represents a step toward totalitarian social control. Indefinite sentences also unfairly penalize the person accused of crimes which normally carry light sentences.

3. Once committed, a person loses all civil liberties and is even more vulnerable to enforced treatment and mistreatment than the incarcerated prisoners.

4. Psychiatry and clinical psychology contain inconsistent, contradictory views of human functioning, so that any psychiatric stance in a legal proceeding is capable (in good faith) of being opposed by another psychiatric stance.

5. Treatment programs are widely carried out without theoretical rationale, or solid empirical support. Little is known concerning the relative efficacy of various treatment programs, if, indeed, they even work. An especially problematic area is physical intrusion into the body as a way of changing behavior, such as occurs with electroconvulsive shock treatment, electrical stimulation of the brain, injections of noxious substances during aversive conditioning, and psychosurgery of one kind or another.

6. "Mental health" concepts, as uncritically applied to convicted persons, are not based on medical considerations, but rather on social and ethical value systems.

7. Coercive treatment programs stand little chance of success precisely because they are coercive.

8. Psychiatrically oriented institutionalized treatment programs extant have failed dismally, yet are "total institutions," as are prisons, and are often even more degrading and dehumanizing than prisons. The social stigma of the label *mentally ill* is at least as bad and enduring as being labeled *criminal.*

These objections leave unsolved the problem of what to do with and for the convicted offender so as to provide correctional rather than retributive experiences during imprisonment. And they completely ignore the question of whether the individual criminal is in a position to perceive what is best for himself.

An indirect result of these arguments, however, is that they make it appear that treatment and therapy are the order of the day in correctional facilities. Professionals and the general public alike tend to believe, as does Antilla (1972), that "treatment ideology has achieved a kind of breakthrough within the last few decades" [p. 287]. Bazelon (1972) has criticized psychologists for failing to change the majority of offenders, after making the explicit assumption that "the experts—you—are minding the store" [p. 151]. This is not a fair attack because it is not true. Mental health workers in the adult correctional system are few and far between, and treatment is the exception, rather than the rule. The rest of this article will examine what ought to be the role of the mental health worker in the criminal justice system, what activities might be expanded, and what avenues for staffing might prove fruitful.

ROLES FOR MENTAL HEALTH WORKERS IN
THE CRIMINAL JUSTICE SYSTEM

In view of the foregoing, it is quite clear that mental health workers in the criminal justice system must examine and question what their role ought to be. This section proposes limits and reiterates some areas where increased efforts and programs can be developed.

First, mental health workers should become very leery about testifying in court. Almost all writers, including Menninger, have complained about psychiatric testimony, yet psychologists and psychiatrists continue to march to the witness box with increasing frequency. Interestingly, the pressure may come more from the prosecution than the defense. Kittrie (1971) quoted a study done in the criminal courts of the District of Columbia which found this to be the case. In such instances, where psychiatric workers are directed to testify, reports ought to be limited to the current mental status of the defendant. If the defendant is suspected of being acutely psychotic (and thus unable to participate in his own defense), the determination ought to follow from a formal civil commitment procedure. In other situations, the mental health worker ought to avoid doing what he patently cannot: that is, render a post hoc judgment of psychological status. Since the major grounds of exculpation are now via the M'Naughton rule, evidence in support of it should come from people who observed the defendant at the time of the offense. To qualify as a defense under M'Naughton, a person would have to be so overtly psychotic as to appear so even to untrained observers. Another reason for allowing adjudication to follow from legal considerations has been stressed by Rubin (1965): Treatment can be as meaningful and successful in a prison facility as a mental hospital or special treatment program. Mental hospitals have the wrong "set" for treating felons; they perceive the patient as helpless and disturbed. Most criminals are not out of contact with reality, but rather are deviant in social values and behaviors.

Similarly, mental health workers ought to invoke extreme caution before suggesting mandatory treatment programs as substitutes for imprisonment. Removal from society is punishment, and mandatory treatment programs, with indefinite commitments, constitute potentially greater punishment to the individual than determinate imprisonment. Even the fact that such treatment programs would be controlled by the state health or social welfare agency is a questionable advantage, because abuses to patients could more easily masquerade as "treatment" and elude legal detection. An example of the dangers to civil liberty is the project outlined in the American Psychological Association *Monitor* of August 1972 ("Treatment Camps for Addicts"). The plan would call for mandatory treatment of addicts in special camps, in order to protect society from drug-occasioned crime and speed the addict's "recovery." There was no mention of how the incorrigible addict would be identified or adjudicated, what legal safeguards would be present during or after commitment proceedings, or what treatment modalities would be used. It is clear from the article that the recalcitrant or negative inmate would face long-term confinement indistinguishable from a prison setting except for the lack of an expiration date.

Research into effective methods of treatment ought to be encouraged, but the research personnel should be drawn from staff outside of the correctional setting. The mental health worker in the correctional institution ought to function as an ethical watchdog to discourage dangerous programs. There are enough innocuous techniques available which have not received adequate scrutiny so that such methods as, for example, aversive conditioning using anectine (Spece, 1972), can be eschewed for a very long time.

Finally, in deciding where the role of the mental health worker ought to be, it can be argued that prisons are not necessarily any more static than other institutions of society. In addition, correctional programs have the practical advantages of being already in existence, having avowedly rehabilitative goals, and having (in most states) a central coordinating office. In general, the mental health worker ought to stay out of the adjudication process and in the correctional system.[2]

TREATMENT IN CORRECTIONAL SETTINGS

Most prisoners receive little or no systematic treatment of any kind. Even in the Lewisburg Federal Penitnetiary, this has been found to be so (Rother and Ervin, 1971). There seems to be three major reasons for this: First, the staffs of most correctional facilities are woefully inadequate. In 1967, it was estimated that the ratio of professional staff to prisoners was 1:179 nationally (Task Force on Corrections, 1967). Smith (1971) quoted a survey that listed only 60 full-time psychiatrists for 230 adult correctional facilities in the United States. Clearly, the experts are not "minding the store."

Second, most prisoners do not manifest "traditional" forms of psychopathology. Using data quoted by Brodsky and Vandiver (Brodsky, 1972), Smith (1971), plus Brodsky's survey (1970), it is clear that the percentage of psychotic and neurotic individuals is quite low (ranges of 1%-3% and 4%-7% respectively). The major diagnostic category was some variation of the character disorder/psychopathic personality label. Such prisoners are hostile, suspicious, and immature and tend to identify with subcultural values that are legally proscribed. They usually perceive their personality functioning to be acceptable. They are not, in general, likely to clamor for individual psychotherapy and usually are seen on referral. Thus, there is no strong sustained interest on the part of prisoners themselves for treatment.[3]

Finally, the custodial staffs of prisons usually view the professional staff with ambivalence or outright hostility. They worry about the possibility of riots, believe that prisoners are generally incorrigible, and suspect that therapy is a form of mollycoddling. Guards usually have little or no formal training in psychology or human relations, often fear and dislike the prisoners they are charged with guarding, and may resent the professional because of his higher status. They therefore are often reluctant to encourage the

---

[2] There is a valuable service that mental health workers can render without infringing civil liberties: to protest against laws which define psychologically abnormal or unusual behavior as criminal, for example, laws against homosexual behavior between consenting adults.

[3] The opposite view is that prisoners recognize the low quality of treatment services and stay away for that reason (American Friends Service Committee, 1971).

expansion or initiation of treatment programs within the correctional setting and may passively oppose ones already present.

Thus, it is one of life's little ironies that treatment is attacked because it does not help prisoners (Antilla, 1972; Bazelon, 1972), when in fact the prisoner's chance of receiving treatment is almost zero. Therapy has not been given the chance to work, and it ought to have that chance before being written off as worthless. Treatment has been identified with psycho-analytically oriented individual psychotherapy, an error that has gone largely unchallenged; obviously, there are more and newer techniques in use. Let me now suggest some specifics concerning treatment in corrections.

The Diagnostic and Reception Center

Increasingly, prisoners are being sent first to these centers. To have an impact on the prison career of the inmate, diagnosis and classification should occur as soon as the offender is incarcerated. The same panoply of professionals as in a well-run mental hospital should have contact with the prisoner, and the results should be discussed at a case conference. Major decisions concerning diagnosis, therapy, and placement with the system would be made there, and a particular "package" tailored to the individual would be arrived at. The inmate should be given feedback; diagnosis is too often a one-way street. This is a particular danger in corrections, where hostility and suspicion are excessively present anyhow. The center staff ought to use the feedback technique to motivate the prisoner to get involved in his own rehabilitation. Enough general evidence exists to conclude that if a prisoner is treated as a dignified and reasonable human being, he will more often than not respond in a like manner. A similar procedure has been in operation in North Carolina, which seems to offer some sort of crisis intervention aid, such as found in a neighborhood community mental health center, for prisoners with acute disturbances.

The Traditional Prison Setting

Within the penitentiary and reformatory, the mental health worker can be a treatment source and "system challenger" (Brodsky, 1972). As a system challenger, he ought to goad the administration to eliminate retrogressive and abusive regulations; as a positive contribution, he should intervene to work on the attitudes and behaviors of the custodial staff toward the offender. Such activities would include in-service training for current staff, human relations instructions to new guards, role-playing sessions, and psychological instruction. To explicate the viewpoint implied above: The mental health worker stands outside the institutional hierarchy. I would argue that the first concern of the therapist is the client, and by staying on the periphery the mental health worker can make his contribution most effectively. This is neither "radical" nor antiestablishment, but simply the recognition that treatment works best when the therapist is not identified as a cog of the system by the inmate. Thus, activities such as sitting on disciplinary boards, writing parole recommendations, or acting as an information conduit to the administration are not properly within the treatment worker's purview.

The backbone of the mental health worker's activities ought to be as a purveyor of therapeutic services. The immediate questions that arise are, What sort of therapy and with whom? Usual guidelines applied to nonincarcerated patients are meaningless, given the behaviors and personality configurations of prisoners. Practical considerations dictate that the cheapest and most intensive methods be used most often, such as group therapy, behavioral techniques, and marathon therapy groups. The few published reports available suggest that intensive therapy can be effective (Sindhu, 1970), as can therapeutic community organization (Miles, 1969), marathon-type retreats (Carrol and McCormick, 1970), and behavior techniques and token economies (DeRisi, 1971; Wright, 1968). Experience suggests that intensive, Synanon-type marathon groups are particularly effective when embedded in the context of regular group sessions.

Simply reducing defenses or eliminating undesirable attitudes and symptoms is not enough, considering the environment to which the prisoner usually returns. Treatment legitimately includes teaching the prisoner ways of putting the institutions of society to work for him (a point suggested by Warden R. Williams, 1970, of the Maryland House of Corrections) and ways to either change or avoid negative environmental influences.

Ideally, the report of the diagnostic center will accompany the prisoner, so treatment—if desirable—can start immediately. If, however, we really take seriously the issue of individual civil rights, prisoners should not be coerced directly or indirectly into participating. Thoughtful explanations of method and desirability are indicated, especially in instances where noxious stimuli or stress methods are used (e.g., in Synanon-type encounters).

Mental health workers can serve as informal counselors to self-help groups such as Alcoholics Anonymous or the Black Muslims. Ethnic-pride groups such as the Black Muslims can have a profound effect on prisoners, and mental health workers should feel free to offer aid. There are two other activities that the treatment worker should do, but probably will not be allowed to do: (a) arrange human relations seminars between inmates and guards, and (b) arrange couples groups in the prison which include both inmates and their spouses (or fiancees).

Partial-Release and Postrelease Settings

The need to confront the social realities and pressures on ex-offenders in their readjustment to street life marks the partial-release and postrelease efforts as perhaps the most important correctional and treatment settings. Two important innovations in the recent past have been the halfway house (usually in an urban setting) for nondangerous offenders and the work-release program (usually operated out of an honor camp). Counseling, and especially experientially oriented group therapy, can be crucial here in alleviating the great strain placed on someone who is *in* a free environment, but not *of* it. The therapist will have to handle complaints and frustrations, help control impulsiveness, defuse defenses, and serve as a stable model—all without appearing smug or saintly. Immediate family can be brought into the treatment at this point, in combined family groups.

Currently there are almost no programs of post-release treatment. This is extraordinarily unfortunate, as the first postrelease year is apparently the hardest; something on the order of 40 percent are rearrested within the first year (Federal Bureau of Investigation, 1970). Aftercare programs run by the correctional system should be quickly established, so that treatment can either be continued or be available if needed. I stress the need for these to be under the aegis of the correctional system because its professionals are probably most qualified to perceive the special problems of ex-offenders in making a satisfactory postrelease adjustment.

All of the foregoing makes no sense at all, given the current staff situation in the correctional system. In addition, it is no secret that many are incompletely trained or marking time until something better comes along. Recruitment is hampered because salaries are relatively low (Task Force on Corrections, 1967), prestige is low, and prisons are frequently away from the urban scene, where professionals like to locate. There are, however, a number of pragmatic, relatively inexpensive remedies available. Perhaps the single most neglected resource is the university-based professional training program. All programs in clinical psychology, social work, and psychiatry require significant amounts of field experience. There is no reason why correctional facilities cannot function as training centers (as, for example, does Jackson State Prison in Michigan). State universities in particular ought to be approached, given their common funding source. To give the correctional-system professional more status as a supervisor, those who meet licensing requirements could be appointed as adjunct clinical staff (a current practice for hospital staff supervisors). An even more innovative plan is in practice in North Carolina, where mental hospital psychologists are hired by the University of North Carolina itself, then assigned to field placements in hospitals and clinics. Something like this could be done with correctional staff as well, thus providing them with perceived prestige, as well as resolving some staffing problems.

A second possibility is for departments of corrections to underwrite the cost of professional education in return for a commitment to work for a number of years following graduation. This system seems to work for the armed forces and the Veteran's Administration, many of whose career professionals were recruited that way. Within the system itself, employment would be more attractive if the duties of the mental health worker were split between various institutions. Or, if not practical, some sort of biyearly rotation between institutions could be offered. Finally, professionals could be enticed by the offer of five-fourths pay; that is, they would be allowed to take one full day per week for outside consulting while receiving full pay and benefits.

Interrupting the cycle of arrest, conviction, and rearrest is crucial; as New York City Police Commissioner Murphy (1972) said, the correctional systems must be changed and changed rapidly. Offering full mental health services at every state of the prison experience—from sentencing to and after release—can help achieve this goal while offering satisfying roles for mental health professionals within the criminal justice system.

REFERENCES

Abrahamsen, D. *The psychology of crime.* New York: Columbia University Press, 1967.

Alexander, F., and Healy, W. *The roots of crime.* New York: Knopf, 1935.

Alexander, F., and Staub, H. *The criminal, the judge, and the public.* (Rev. ed.) Glencoe, Ill.: Free Press, 1956.

American Friends Service Committee. *Struggle for justice.* New York: Hill & Wang, 1971.

Antilla, I. Punishment versus treatment—Is there a third alternative? *Abstracts on Criminology and Penology,* 1972, **12**, 287-290.

Bazelon, D.L. Psychologists in corrections. Are they doing good for the offender or well for themselves; In S.L. Brodsky (Ed.), *Psychologists in the criminal justice system.* Marysville, Ohio: American Association of Correctional Psychologists, 1972.

Brodsky, S. L. Mental disease and mental ability. In S. L.Brodsky and N.E. Eggleston (Eds.), *The military prison: Theory, practice and research.* Carbondale: Southern Illinois University Press, 1970.

Brodsky, S. L. *Psychologists in the criminal justice system.* Marysville, Ohio: American Association of Correctional Psychologists, 1972.

Carroll, J.L., and McCormick, C.G. The Cursillo movement in a penal setting: An introduction. *Canadian Journal of Corrections,* 1970, **12**, 151-160.

Christie, N. Law and medicine: The case against role blurring. *Law and Society Review,* 1971, 5 357-366.

DeRisi, W. J. Performance contingent parole: A behavior modification system for juvenile offenders. Paper presented at the meeting of the American Psychological Association, Washington, D.C., September 1971.

Federal Bureau of Investigation. *Uniform crime reports—1970.* Washington, D.C.: U.S. Government Printing Office, 1971.

Glueck, S. *Law and psychiatry: Cold war or entente cordiale?* Baltimore, Md.: John Hopkins University Press, 1962.

Halleck, S. *Psychiatry and the dilemma of crime.* New York: Harper, 1967.

Kittrie, N. *The right to be different.* Baltimore, Md.: Johns Hopkins University Press, 1971.

Lindner, R. M. *Stone walls and men.* New York: Odyssey, 1946.

Menninger, K. *The crime of punishment.* New York: Viking, 1968.

Miles, A. E. The effects of a therapeutic community on the interpersonal relationships of a group of psychopaths. *British Journal of Criminology,* 1969, **9**, 22-38.

Murphy, P. V. America must learn correction needs. *American Journal of Corrections,* 1972, **34**, 22-24, 47.

Rother, L.H. and Ervin, F.R. Psychiatric care of federal prisoners. *American Journal of Psychiatry,* 1971, **128**, 424-430.

Rubin, S. *Psychiatry and criminal law.* Dobbs Ferry, N.Y.: Oceana, 1965.

Sindhu, H. S. Therapy with violent psychopaths in an Indian prison community. *International Journal of Offender Therapy,* 1970, **14**, 138-144.

Smith, C. E. Recognizing and sentencing the exceptional and dangerous offender. *Federal Probation,* 1971, **4**, 3-12.

Spece, R. J. Conditioning and other technologies used to "treat?" "rehabilitate?" "demolish?" prisoners and mental patients. *Southern California Law Review,* 1972, **45**, 616-684.

Szasz, T. S. *Law, liberty and psychiatry.* New York: Macmillan, 1963.

Task Force on Corrections. *President's Commission on Law Enforcement and Administration of Justice.* Washington, D.C.: Government Printing Office, 1967.

Williams, R. L. The effects of social change and community involvement on modern day correctional practices and processes. In D. E. Silber (Chm.), The personality of the offender and the correctional system: Are the right needs being met? Symposium presented at the meeting of the American Psychological Association, Miami Beach, Florida, September 1970.

Wright, W. F. Treatment program at the reception, diagnostic, and treatment centre, Grandview School, Galt, Ont. *Canadian Journal of Corrections,* 1968, **10**, 337-345.

20
The Criminalization of Mentally Disordered
Behavior: Possible Side-Effect of a
New Mental Health Law *

MARC F. ABRAMSON

On July 1, 1969, a new mental health act went into effect in California. The Community Mental Health Services Law consisted of a revision of the Short-Doyle Act of 1957 and an entirely new law, the Lanterman-Petris-Short Act (hereafter abbreviated LPS). The original Short-Doyle Act of 1957 was a pioneering effort by the state to stimulate mental health programs on the county mental health program costs. The revised Short-Doyle Act was intended to increase the local community's role in providing mental health services by making community mental health centers mandatory in counties with a population of 100,000 or more, increasing the state reimbursement to 90 percent (it had already been increased to 75 percent in 1968), and establishing the principle of a single coordinated system of care for the mentally ill by making the counties pay for the inpatient treatment of county residents at state hospitals.

LPS was intended to increase the legal rights and reduce the legal disabilities of mentally ill persons involuntarily detained and treated in mental hospitals. The previous provisions for indeterminate judicial commitment of the mentally ill were repealed, and a new mental health certification procedure was substituted. The criteria for initial involuntary treatment were made more stringent, and a graded series of standards was established; it requires the demonstration of increasingly severe impairment or dangerousness from mental disorder or chronic alcoholism in order to justify longer periods of involuntary detention and treatment. In general, these longer

*Reprinted from Hospital & Community Psychiatry, 1972, 23, 101-105, with permission. Copyright 1972, the American Psychiatric Association.

periods of involuntary treatment follow mandatory judicial hearings. In contrast, the initial, shorter periods merely require a less formal mental health certification procedure, with formal judicial hearings only on request of the patient. Some observers considered LPS the Magna Carta of the mentally ill.

Prior to LPS, emergency apprehension and 72 hours of involuntary detention and treatment were permitted if a person were "so mentally ill as to be likely to cause injury to himself or others and to require immediate care, treatment or restraint." The minimum standard for involuntary treatment beyond 72 hours was that the mentally ill person be "in need of supervision, treatment, care, or restraint"—in effect, that he need further hospitalization. There had to be a judicial opinion of that need, and the patient was then committed by the court for an indeterminate period of time. The need-for-hospitalization standard sufficed for indeterminate commitment, and there was no requirement that the mentally ill person be dangerous to himself or others.

In contrast, LPS permits initial involuntary detention and treatment for 72 hours if a person is dangerous to self or others, or gravely disabled as a result of mental disorder or impairment by chronic alcoholism. In LPS, the need-for-hospitalization standard is omitted. Dangerousness to self or others is not further defined in LPS, but "gravely disabled" is defined as being "unable to provide for one's basic personal needs for food, clothing, or shelter." These same criteria permit an additional 14 days of involuntary treatment beyond the initial 72 hours, and a further 14-day extension is possible for suicidal persons.

Thus, after 17 days (72 hours plus 14 days), involuntary treatment is no longer possible for a patient merely "dangerous to others." However, there is available a judicial commitment for 90 days for an "imminently dangerous person" who presents "an imminent threat of substantial physical harm to others." At the end of 90 days of this post-certification involuntary treatment, such an "imminently dangerous person" must be released. Repeat 90-day commitments are possible if the patient is demonstrably assaultive during inpatient treatment. However, very few patients receiving adequate amounts of modern tranquilizing drugs meet that criterion.

Suicidal patients must be released upon demand after 31 days of involuntary treatment, unless a judicial opinion of "grave disability" is obtained. In that case, a conservator is appointed for the gravely disabled patient, who can then be involuntarily detained and treated indefinitely with periodic judicial review of continuing "grave disability."

How did LPS come into being? Some of the reasons are described in a background report prepared for the California legislature, *The Dilemma of Mental Commitments in California.* As described in the report, a widespread feeling existed that patients were being "railroaded" into state hospitals, that indeterminate commitment permitted and encouraged unnecessarily long warehousing of patients made chronic by the system, that patients suffered unnecessary legal disabilities because of being committed, that the "treatment" part of involuntary detention and treatment was grossly deficient, and that although the court did the committing, actual judicial attention to the commitment process was *pro forma* and perfunctory.[1]

The report's documentation for those allegations is at times misleading. For example, much is made of the observed brevity of formal commitment hearings, which often took only a few minutes of the judge's time. However, no mention is made of the careful and prolonged examination of the patient and the considered exploration of alternatives to commitment that may have gone into the preparation of the psychiatric report to the court.

However, the extensive bibliography in the report does suggest that the above allegations were a substantial part of the written conventional wisdom of the 1960s. Works of Goffman[2] and Scheff[3] are cited. When LPS was being considered, some civil libertarians agreed with some right wingers that the then-existing mental health commitment system was a possible instrument of state control and suppression of the individual. The voluminous writings of Thomas Szasz must have had an influence.[4]

Many psychiatrists have always been uneasy about the social control function of institutional psychiatry. It is unpleasant to be responsible for depriving another person of his liberty. It is more comfortable to deal only with voluntary patients. Also, some mental health professionals may have covertly wanted to avoid responsibility for dealing with nasty, unruly, involuntary patients. When the LPS legislation was being considered by the California legislature, the lay and professional community interested in mental health legislation gave the proposed act widespread support and acclaim.

In many respects, the new law seems to be working. The inpatient population of state hospitals is down, and the community is apparently providing local care for the mentally ill.[5,6] However, one possible consequence

[1]California Legislature, Assembly Interim Committee on Ways and Means, Subcommittee on Mental Health Services, *The Dilemma of Mental Commitments in California,* California Legislature, Sacramento, 1966.

[2]E. Goffman, *Asylums,* Doubleday, New York, 1961; *Stigma,* Prentice-Hall, Englewood Cliffs, New Jersey, 1963.

[3]T.J. Scheff, *Being Mentally Ill: A Sociological Theory,* Aldine, Chicago, 1966.

[4]T. Szasz, *The Myth of Mental Illness,* Harper & Row, New York, 1961; *Law, Liberty, and Psychiatry,* Macmillan, New York, 1963; *Psychiatric Justice,* Macmillan, New York, 1965.

[5]J. Spensley *et al.,* "LPS and the Mental Health Center," *California Medicine,* Vol. 114, January 1971, pp. 49-51.

[6]J.M. Stubblebine and J.B Decker, "Are Urban Mental Health Centers Worth It?" *American Journal of Psychiatry,* Vol. 127, January 1971, pp. 908-912.

of the new law was never mentioned in the background report. There may be a limit to society's tolerance of mentally disordered behavior. If the entry of persons exhibiting mentally disordered behavior into the mental health system of social control is impeded, community pressure will force them into the criminal justice system of social control.[7] Further, if the mental health system is forced to release mentally disordered persons into the community prematurely, there will be an increase in pressure for use of the criminal justice system to reinstitutionalize them.

From my own vantage point as a psychiatric consultant to a county jail system, county courts, and the adult division of a county probation department, I believe that as a result of LPS, mentally disordered persons are being increasingly subjected to arrest and criminal prosecution. They are often charged with crimes such as public drunkenness, disorderly behavior, malicious mischief, or, interestingly, possession of marijuana or of dangerous drugs. Frequently, mentally deranged youth come to police attention becausy of their disorderly public behavior, and are found to have some marijuana in their possession. Illegal barbiturates are sometimes found on a comatose or groggy person following a suicide attempt or gesture. On occasion, concerned friends or relatives inform police that a mentally disordered person has a stash of marijuana in his room in order to secure his involuntary detention and treatment.

Mental health professionals in California have tended to use a rather narrow definition of the criteria "dangerous to self or others" and "gravely disabled." The removal of the need-for-hospitalization standard in LPS as a sufficient criterion for involuntary treatment was interpreted by many mental health professionals as a rebuke to their previous exercise of professional discretion. At times, there seems to be an almost passive-aggressive strictness to the way they have interpreted these new criteria for involuntary detention and treatment. This may be particularly true of those involved almost exclusively in giving outpatient treatment.

However, even institutional psychiatrists who are long used to treating the involuntary patient apply the LPS criteria strictly. Habeas corpus appeal is possible at all stages of LPS procedures, and few institutional psychiatrists are eager to argue with attorneys in court about the applicability of the criteria to a patient who demands his release. Some public-defender agencies in California are quite conscientious in providing aggressive representation for any involuntary patient who "wants out."

Police seem to be aware of the more stringent criteria under which mental health professionals are now accepting responsibility for involuntary

[7]R.S. Rock *et al.*, *Hospitalization and Discharge of the Mentally Ill,* University of Chicago Press, Chicago, 1968.

detention and treatment, and thus regard arrest and booking into jail as a more reliable way of securing involuntary detention of mentally disordered persons.

Once the criminal justice machinery is invoked, it is frequently hard to stop. There seems to be a marked pressure in the criminal justice system to justify an arrest by carrying the process through to conviction and sentencing. In the report of the President's Commission on Law Enforcement and Administration of Justice, it is frequently suggested that persons who commit minor, nuisance offenses be diverted, as much as possible, from the criminal justice system.[8] In contrast, the main effect of LPS commitment criteria is completely opposite in direction.

Long-term commitment to a mental hospital is possible for some mentally disordered persons who are not considered gravely disabled, provided they have already been arrested. California statutes still permit long-term civil commitment for users of hard narcotics; however, this procedure is usually invoked only after criminal conviction, prior to sentencing. Abusers of habit-forming nonnarcotic drugs are no longer vulnerable since provision for their civil commitment was repealed about one year after LPS went into effect.

The only completely indeterminate commitments still existing in California are those for mentally disordered sex offenders (again applicable only after criminal conviction), and penal-code commitments that follow the adjudication of mental incompetency to stand trial or of being not guilty by reason of insanity.

If a mentally disordered person is arrested, these penal-code commitments can be used to secure long-term hospitalization. Raising the question of mental incompetency to stand trial sometimes permits psychiatric examiners to reintroduce covertly the old need-for-hospitalization criterion to secure involuntary treatment of the mentally disordered person for an adequate length of time, beyond the LPS time limits. However, the inherent duplicity of this stratagem has an antitherapeutic effect on the patient and introduces artificial and irrelevant criteria for release from the hospital. This stratagem also forces legal and psychiatric decision-makers to twist the accepted criteria for mental incompetency to stand trial. This undermining of the criteria for incompetency to stand trial by the forced reintroduction of the need-for-hospitalization standard is in marked contrast to efforts in recent years to make criteria for mental incompetency to stand trial more explicit and

[8] President's Commission on Law Enforcement and Administration of Justice. *The Challenge of Crime in a Free Society,* U.S. Government Printing Office, Washington, D.C., 1967.

operational.[9-12]

Here in San Mateo County there are some data suggesting that adjudications of incompetency to stand trial have increased since LPS. In 1968, before LPS went into effect, there were 16 commitments to mental hospitals because of incompetency to stand trial, out of approximately 11,000 criminal complaints issued by the district attorney. In 1970, the year after LPS went into effect, there were approximately 15,000 criminal complaints issued, an increase of 36 per cent over 1968, and 33 mental commitments because of incompetency to stand trial, an increase of more than 100 per cent.

In San Mateo County there are many young men who are borderline psychotic drug abusers. Many of them are on probation for drug-related offenses. Frequently, with or without an assist from some mind-altering drugs, these young men are assaultive or make public disturbances and thus come to the attention of the police. They may be taken to a local mental hospital to be held up to 72 hours, often after being arrested and jailed. While hospitalized, their disordered behavior is often controlled by psychotropic medication. They may be detained for two more weeks, but after the total of 17 days of inpatient care they are usually not felt to meet the LPS criteria for further involuntary treatment. They are then returned to the community or to jail under the supervision of their probation officers, who try to help them, only to experience extreme frustration because the patients refuse voluntary mental health care.

Sometimes, if prematurely released under LPS criteria, these patients may be rehospitalized via the incompetency-to-stand-trial statute. That may get tortuously complicated. For example, if the young man already was on probation, it probably was on the condition that he abstain from using drugs again. If he is caught using drugs, the probation officer may start the legal procedure to revoke probation because of violation of a condition of probation, and may then raise to the court the question of the patient's mental competency to stand trial, in this case the "trial" being the probation revocation procedure itself. Psychiatric examiners may then find the patient incompetent to stand trial, and he can be rehospitalized. The time consumed is considerable, and there are many trips to and from jail, hospital, and court.

[9] A. Robey, "Criteria for Competency to Stand Trial: A Checklist for Psychiatrists." *American Journal of Psychiatry,* Vol. 122, December 1965, pp. 616-623.

[10] J.H. Hess and H.E. Thomas, "Incompetency to Stand Trial: Procedures, Results and Problems," *American Journal of Psychiatry,* Vol. 119, February 1963, pp. 713-720.

[11] A.L. McGarry, "Competency for Trial and Due Process via the State Hospital," *American Journal of Psychiatry,* Vol. 122, December 1965, pp. 623-631.

[12] B.A. Bukatman, J.L. Foy, and E. Degrazia, "What Is Competency to Stand Trial?" *American Journal of Psychiatry,* Vol. 127, March 1971, pp. 1225-1229.

There may be one or more intervening stints of 17 days of hospitalization under LPS, with the patient being sent to the hospital from the jail, and then returned to jail, and perhaps to the hospital again, all the while awaiting final disposition of the incompetency-to-stand-trial proceedings. The same process can occur after conviction, but before sentencing, in which case the allegation is of incompetency to continue with sentencing.

An alternative form of control, without attempting to secure hospitalization, is probation revocation and a lengthy sentence in the county jail. Unfortunately, county correctional programs at present usually offer little in the way of rehabilitation or treatment. Even in affluent California, county jails have long been the poor stepchild in the correctional system. State prisons are also too woefully under-staffed to provide adequate mental health treatment to offenders.

There is no easy way to know how many mentally disordered persons are being routinely processed by the criminal justic system into jail and prison, persons who before LPS could have been detained and treated in mental hospitals. Those diverted to hospitals by being considered incompetent to stand trial may be only a tiny fraction. A California prison psychiatrist said in a recent newspaper interview, "We are literally drowning in patients, running around trying to put our fingers in the bursting dikes, while hundreds of men continue to deteriorate psychiatrically before our eyes into serious psychoses. . . . The crisis stems from recent changes in the mental health laws allowing more mentally sick patients to be shifted away from the mental health department into the department of corrections. . . . Many more men are being sent to prison who have serious mental problems."[13]

The criminalization of mentally disordered behavior is not totally without its positive aspects. It may create a pressure to upgrade the quality of mental health treatment in correctional programs. It may also help some mentally disordered persons by encouraging them to feel responsible for their behavior, and making them aware of precisely what behavior society permits and what it proscribes. Some paranoid patients may do well on probation for the additional reason that they do not have to damage their self-esteem by admitting to mental illness.

However, despite these occasionally useful consequences, I think the general impact of this criminalization of mentally disordered behavior has been negative. Clearly, here in California a great experiment in social policy is under way that deserves careful observation and research beyond the impressions in this brief article. It would indeed be ironic if the Magna Carta of the mentally ill in California led to their criminal stigmatization and incarceration in jails and prisons, where little or no mental health treatment

[13]*Sacramento Bee,* February 13, 1971, p. A4.

is provided. Those who castigate institutional psychiatry for its present and past deficiencies may be quite ignorant of what occurs when mentally disordered patients are forced into the criminal justice system.

21
The Psychiatrization of Criminal Behavior*

In a thoughtful paper in the April 1972 issue of this journal, Dr. Marc. Abramson discussed California's 1969 Lanterman-Petris-Short Act (LPS0, which, among other things, made the criteria for involuntary civil commitment more stringent. While acknowledging some beneficial aspects of the legislation, Abramson argued that it has one side-effect, which he called "the criminalization of mentally disordered behavior," that has made the law's over-all impact negative.[1]

In reply to Abramson's arguments, I advance the position that rather than going too far in restricting the power of mental health professionals in civil commitments, LPS has not gone for enough.

Abramson's arguments proceed in three stages:

First, there may be a limit to society's tolerance for deviance.

Second, if certain types of deviants (namely, "mentally disordered" offenders) can no longer be processed through the mental health system of social control because of laws like LPS, community pressure will force them into the criminal justice system.

Third, as a rule, these mentally disordered offenders would be better off in the mental health system (mental hospitals) than in the criminal justice system (jails and prisons), because commitment as a mental patient carries

---

*Reprinted from *Hospital & Community Psychiatry,* February 1973, **24**, 105-107, with permission. Copyright 1973, the American Psychiatric Association.

[1]M.F. Abramson, "The Criminalization of Mentally Disordered Behavior: Possible Side-Effect of a New Mental Health Law," *Hospital & Community Psychiatry,* Vol. 23, April 1972, pp. 101-105.

less stigmatization and more chance for treatment than does conviction as a criminal.

I believe that Abramson's first two points are subject to severe qualification in a democratic society, and that his third point is false. In the interests of smoothness, let me take up the third point first.

The mentally abnormal offender is a source of irritation for both the criminal justice and mental health systems. The assumption of free will upon which criminal law is built seems somehow inappropriate when that system is dealing with psychologically abnormal persons, and mental health professionals are much more comfortable handling neurotic parents than their "acting-out" delinquent children. Yet the mentally abnormal offender, by definition, qualifies for entrance into both systems, and each system asserts priority for controlling and correcting him. A paradigm clash occurs, to which the traditionally acrimonious relations between law and psychiatry bear witness.

Abramson believes that where the mental health and criminal justice paradigms overlap, priority should be given to the mental health system, because it is in the individual's best interests to be in a hospital rather than a jail. Yet the two reasons given for this alleged superiority of mental hospitals over jails—the increased treatment opportunity and decreased stigmatization associated with hospitals—are open to grave doubt.

Despite frequent dataless assertions to the contrary, we do not now have an effective way of treating antisocial behavior. The enduring effects of any form of treatment are exceedingly difficult to document. The vast majority of research on behavior change has used voluntary, motivated, and middle-class patients. To extrapolate from these weak findings to the involuntary treatment of unmotivated individuals with serious behavior problems is impossible. While certain psychotropic medications may alleviate psychotic states, this fact has no bearing on whether a hospital or a jail is the preferred disposition for a mentally abnormal offender, since medication could be made equally available in both situations.

As for stimatization, all available evidence indicates that the stigmatization acquired by residence in a mental hospital is at least as severe as that attached to a criminal record. This finding applies to self-perception,[2] interpersonal relations,[3] and societal acceptance.[4]

[2] A. Farina et al., "Mental Illness and the Impact of Believing Others Know About It," Journal of Abnormal Psychology, Vol. 77, February 1971, pp. 1-6.

[3] A. Farina, C.H. Holland, and K. Ring, "The Role of Stigma and Set in Interpersonal Interaction," Journal of Abnormal Psychology, Vol. 71, December 1966, pp. 421-428.

[4] B. Ennis, "Civil Liberties and Mental Illness," Criminal Law Bulletin, Vol. 7, March 1971, pp. 101-127.

Given the conclusions that hospitalization offers no increased opportunity for treatment and no refuge from stigmatization, it is my preference that mentally abnormal offenders be processed through the criminal justice system. While both systems are likely to be equally ineffective in inducing desired changes in behavior and while both share equal potential for damaging labeling, the criminal justice system has one important advantage.

This advantage has been called "the rule of law,"[5] "the principle of legality," [6] and "the positive side of the criminal law."[7] It is what qualifies the first two points of Abramson's argument. Briefly, the terms refer to the proposition that behavior that society wishes to prohibit must be clearly and legally defined before it occurs, and that the state may intervene only after a citizen has been legally convicted of performing the prohibited behavior.

Society, as Abramson says, may well have a tolerance level for deviance and may wish to shunt deviants into the criminal justice system when they can no longer be processed as freely through the mental health system. But the criminal justice system forces society to confront its tolerance level, to think out, evaluate, and agree upon exactly what behaviors are so deviant that their perpetrators should be incarcerated. By holding up for public debate in the courts and the legislature such issues as homosexuality, prostitution, abortion, and marijuana use—all of which have mental health aspects—the system forces society to come face to face with its norms and values.

All the advantages associated with open airing of issues and democratic problem-solving are lost when the designation of deviance is made behind consultation-room doors by unelected mental health personnel who offer dubious diagnosis of "need for hospitalization." Gone too are many of the careful protections of individual rights that the criminal justice system affords the defendant but that the mental health system considers unnecessary.

It can be argued that the rule of law is more apparent than real, that so much *sub rosa* discretion is being exercised at every stage of the judicial process that considerations of legality are essentially meaningless. As long as discretion must be exercised, so the argument goes, better that it be exercised by mental health professionals, with their superior training and abilities, than by the great unwashed.

It is true that the amount of discretion exercised in the legal system is enormous. When the discretion used by the police in deciding whether to make an arrest and the prosecutor in whether to press charges is added to the discretion of the judge in determining sentence and the parole board in

---

[5] T. Szasz, *Law, Liberty, and Psychiatry,* Macmillan, New York City, 1963.
[6] J. Hall, *General Principles of Criminal Law,* Bobbs-Merrill, Indianapolis, Indiana, 1960.
[7] S. Kadish, "The Decline of Innocence," *Cambridge Law Journal,* Vol. 26, 1968, pp. 273-290.

releasing, it would seem that what actually happens to the accused depends more upon the caprice of the system than upon any concern for his welfare. Nevertheless, the excess of potentially abusive discretion currently existing in the legal process is hardly an excuse for further expanding the bases of discretion, unless it can be conclusively demonstrated that judgment exercised by mental health professionals is somehow "wiser" than that of police, prosecutors, judges, and parole boards. Yet research on one of the most important and frequent problems addressed to psychiatrists and psychologists by the criminal justice system—the prediction of dangerousness —suggests that this increment in wisdom is nowhere to be found.[8]

As in the case of rival scientific theories, the current paradigm clash between criminal justice and mental health may be a portent of true progress, a sign that revolutionary advances in our ways of conceptualizing and responding to antisocial behavior are in the offing. Clearly both systems are inadequate for the tasks they have set themselves. Both are in great need of redefinition and overhaul.

Ultimately a single system for the state control of human behavior is enough. While this system could incorporate mental health concepts much more than the present criminal justice system—such concepts as easy access to voluntary therapy, medication, and training, in an environment conducive to prosocial behavior—the system must be basically legal rather than psychological or medical. It must have a firm commitment to the rule of law and due process. The Lanterman-Petris-Short Act was one step in this direction.

I do not doubt that on a purely humane level mental hospitals may be preferable to jails in many jurisdictions. Becausyof funding discrepancies or differences in staff competence, hospitals that offer a variety of treatments in an atmosphere of relative respect for the individual may exist alongside jails where the accused and the convicted alike are herded together in an environment seemingly designed to destory whatever remnants of human spirit and psyche are left.

When this situation exists, the mental health professional may feel a moral obligation to save as many mentally abnormal offenders as possible from the brutalizing effects of the criminal justice system, and may feel frustrated when laws like LPS inhibit him. He may even try to subvert the intent of the law, as is suggested by Abramson's data that findings of incompetence to stand trial have increased since the inception of LPS.

But how can the compassion of mental health personnel be limited to those who are mentally abnormal? If the effects of jail or prison are brutalizing, are they not equally so for the "normal" as well as the

---

[8] A. Dershowitz, "The Psychiatrist's Power in Civil Commitment," *Psychology Today,* Vol. 2, February 1971, pp. 43, 44.

"abnormal" offender? Can genuine concern for humane treatment be restricted to those susceptible to diagnosis, when being born in a ghetto is more criminogenic than being "mentally ill?" If community mental health personnel are to remain true to their stated goals of adopting a population perspective and a preventive set, they would do well to redirect their energies from rescuing a relatively few individuals from the criminal justice system to improving that system until it at least reaches a level of psychological neutrality for all concerned.

Community Mental Health and the Criminal Justice System: Future Directions

JOHN MONAHAN

As increasing numbers of community mental health professionals begin to interact with the agencies of the criminal justice system, it can be expected that major developments in the field will take place. The purpose of this volume has been to serve as a catalyst for such developments. The practice of mental health—criminal justice collaboration has revealed much about the potentialities and the limitations of such an approach to human problem solving. It remains for us to consider the directions in which the field should venture as it enters its second decade of existence.

I would like to propose that the future of community mental health interaction with the criminal justice system be characterized by four terms: experimental, preventive, ecological and safeguards (*cf.* Heller and Monahan, 1975).

EXPERIMENTAL

If the field of community mental health in general, and in its application to the criminal justice system in particular, is ever to fulfill its promise, it will do so only if it seriously adopts an experimental ideology. By this I do not mean an inappropriate reliance upon laboratory methodology or a reverence for data *uber alles,* but rather a genuine commitment to innovation and the evaluation of innovation—a stance of "let's try it out and see if it works." All too often in the past, community programs have run the course of their funding with nothing to show for it but narrative descriptions and glowing press releases. Others interested in the problem area are condemned to repeating mistakes which have already been made, and those who must decide which programs are to continue or be expanded are left with only their intuition to guide them. Perhaps the most lamentable facet of this situation is that it is almost always avoidable. Sophisticated and meaningful evaluations of programs in the area of mental health and criminal justice *can* be done, as many of the authors in this volume have demonstrated. They *must* be done if we are to learn by our experience.

PREVENTIVE

Two facts relevant to the provision of mental health services seem clear. The first is that only by emphasizing the prevention of human behavior problems through system-level intervention will a substantial impact on the prevalence of those problems be obtained. The second is that there are now, and in all likelihood always will be, persons who are past the point of prevention and who are in need of remedial treatment. To neglect prevention and to put all mental health resources into treatment services is surely a short-sighted strategy, one which will never succeed in reducing rates of psychological difficulties. To neglect treatment, on the other hand, and to put all resources into prevention is an equally ill-advised tack. One cannot step over the bodies on the community mental health center doorstep on one's way to consult to a police department, at least not all the time.

What mental health professionals must offer the criminal justice system (among other community agencies) is a *balance* between prevention and treatment services. Given the current preponderance of effort at the treatment level, what this means is a decided shift toward prevention. In reviewing the vast amount of literature on community mental health interaction with the criminal justice system prior to editing this volume, the editor was confronted with scores of reports of mental health treatment programs for convicted offenders, yet a paucity of work in primary and secondary prevention. A balance must be achieved in the future.

Lack of preventive efforts at the interface of mental health and criminal justice are hampered by a lack of knowledge concerning the etiological factors giving rise to psychological disorder. This has led many to write off prevention as a wishful pipe dream.

Etiological knowledge, however, while certainly useful, is not a necessary prerequisite for mounting effective prevention programs. Many forms of physical disease were effectively prevented with incomplete or nonexistent knowledge of their etiology. At the end of the 18th century, long before the microbial nature of the causative agents had been demonstrated, Edward Jenner validated a belief prevalent among rural people in parts of

England that human infection with cowpox created resistance to smallpox. Without any knowledge of etiology, one of the most successful prevention programs of all times was launched.

ECOLOGICAL

Since most current practitioners in the field of community mental health come from a background in clinical work, it is not surprising that they would bring with them their clinical perspectives to guide the development of theory and intervention on the community level. There is a noticeable tendency in the literature for formerly psychoanalytic therapists to assess community problems in terms of the dynamics of unconscious conflicts. Others, when they leave the clinic for the community, find negative reinforcement lurking on street corners or quickly come to believe that the community is as much in need of "growth" as is the individual client.

While analogies derived from the clinical study of individuals or small groups may have much to offer community work, there may be virtue in searching for new analogies which have more direct relevance to community functioning. Such analogies could open community practice to new schema of analyses and interventions, which would be concealed by reliance upon insights gleaned from the study of the individual.

Heller and Monahan (1975) suggest a prime candidate for a basic metaphor to guide community work—the concept of ecology, or the science of the relationship of people to their environment. The selection in this volume by Wenk and Moos suggests some of the possibilities of an ecological orientation to work in the criminal justice system. A primary implication of adopting an ecological position is the necessity for interdisciplinary cooperation. It is the nature of services provided and interventions planned, rather than their disciplinary labels, which must be dealt with.

The Legal Clinic at the York-Finch General Hospital in Toronto is an excellent example of an ecological and interdisciplinary approach to problems on the border of mental health and criminal justice. Recognizing that the mental health unit of the hospital often saw patients whose problems were as much legal as psychological, the unit staff secured the services of an attorney with whom clients could consult on the legal aspects of their problems. In the first six months of its existence, the Legal Clinic has seen over 200 clients, with 75 percent of them having domestic difficulties, 10 percent landlord-tenant problems, and the rest miscellaneous (J. Cooper, 1974, personal communication). One would hope that the future would see a great expansion of such efforts.

SAFEGUARDS

As was stated in the Introduction, the issue of individual liberty is one of the most controversial topics in the interface of mental health and criminal justice. The last few years have witnessed a remarkable and laudable judicial turn-around concerning the mental health system. After decades of a "hands off" policy with regard to the protection of patients, courts and legislatures are now enacting strict limits on civil and criminal commitment, and are increasingly finding that a "right to treatment" exists within institutional walls.

Considering that the values of self-direction and human autonomy are professed by mental health professionals of many orientations, it is both ironic and lamentable that community mental health personnel are not more often in the forefront of the movement for the right to remain free from unnecessary intervention, and the right to decent treatment when it is mandated. Especially in the nebulous area where the mental health and criminal justice systems overlap, *simultaneous* with the development of prevention and treatment programs, the mental health professional must adopt *explicit* positions vis a vis the rights of the targeted population to decline intervention. It is becoming increasing clear that if community mental health programs do not police themselves, society will assume the task. And it should.

If the second decade of community mental health interaction with the criminal justice system adopts a stance that values innovation and experimentation while stressing the prevention of problems rather than their remediation, that considers problems in their ecological context and pays heed to the distinction between *offering* help and *imposing* it, then a productive and exciting period awaits us.

REFERENCE

Heller, K. and Monahan, J. Unpublished text in community psychology, 1975.

Author Index

Grunebaum, H. 112, 129
Grusec, J. 242, 251
Guberman, M. 52, 81-88
Guillon, M. 134, 140, 243, 251
Gulevich, G. 26, 31
Gump, P. 190
Gupta, R. 25, 32
Gurin, A. 50
Guttridge, F. 13

Hagardine, J.E. 231
Haley, J. 251
Halfon, A. 19, 31, 34
Hall, J. 315
Halleck, S. 7, 8, 254, 293, 303
Hammond, K. 66, 78
Harlow, E. 209
Harris, M. 77, 78
Hawkins, G. 23, 33, 285, 291
Healy, W. 293, 302
Heller, K. 3, 6, 7, 8, 13, 29, 31, 319, 321, 322
Hellman, D. 16, 31
Herrera, A. 227
Hess, J.A. 291, 310
Hickey, J. 175-185, 186
Hobbs, N. 271, 291
Hodges, E. 18, 31
Hollingshead, A.B. 291
Houts, P.S. 203
Howard, J. 4, 8
Hudson, J. 221
Hughes, J.J. 52, 89-98
Hunt, R. 19, 31, 289, 291
Hutschnecker, A. 26-27

Inhelder, B. 178, 186
Insel, P. 28, 29, 31, 33, 172, 173
Iscoe, I. 51, 53
Ittelson, W. 172, 173

Jackson, D.D. 241, 251
Jaman, D.R. 208
Jarvis,.P.E. 57, 64
Jesness, C. 171, 173
Jew, C. 171, 173
John, V. 190
Johnson, B.M. 212
Johnson, D. 52, 53, 65, 78
Jones, H. 50
Justice, B. 16, 31
Justice, R. 16, 31

Kadish, S. 315
Kahneman, D. 25, 31
Kaplan, H.A. 253, 257-275, 277

Kassebaum, G. 171, 173
Katkin, E. 172, 173
Katz, J. 291
Kelley, H. 116, 129
Kelly, C. 24, 31
Kelly, F.C. 52, 81-88
Kennedy, J.F. 11
Kennedy, P. 153, 160
Keveles, G. 19, 34
King, M.L. 42
Kittrie, N. 6, 9, 15, 23, 32, 171, 173, 295, 296, 303
Klapmuts, N. 52, 53, 172, 205-238
Klein, M.W. 50
Kohlberg, L. 172, 175-185, 186
Kozol, H. 17, 18, 20, 32
Kraft, J. 16, 31
Kumasaka, Y. 25, 32
Kutner, L. 291

Lamb, H.R. 172, 173
Langer, J. 178, 186
Leenhouts, K. 291
Lehman, W. 169
Lemert, E. 131, 132, 138, 140
Lerman, P. 223
Levy, J. 66, 78
Liberman, R. 88
Liebman, D. 51, 52, 53
Linder, R.M. 293, 294, 303
Lion, J. 14, 31
Lipset, S.M. 55, 56, 64, 103, 109
Lipsitt, P. 87
Lipton, D.S. 220
Livermore, J. 24, 32, 291
Llewellyn, L.G. 66, 190
Lonkes, G.A. 87
Lubeck, S.G. 50, 175, 186

MacNamara, J.H. 88
Malmquist, C. 24, 32, 291
Mann, P. 51, 53, 55-64, 65, 78
Martinson, R. 171, 173, 207, 208, 220
Massey, F.J. 246, 251
Matthews, R.A. 87
Mattocks, A. 171, 173
Maynard, R. 27, 32
McCann, R. 101, 109
McCarthy, D. 153, 160
McClosky, C.C. 101, 109
McCorkle, L.W. 226
McCormick, C.G. 300, 302
McDermitt, R. 131, 140
McDevitt, R. 66, 79
McDonough, L.B. 51, 53, 65-77, 78
McEachern, A.W. 87

Subject Index

TITLES IN THE PERGAMON GENERAL PSYCHOLOGY SERIES (Continued)